Fertility and Kinship in the Philippines

Fertility and Kinship in the Philippines

Elena Yu
and
William T. Liu

UNIVERSITY OF NOTRE DAME PRESS
NOTRE DAME / LONDON

Library of Congress Cataloging in Publication Data

Yu, Elena S. H
Fertility and kinship in the Philippines.

Bibliography: p.
1. Family—Philippine Islands—Cebu (Province)
2. Family size—Philippine Islands—Cebu (Province)
3. Fertility, Human—Philippine Islands—Cebu (Province)
4. Ethnology—Philippine Islands—Cebu (Province)
I. Liu, William Thomas, 1930- joint author.
II. Title.
HQ680.Y8 306.8'09599'5 80-50269
ISBN 0-268-00949-X

Manufactured in the United States of America

This book is dedicated to
the memory of
Dr. George N. Shuster

Contents

Foreword

When William T. Liu came to Chicago from Notre Dame a decade and more ago to discuss his proposal to carry out a large-scale study of fertility and its problems in the province of Cebu in the central Philippines, I gave him only one suggestion—that he and his staff remain long enough to get beneath the surface organization and discover the underlying structures of Filipino society which controlled the solution of population problems. The present volume, *Fertility and Kinship in the Philippines*, by Elena Yu and William T. Liu, which culminates a decade of research and writing, not only does what I hoped it might do, but goes beyond the central Visayas to illuminate the Philippines as a whole.

The writers of this volume and their associates, both Filipino and American, not only bring different perspectives to bear on the problems of fertility, but have integrated the methods and procedures of modern sociology and social anthropology in admirable fashion. They not only provide the requisite statistical tables on the Cebuano population and its reproductive behavior, but illustrate that behavior with verbatim accounts from intensive interviews carried out over a period of some eighteen months by a trained group of college-educated Filipino field workers and research assistants. The conclusions that the authors reach are not only convincing, but are relevant beyond the Philippines to most developing countries.

Philippine population grew slowly during the Spanish period from an estimated half-million at the time of Magellan's visit in A.D. 1521 to around seven or eight million at the beginning of the American period. When I was first in the Philippines in 1934–35, this figure had doubled to around fifteen million and currently stands at about forty-five million. Demographic projections for the end of this century double this figure at a minimum. The rate of population growth is one of the highest of modern countries, and faced with these figures, the political leaders and the Catholic hierarchy have begun to cooperate in a program of family planning, and the legal restrictions on contraceptive information have been largely removed.

Once the investigators probed beneath the surface they discovered that the Filipinos had been concerned with population problems for many years and had developed a complex system of fertility coping mechanisms, operating through traditional midwives and healers and including a rich body of folk contraceptive knowledge. But for the most part this "folk wisdom" turned out to be inadequate and the birth rate continued to be high, with the resulting children being supported in part by the extended family and kinship networks.

The authors' analysis of the Cebuano social system is exemplary. The social system is basically similar throughout most of the Philippines, and everywhere children occupy a central position, both structurally and in actuality. A large family has both advantages and risks, and how the members make decisions with regard to procreation, and how the children are distributed through the larger kinship system is one of the major contributions of this study.

The writers have some important conclusions with regard to the Philippines, and some suggestions as to policy which are relevant to all efforts to control population growth: "an emphasis on disseminating contraceptive methods alone without accompanying changes in the masses' economic conditions, health care, sociocultural values, and psychological perceptions will be inadequate." The study as a whole is admirable; I recommend it to all who are interested in the Philippines as the best account we yet have of Philippine society and its behavior. All those who participated in a decade of research are to be congratulated on the results.

FRED EGGAN
Director, Philippine Studies Program
University of Chicago

Preface

The idea of studying the relationship between family processes and marital fertility had its origin in a series of conferences held at the University of Notre Dame in the mid-sixties. The principal aim of those meetings, which resulted in half a dozen volumes,[1] was to bring together eminent scholars in diverse fields to discuss the implications of social change, world population growth, and the Catholic Church's position on birth control.

A number of significant developments triggered the Notre Dame conferences. The first was the painful transition of the institutional church during and immediately after Vatican II. Inspired by the late Pope John XXIII, the Council aimed to modernize an old institution by encouraging the expression of divergent theological opinions, particularly on the role of the Church in a rapidly changing world. The second development was the challenge to the secular establishment posed by student activism in major American universities—a challenge which was intermixed with the surging anti-Vietnam war movement and which led to persistent questioning of such traditional values as premarital abstinence, the drive to achieve, and the institutions of marriage and the family *per se*. From coast to coast, the popular cultures exhibited the triumph of the senses against both traditions and reasons. Finally, a third development in that decade was the dissemination of the Pill and the Intrauterine device. To be sure, such discoveries of more efficient, female-controlled contraceptive methods did not in and of themselves start the worldwide birth control movement. They did, however, provide the needed technological structure for the idea of family planning policies. As a result of the diffusion of these biomedical discoveries, sex and pregnancy were no longer a unitary process, but two separate decisions. The woman was able to gain control of her own body, since use of the new contraceptive methods required neither the consent, the cooperation, nor the knowledge of her partner. Thus, it was not coincidental that the sixties also brought the feminist movement to fruition and introduced the world to a more personalistic view of morality as against the traditional community control of sex. Concurrently, there was renewed confidence in technological solutions to the population crisis. Some regarded reproduction as a "disease." And, like a disease, it could be checked by a chemical substance, by surgical intervention, or, if necessary, by mass immunization. Incredible as they may sound today, such "solutions" were nevertheless proposed in some circles.

Social scientists for their part were more interested in understanding the conditions under which fertility rates increased or decreased. It was not difficult for the experts on fertility research to agree that the links between sociodemographic factors on the one hand, and family size and structure on the other hand, were inextricably interrelated. However, what constituted the proper unit of observation or the critical variables for systematic research remained to be established. It was in the context of this search for new knowledge and new methods of studying human fertility that the idea for conducting a study in the Philippines was conceived.

Initially, the Philippines was selected as a research site because, at that time, a group of social scientists at Notre Dame was planning to conduct a similar project in three Latin American countries. An Asian country with four centuries of Hispanic influence would thus provide a rare opportunity for cross-cultural comparisons. Moreover, William T. Liu had conducted research into the family in several Southeast Asian countries. The Philippines offered an interesting contrast not only because it is a Catholic country, but also because it has a bilateral, rather than a unilineal, kinship system.

Unfortunately, the Notre Dame Latin-American project was aborted shortly after the field work began for reasons extraneous to the research itself. The Philippine project, however, was carried out in the field according to the original plan. Field work was conducted from 1967 through 1969. Organization of the field materials, coding, and the preparation of preliminary drafts followed. In 1971, with the assistance of the International Census Division of the United States Bureau of the Census, tabulations of the fertility data were made. These operations revealed some coding inconsistencies which required further checks and recoding. The tedious work of "cleaning up" and re-editing the data file was ably performed by Igbal Alam, who was then a graduate student in the Department of Population Dynamics at Johns Hopkins University. Due primarily to insufficient funds, the validity and reliability checks of the data file took one year to complete. The final edited tape was used for data analysis in the spring and summer of 1974, after a lapse of one full year during which additional funding was being sought to complete the work. Thus, even though several preliminary chapters had been drafted by this time, the preparation of this volume did not gain momentum until 1975 when Elena Yu, having completed her Ph. D., was able to devote relatively uninterrupted attention to several thousand pages of field notes, interview protocols, reports, publications, dissertations, and computer printout sheets. Publication procedures and critical reviews of the completed chapters by several readers further delayed the publication date. Consequently, a decade has passed since we first visited and interviewed the Cebuano families.

In retrospect, however, the delay was fortuitous. It provided our colleagues and collaborators opportunities individually to publish the portions of the Cebu data which were of primary interest to them, and, at the same time, it gave us enough time to examine carefully what remained to be published. As a result of this delay, we were also able to test our perceptions, findings, and conclusions from the unpublished data against the realities of current sociodemographic literature and Philippine family-planning developments. After months upon months of heated arguments, mutual criticisms, and persistent teamwork, we are pleased to share without hesitation the product of our labor.

In conducting this research, which was called the Cebu Family Health Project, we owe much to the goodwill and efforts of numerous individuals from diverse disciplines and backgrounds, not to mention the thousands of Cebuano families who allowed us to share vicariously in their private lives.

It was Dra. Virginia Pato, now a faculty member of the Cebu Institute of Medicine, who first suggested to William T. Liu the choice of Cebu over Manila as an ideal research site for his proposed project. With her assistance as Co-Investigator of the Cebu Project, we were able to initiate a public health program for fourth-year medical students at the C.I.M. The latter, in turn, developed an Interns Training Program in Pakna-an, a barrio outside the city. The Pakna-an Project was ably supervised by Dr. Francisco Diy, Chairman of the Department of Public Health at the Cebu Institute of Medicine, and by Dr. Florentino Solon, Chief Medical Officer of the Regional Health Office, who was also on the faculty of the Nutrition Department at C.I.M. The Cebu Project and the Pakna-an Project introduced social science training into the medical education programs in Cebu, for which the C.I.M. Director, Dr. Jacinto Velez and the Dean, Dr. Uldarico Bacay, should also share the credit.

During the first year, on the senior investigating team, besides William T. Liu, there was also Bernadine Allen, a psychologist who initially helped to train research assistants and took charge of day-to-day supervision of the field work. She left the project at the end of the first year and was succeeded by Ira Hutchison III and Leo Pinard II, both of whom were graduate students from Notre Dame. In addition, Ernest Brandewie, then Chairman of the Department of Anthropology at the University of San Carlos, was particularly helpful in selecting and training his top graduate students to work for the project. Dr. Brandewie faithfully attended every weekly field seminar and led the discussions on a number of occasions. Father Joseph Goertz, S.V.D., and Dra. Lourdes R. Quisumbing, Chair of the Psychology Department at San Carlos and Dean of the St. Theresa's College respectively, were helpful in giving us generous suggestions. Father Rudolf Rahman, S.V.D. and Father R. Kolk, S.V.D., President and Academic Vice President respectively of the University of San Carlos, had been particularly enthusiastic about the project. Together, they did more than what one could expect to accommodate our research team.

During the second year, Robert Duff, then a graduate student at Notre Dame, joined the research staff and conducted a separate survey to ascertain the particular ways in which birth control information was transmitted in Cebuano neighborhoods. The following summer, Professor Arthur J. Rubel, working with Professor Mimi Trosdal of the Linguistics Department at San Carlos, and other assistants, conducted a special study on the folk midwives in Cebu.

We are also very thankful for the contributions of several capable research assistants and interviewers. Leonisa Ramas, Manolita Campos, Agnes Demetria, and Angelina Lagcao were most helpful in the formulation of research instruments. In addition, the skillful interviewing work carried out by our team of interviewers is deeply appreciated. These interviewers were: Amparo Regaña, Leo Enilog, Susan Alonte, Concepcion Avancena, Josefina Bago, Eleonore May Bessario, Filomena Borromeo, Josefina Camomot, Lillian Cui, Nieva Damo, Edith Escano, Bernadette Labaria, Marietta Lim, Bernardina Lucero, Ruperta Lamapas, Silvia Maambong, Elena Moreno, Emiliana Ocanada, Beatriz Santiago, Jesusa Torres, Gliceria Ybanez, Wilfredo Andrya, Rigoberto Blanco, Gregorio Torres, Jose B. Fuliga, and Melinda Bacol.

To Dolores Lozada Gacasan we owe a special note of gratitude. She not only served ably as secretary, office manager, bookkeeper, and personnel counselor, but also functioned as an important cultural "broker" between the American and the indigenous researchers. Her presence facilitated cross-cultural communications and understanding.

Furthermore, there were many community leaders and medical practitioners in Cebu whose help was so crucial that no project of this magnitude could have been conducted without their support. These community leaders and medical personnel were Uldarico Bacay, M.D., Dean of the Cebu Institute of Medicine; Guillermo Blanco, M.D., President of Philippine Pediatric Society, Cebu Chapter; Venustiano H. J. Borromeo, M.D., President, Cebu Medical Society; Hugo Cruel, Assistant City Health Officer; Horace DeLien, M.D., Director, Public Health Division, USAID/Philippines; Francisco Diy, M.D., Chair, Department of

Public Health, Cebu Institute of Medicine; Cesar Estalilla, M.D., President, Catholic Physicians Guild; Luz de la Paz Pelaez, M.D., Cebu Institute of Medicine; Manuel Segura, M.D., Cebu City Health Officer; Florentino Solon, M.D., Regional Health Officer; and Jacinto Velez, M.D., Cebu Velez General Hospital.

We should add that a number of social scientists both as colleagues and as critics were also particularly supportive of our research. These were: Dr. Mercedes Concepcion of the Institute of Population Studies, University of the Philippines; the late Father Frank Lynch, S.J., then the Director of the Institute of Philippine Culture; Father J. Bulatao, S.J., Ateneo de Manila University; Father Francis Madigan, S.J., Cagayan de Oro University, and Father Wilhelm Flieger, S.V.D., University of San Carlos.

Several American social scientists who had constantly given us their support and suggestions also deserve mention here. Fred L. Strodtbeck, Philip Hauser, Fred Eggan, and Morris Janowitz of the University of Chicago; William D'Antonio, now at the University of Connecticut; the late John Kosa of the Harvard Medical School; the late Irene Taeuber of Princeton University; John Kantner and Melvin Zelnik of the Department of Population Dynamics, Johns Hopkins University; Reuben Hill of the University of Minnesota; and Ronald Freedman of the University of Michigan were particularly helpful in the early stages of research design. Tom Sasaki at the University of Notre Dame; Alan Schneiberg at Northwestern University; Kristin Luker at the University of California, San Diego; and Chester Hunt at Western Michigan University have read portions of this volume in its preliminary draft stages and have contributed to our thinking through the kinds of questions they raised.

To our colleagues on the Cebu Project we would like to mention specifically Virginia Pato, Arthur J. Rubel, Robert Duff, Ira Hutchison, and Leo W. Pinard for their individual and collective contributions.

At this juncture, we cannot resist the temptation to interject some personal notes of deep gratitude. For William T. Liu, the friendship and guidance of the late George N. Shuster has been invaluable. It was the leadership of Dr. Shuster, former President of Hunter College of the City University of New York, who after retirement came to Notre Dame, that provided the impetus for the Notre Dame Conferences on Population in the sixties. Both the Population Conferences and the Center for the Study of Man established by Dr. Shuster fell on the shoulders of William T. Liu upon Dr. Shuster's second retirement.

Elena Yu would like to express her *utang-na-loob* to her Filipino godmother, Rufina Ouano, in whose house she grew up as a child. It was through her godmother and other members and servants in that unforgettable household that Elena Yu learned to speak Cebuano, which proved valuable in the course of writing parts of this book.

Last but not least, the Cebu project was initially funded by the United States Agency for International Development between 1967 and 1969, and subsequently by the Ford Foundation, from 1974 until the manuscript was nearing completion. During the interim, the University of Notre Dame, through the O'Brien Fund for faculty research awarded to William T. Liu and the University of Victoria, through the Canada Council Faculty Research Grant awarded to Elena Yu, had contributed to the continuation of research efforts that made possible the final completion of this book. We are also most appreciative of the patient editorial assistance rendered by Ann Rice, Richard Allen, Beth Luey, Barbara Millward and James Langford. Needless to say, we alone are responsible for any errors that may be contained herein.

1 / Introduction

Sprawled on the Pacific fringe of Southeast Asia is a swarm of some 7,100 islands which constitutes the *Republika ng Pilipinas*. Once the oriental entrepôt of a far-flung Spanish empire, it was the first country in Southeast Asia to achieve independence after World War II and is the only Christian country in all of Asia.

Only 2,870 of its islands and islets have been named; not all are inhabited. Its two largest ones, Luzon to the north and Mindanao to the south, together comprise almost two-thirds of the nation's total land area of 300,000 square kilometers. Between Luzon and Mindanao are legions of scattered land masses which are collectively called the Visayas or the Bisayan area. The country as a whole exhibits marked regionality in social, economic, and religious life. Its riparian geography is graced with tropical forests, volcanic peaks, lush valleys, and rice terraces; its landscape, bordered with fishing villages, is dotted with Spanish cathedrals, Islamic mosques, Hollywood houses, and nipa huts. Its mountain ranges contain rich deposits of gold, copper, lead, zinc, manganese, iron ore, nickel-bearing laterites, refractory chromite, and coal. Other minerals found are salt, sulphur, clay for brickmaking and pottery, adobe stone, marble, petroleum, cement materials (limestone and shale), glass sand, guano, phosphate rocks, gypsum, asphalt, asbestos, barite, and magnesite—much of which has yet to be exploited.

Such contrastive topography and abundant resources belie the plethora of social and economic problems that beset the nation, as in other less developed countries. In the Philippines, however, these problems have been so intertwined with population growth over the decades that it is futile to try to separate the antecedent from the consequent factors, or even to untangle the chain of complex interrelations.

In this book, we make no pretense of diagnosing the entire gamut of socioeconomic ills that plague the Philippines, nor do we purport to present a comprehensive analysis of the staggering population increase in the country. Rather, we seek only to unravel a small but potent aspect of the human reproduction problem: family, kinship, and fertility-coping behavior. Our objective is to describe how the people from one area of central Philippines (Cebu Province) have coped with the realities of large family size: What have they done to limit their number of births?

What do they know about contraceptive methods? How successful have they been in using them? And how do lower-class people cope with the psychic and economic burden of raising children? We are interested in how the family, serving as an intermediary between the cultural system and the individual, shapes the latter's perception of kinship duties and obligations, assists her or him in coping with the exigencies of sheer survival and reproduction, and in turn influences his or her family-building processes. In searching for answers to these questions, we will attempt to identify some of the social institutions and value systems that encourage the propagation of large families, and try to provide a preliminary understanding of the patterns of interaction between husband and wife, families and relatives, as well as friends and neighbors—in addition to a brief description of folk contraceptive practices—all of which form part of the reproductive context of the Cebuanos.

Magnitude of the Population Problem

Just a decade before the present study was conducted, a few demographic researchers attuned to the Philippine situation had maintained that the country was *not* overpopulated (Hawley, 1954a; Madigan, 1959), that it was "more in the category of underpopulation" (Madigan, 1959:20). What they recognized were maldistribution of population and insufficient exploitation of natural resources. The argument was also advanced that not only was the growth trend *not* a cause for alarm, but that it would "undoubtedly be good for the agricultural industry" and "good for the already established light consumer industry," and that "there is bound to be some increase in jobs because more persons mean more jobs to take care of them" (Madigan, 1959:21).[1] Such views were sharply questioned by other analysts (Aromin, 1959; Carroll, 1959) and stood in striking contrast with the unsubstantiated impressions afforded by historians, geographers, travelers, and others whose interest in Philippine population and fertility was merely peripheral. Despite their divergent disciplinary orientations and investigative purposes, these investigators were convinced that explosive population growth was imminent in "the Pearl of the Orient." Finally, when the foreboding projections made by the Bureau of Census and Statistics Survey of Households (BCSSH, now called National Census and Statistics Office) were followed by the census count in 1970, the message was unequivocal. Starting with a population of only 7.6 million in 1903, the country had an observed total population of 19,234,182 by 1948. This increased to 27,087,685 in 1960, and on May 6, 1970, it stood at 36,684,486. Concepcion (1966:192) stated the dramatic increase succinctly: "From the time of Magellan's voyage to these islands in 1521 where there were about half a million Filipinos, it took four and a half centuries to add over 30 million people—the increase now anticipated in about two decades!" The figure is even more startling when it is gauged on an international yardstick. The Philippines, with a land area roughly twice that of the state of Ohio, ranks fifteenth in population among the countries of the world. Of these fifteen countries, only Germany and Bangladesh have smaller land areas than the Philippines. In terms of population density, however, the Philippines has about 148 persons per square kilometer, as compared to 64.1 in 1948 and 90.3 in 1960. Such a measure of population concentration is admittedly crude, for it assumes that the people are evenly distributed across the country and it fails to exclude the mountainous, swampy, and other nonarable regions. However, it does give a quick comparison of the increase over the years and across countries. If we rank-order the U.N. midyear 1977 estimates for all the countries in the world with a population of at least 500,000, the magnitude of population growth in the Philippines becomes readily apparent. Its estimate of 44.3 millions is nearly twice that projected for Canada, whose land area is more than thirty-three times the size of the Philippines. Compared to populations in countries of the Western Hemisphere, the Philippine population is exceeded only by those of Brazil, Mexico, and the United States.

An alternative method commonly used to ascertain the magnitude of population growth is to evaluate the data on live births and deaths. Unfortunately, the collection of such statistics for the Philippines is shrouded in confusion (cf. Hawley, 1954b; Valenzuela, 1954; Morrison, 1956; Carroll, 1959; Concepcion, 1966; Mortel and Nazaret, 1971; Flieger, 1974). For instance, Hawley (1954b; 1954c) has criticized the 1948 census enumeration effort and hinted that more than one census taker must have *estimated* the population in potentially dangerous or inaccessible areas of the countryside rather than *count* it as they were instructed. That these suspicions have not been dispelled even in the most recent census (1970) is well articulated in Flieger's paper (1974), where he meticulously presented his arguments as to why the census age structure is incorrect for either the 1960 or the 1970 census material, or both. In that same paper, he also questioned the accuracy of the *Vital Statistics Report 1970* (BCS, 1973)—the most recently available publication—since it gave an "implausible" national crude death rate of 7.33 per thousand males, and of 5.47 per thousand females. Even the data collected through a dual record procedure in the Sample Vital Registration System set up by NCSO in 1971 to overcome these errors are of dubious quality (Flieger, 1974:4–8). Among other reasons, it was reported that deaths which occurred in nonsample areas or among transients were included in the reports of vital events in the sampled areas; the requisite of independence in dual record-keeping was said to have been violated by the facts that there was considerable overlapping of personnel in both collecting systems and that the same reporters were often employed at both chores of record-keeping enumeration. The field personnel's naïveté about sampling procedures and demographic research only exacerbated the problem.

Consequently, fertility researchers must labor under the constraint of these methodological limitations. By and large, the consensus seems to be that the high death rate from the beginning of the century until 1930 had declined rapidly thereafter, especially after World War II, when health conditions improved considerably. It is also generally agreed that the estimated crude birth rate between the end of the nineteenth century and the years immediately after World War II is around 49 per thousand population, the same figure as the birth rate estimated for the country from 1876 to 1903 (Aromin, 1959, 1963; cf. also Morrison, 1957:17; United Nations, 1959). By the late fifties, the United Nations and ECAFE office still calculated the same estimated birth rate of 49 per thousand per year (Aromin, 1959:28), whereas Jupp (1960:17) supplied an estimate of a little over 47 per thousand for different intervals between 1930 and 1952. All in all, refined estimates of the birth rate for the period between 1948 and 1962 varied from 42.6 to 56.4 per thousand population (Adams, 1958; Pascual, 1966; Madigan and Avancena, 1964; De Los Angeles, 1965; Madigan, 1965) and ranged from 38.6 to 50 per thousand between 1968 and 1975 (United Nations, 1977; Lorimer, 1966; Keyfietz and Flieger, 1971; Concepcion, 1974). The most recently published report on the levels and trends of fertility throughout the world released by the United Nations (1977:200) offered the hypothesis that the crude birth rate, ranging between 45 and 50 per thousand "had probably not changed for the past seventy years."[2]

Depending upon the kinds of assumptions made and the source one most trusts, the projections for 1980 range from a low of 49 to 54.3 million estimated by Lorimer (1966) to a high of 55 to 59 million calculated by the Inter-Agency Committee on Demography, National Economic Council of the Philippines. By the year 2000 the population figure may increase to as high as 111 million (Concepcion and Flieger, 1968:714).[3] To be sure, the accuracy of these predictions depends heavily on the veracity of the population censuses and the sample surveys of households,[4] other things being equal. Yet there is reasonable evidence to suspect that the error in these sources may have been in the direction of an *under*estimate.[5] If this is true, the actual Philippine population may be larger than the experts have calculated and projected.

Fertility Studies in the Philippines

Amidst the global concern and pressing national need to stem the onrushing tide of accelerating population increase, the first fertility survey was launched in 1956, when a few questions were inserted into the interview schedule of the Philippine Statistical Survey of Households (PSSH). By May 1963, it was learned from the PSSH that the average number of children born per ever-married woman with completed fertility (forty-five years and over) in the rural areas was 6.4; in May 1965 this stood at 6.7 (BCSSH, 1968b). Furthermore, the 1963 survey showed that 42.1 percent of the urban and 48.1 percent of rural ever-married women forty-five years or older had seven or more children. By 1965 these figures had increased somewhat: 43.6 percent for women in the urban sector, and 48.1 percent for the rural areas. These facts did not appear to deviate significantly from Taeuber's report (1960:108) that in 1939, 53 percent of all women aged forty-five to fifty-four who provided information on children ever born had stated having seven or more children.

Beginning in 1963, a series of fertility inquiries was conducted under different auspices in selected areas of the country (Concepcion and Flieger, 1968; Concepcion and Hendershoot, 1969). Of these, the ones conducted in Imus, Cavite (1963), Tiwi, Albay (1964), Calasiao, Pangasinan (1964), Miagao, Iloilo (1966), Manila (1967), and lowland Philippines (1967) are noteworthy since they preceded the Cebu Family Health Project. Their significance rests not on methodological rigor but on their pioneering effort to appraise the knowledge, attitudes, and practice (KAP) of contraception among Filipinos. Analyses of the data from Imus, Tiwi, Calasiao, and Miagao were carried out by Trinidad S. Osteria and Antonio R. Pacheco separately as part of their M.A. theses in demography submitted to the Population Institute of the University of the Philippines. Since these materials were largely unavailable to researchers, a distillation of the two theses was subsequently mimeographed and published under the editorship of Edmund M. Murphy (1968).

Strictly speaking, these surveys are not exactly comparable because the sampling procedures, the types of questions asked, and the instructions given to the interviewers varied. However, sufficiently parallel information was sought from all the surveys to justify a "forced" comparison for the sake of obtaining an overall picture of the Filipino KAP data prior to our study.

The results from the first four fertility surveys in the country indicated that in terms of the number of children ever born, Imus (1963) and

Calasiao (1964) stood apart from Tiwi (1964) and Miagao (1966). Tabulations from each of the latter two places showed that about 55 percent of the married women (aged fifteen to forty-four) had had five or more children at the time of the interview, while in Imus and Calasiao the corresponding figure was about 49 percent (Murphy, 1968:34). Nonetheless, this difference of 6 percent suggests that in general the fertility performance of all the married women interviewed was quite high.

When age and marriage duration were standardized, and the mean number of children ever born tabulated by the various socioeconomic characteristics (Murphy, 1968:36–37), a fragmented consistency is discernible. Across the board, the average number of children ever born hovered around three to four children. Women whose husbands had at least some college education exhibited a slightly lower fertility than those whose husbands were less educated. There was only one exception: the Calasiao women whose husbands had no schooling had had only 2.33 children. Hence, they seem to belong to the low fertility group.

A careful examination of the interrelationship between the wife's education and fertility outcome in each of the four areas yielded no significant variables and showed very little consistency from place to place. In Imus, for instance, women who had no schooling whatsoever, those who had completed high school, and those who had completed college shared a great deal in common. Their average number of children ranged only from 3.14 to 3.56. In Tiwi, however, women who had completed college had only 1.98 children, while the corresponding figures for those with less education ranged from 3.8 to 4.9 children. However, the number of married women who completed college was only 11 out of 1,410 interviewed in that locale, much too small for us to feel confident about that finding.

With respect to the husband's occupation, the picture is equally muddled. Whereas in Imus the average number of children ever born was lower among white-collar workers and proprietors or sales workers, the relationship is exactly inverse in Miagao, where farmers and blue-collar workers had fewer children. All in all, these results do not appear to lend strong support to Concepcion's earlier findings (1963), based on national sample surveys by the Bureau of Census, that fertility (as measured by children ever born) varied inversely with socioeconomic status no matter which of the variables was used to measure status.

Furthermore, in three of the four areas studied (Imus, Calasiao, and Miagao), a large discrepancy exists between the percentage of married women who had knowledge of birth control and those who practiced it. Of the small percentage of ever-married women who knew about birth control,[6] fewer than half in each locale practiced it.[7] The datum from

Tiwi, Albay, is the only exception. There the percentages of women claiming both knowledge and practice of birth control are exactly the same, leading Concepcion and Flieger to speculate that KAP questions on contraception must have been meaningless to this group of respondents (of course, their symbolic significance to the other group of respondents cannot be clearly established, either).

Fear of injuring health was the most frequently cited reason by women in Imus, Calasiao, and Miagao for not trying family limitation methods even though they claimed to have some knowledge of contraception. The second reason cited in Imus and Calasiao, but not in Miagao, was fear of God.

In April and May 1966, the University of the Philippines Population Institute conducted a sample survey of Manila households. A total of 917 wives under forty years of age were interviewed. Pratt (1967) compared the results of this survey with those obtained by the Bureau of Census and Statistical Survey of Households (BCSSH) in 1956. His conclusions were not encouraging. There was no appreciable change in fertility between the two periods. The number of children ever born at successive ages of the respondents was about the same as a decade earlier. Completed family size for those interviewed remained at six children or slightly more. Although 82.1 percent of the married women under forty years of age had some knowledge of birth control and as many as 70 percent expressed approval, only 39.7 percent of these women practiced it.

In a larger family survey in 1967, almost all the noncity dwellers over fifteen years of age in the so-called Lowland Christian areas of the Philippines were designated as the sampling frame.[8] A total of twenty-four respondents per municipality were interviewed from one hundred municipalities selected (Lynch and Makil, 1967). It was found that 62 percent of the married women approved of family planning, while 38 percent disapproved. Age breakdowns indicated that, on the whole, more married women approved than disapproved, with the greatest percentage of approval found among women between twenty-five and thirty-four years of age. In their own words (Lynch and Makil, 1967: 302–03):

> The tendency to favor family planning is associated with high educational attainment, frequent mass-media exposure, upper social status, and being a Protestant. . . . Respondents who disapprove of family planning appeal most often to general norms of religion, morality, and health—but rarely mention the Catholic faith. . . . Among those who approve . . . by far the greatest percentage favor techniques approved by the Catholic church. Both those who approve and those who disapprove of family planning tend to say their pastors agree with them.

In summary, the studies reviewed here have followed the standard KAP survey approach. The investigations were not coordinated with the intention of ensuring a probability sample of the Philippines as a whole, nor were the selected communities meant to represent the provinces from which they were drawn. As Flieger and Concepcion pointed out, their objective was to provide much-needed preliminary empirical data on the prevalence of contraceptive knowledge, attitudes, and practices in diverse areas throughout the country. Aside from raising key issues pertaining to the reliability and validity of KAP measurements, they uncovered evidence of contraceptive ignorance and confusion. It was not uncommon for respondents to mistake contraception for induced abortion.

Because the data gathered in such studies are suited for large-scale coverage and for tabulated numerical summaries, contextual materials are often ignored by the interviewers or lost between the punch holes of IBM cards. Thus, the richness of family, kinship, and social interactional data that might have a bearing on contraceptive decisions and fertility outcome has remained unappreciated.

To be sure, such limitations can partly be attributed to the fact that the parameters of the problem were not entirely known when these studies were initiated, owing to the absence of aggregate data on fertility other than those obtained from the survey of households. Concepcion and Flieger (1968) noted that there was widespread belief at the time—and this was still not dispelled when we conducted our interviews in Cebu—that Filipinos would be too shy to submit to questions on childbirth asked by total strangers, let alone to discuss family planning and fertility-related issues. Hence, the overriding concern at the time was the development of a research instrument applicable to the Filipino culture that would provide the KAP of family planning and not tax the respondents' patience. The conditions in the Philippines thus stood in sharp contrast to what had transpired in the United States, where fertility studies had engaged the attention of sociologists for well over a decade.

The Objectives of This Study

The purpose of this study is threefold: (1) to describe the fertility-related behavior and attitudes of Filipino women against the social-structural constraints and variations in Philippine society, particularly in the Lowland Christian and Visayan region; (2) to understand the cultural elements that shape normative patterns and relations, kinship obligations, and child care; and (3) to describe in detail the role of the

Filipino family in influencing and coping with fertility outcome, by mediating between the cultural system and the individual.

Since published findings on the earlier surveys had to do with regions outside the Visayas, very little was known about Visayan women's fertility when this study began. Consequently, the work was designed primarily to explore as much as possible the parameters of fertility-related behavior in the Cebuano culture, and to unravel profitable areas for more specific and quantitative research. Survey data were supplemented with in-depth interviews on a very small sample of women for the purpose of gaining insights into fertility-related behavior that would not have surfaced had we confined ourselves to a structured instrument administered on a single visit with each respondent.

After thousands of interview hours over nearly eighteen months in Cebu, the task of organizing and reporting theoretically relevant findings in a coherent manner for the general reader proved to be quite a challenge. This volume was preceded by five doctoral dissertations, a specially edited journal published in the Philippines, and more than a dozen journal articles scattered in various fields, including anthropology, sociology, marriage and the family, communication, population and demography, religion and theology, and family planning. These publications involved most of our professional staff members and covered a period from 1968 through 1976. The present volume not only integrates our published findings, but also adds new, unpublished materials we believe are important in understanding Filipino fertility.

In order to summarize our research findings adequately, we believe that it is necessary to give the historical context of Philippine society. Human fertility, like social behavior in general, represents an adaptation to and reflection of the various demands of the sociopolitical system. Changes in society are often accompanied by changes in familial behavior, which are discernible in the variations of fertility behavior over time. Specifically, we believe that the enduring effects of colonization have had an enormous impact on many Filipino institutions. Because of its unique contacts with Spain and the United States, Philippine society cannot be compared with Hispanic societies in the Western Hemisphere, some similarities notwithstanding. It has its unique characteristics, as the reader will appreciate after reading Chapter 2.

In Chapter 3, the procedure of data collection and some of the rarely publicized problems of field research are reported. Viewed from the perspective of standard survey texts used in this country, our field approach in the Philippines may be perceived as unorthodox. But, then, the kind of field problems we encountered were unlike those found in this country, where the sampling frames are available, maps are accurate, telephone appointments can be made, and the respondents are accustomed to being interviewed alone. Because these conditions did not exist when we conducted our study, new procedures had to be improvised, and difficult decisions had to be made.

A profile of Cebuano reproductive behavior is presented in Chapter 4, where some indicators of Filipino fertility are summarized in statistical tables, augmented with textual materials gathered from in-depth interviews. This section is followed by two chapters on the Cebuanos' knowledge of modern contraceptives and folk methods of birth control. We will argue that within the context of Filipino reproduction, the *mananabang*, or indigenous untrained folk midwife, is a creation of the culture and its institutions. In turn, the *mananabang* as a social type creates its own market, develops its own practices, and supports the syndrome of pronatalistic values.

Next, we confront the meaning of pregnancy in male-female relationships, both in and out of wedlock, in Chapters 7 and 8. In a country where the gulf between the rich and the poor is extremely wide, various forms of dependency relationships develop to improve the individual's chances for survival and status attainment. The *querida* or mistress system, which occurs in varying forms in the Philippines and other Catholic countries, can be viewed as an adaptation to social demands and archaic institutions. Because of their unique impact on *societal* fertility, we deemed it important to discuss extramarital relationships in a separate chapter, especially since the majority of demographic studies have dealt solely with marital, rather than societal, fertility.

Finally, we come full circle and ask a different set of questions normally not raised in standard KAP studies. How, for instance, do the Cebuanos cope with their large numbers of children? Do they not realize that children are "expensive" to raise? Why, then, do they not regulate their family size? Three chapters—9, 10, and 11—are devoted to these issues. The first deals exclusively with the relationship between the family system and fertility—how sociologists have traditionally phrased their questions and how one may look at the same sets of variables differently. The second focuses on the web of kinship and its significance for lower-class survival relative to the middle-class lifestyle. The third chapter describes in great detail the Cebuano practice of "spreading their cost" of child-rearing and at the same time maximizing their socioeconomic gains. The coping mechanisms discussed in these three chapters have heretofore not been given due emphasis by family planners. They have, however, worked marvelously to sustain the population growth of the Philippines—as the reader will readily grasp in Chapter 12, where we draw together our findings from each of the chapters in this volume and present our conclusions.

2 / Philippine Society

Because of unique historical circumstances, Philippine society and culture defy sweeping typifications. Racially, the Filipinos are a blend of Malay stocks to which have been added distinctive strains of Chinese,[1] Spanish, American, and some European extractions. The country was settled by Hinduized Malays of the Shri-Visayan and Madjapahit empires, as well as Muslim Malays from Malacca and the ubiquitous Chinese traders, long before Magellan "discovered" it in 1521. His death at the hands of Lapu-Lapu delayed the Spanish conquest of the Philippines by more than forty years. It was not until 1565 that Migual Lopez de Lagaspi took formal possession of some of its islands in the name of King Philip II of Spain.

Spanish Heritage

The arrival of the Spanish conquerors led to the development of a three-tier economy (Wickberg, 1965): (1) a "Western" economy managed solely for and by the Spaniards whose main objective was to trade Mexican silver for Chinese luxury goods, as epitomized in the famous galleon trade that plied between Manila and Acapulco; (2) a "native" subsistence economy which remained largely as it had been before the Conquest because the galleon trade was the primary and sufficient source of income for the Spanish settlers in the Philippines; and (3) a Chinese economy which mediated between the other two systems. Besides engaging in maritime trading and artisanry with the local population, the Chinese acted as middlemen, taking their imports to the villagers in exchange for local crafts and products for the Spaniards. Consequently, three different legal statuses were formulated for the populace: Spaniard, "Indio" (the Spanish term for "natives"), and Chinese, to which a fourth, Mestizo, appeared when interracial marriages became more widespread during the eighteenth century. Using the principle of divide and rule, the Spaniards were always in the upper class, while the Chinese and the Indios were free to move up and down the social ladder. Such a style of colonial administration produced enduring consequences in the Philippines, for the agricultural development of the country was haphazard, if not largely neglected, and the Chinese gradually acquired a virtual monopoly of the retail trade.

Catholicism was the only major unifying force in this fragmented society. Through this ideology, Spain "liberated" the Philippines on the expressed rationale that the pre-Conquest "pagan" religion of the Filipinos was a tyrannical enslavement of the devil, and that the preexisting sharecropping and debt peonage system based on usury was an unjust form of social organization. Thus, in Phelan's view (1959), the Spanish Conquest was "justified" on both "spiritual and social grounds."

Nevertheless, missionary work in the Philippines was not without its problems, a shortage of priests being one of them.[2] The friars' attempt to resettle and congregate the Filipinos in order to maximize religious indoctrination by a few and to keep the people from living *sin policia* (without a polity) was tenaciously resisted, since it was incompatible with the indigenous subsistence economy. Consequently, the external ritual of the church became the principal inducement for gathering the people. In the process, Spanish Catholicism became "Filipinized." Holy Week, Corpus Christi, and *pista sa nayon* (town fiesta), with their colorful pageantry, became splendid occasions for blending the sacred and profane (Phelan, 1959: 72–89). The magical spirits and superstitious beliefs from the pre-Conquest era also became entrenched in the syncretic folk Catholicism still in evidence in many parts of the country.[3] All through the Spanish colonization, the Filipinos' faith in the efficacy of holy water was "almost boundless, and their demand for it was insatiable" (Phelan, 1959:75). Such a demand still exists nowadays, although as one goes up the social ladder its prevalence has been considerably attenuated. The Spanish clergy's ethnocentric stance of restricting Filipino priesthood in the end worked against their goal of hispanization of the islands. In Phelan's opinion, however, Spain's success in colonizing the Philippines stemmed precisely from their failure to acculturate the Indios as much as they had originally expected. The concentration of social, economic, political, and ecclesiastical power in the Spanish theocratic administration produced a polarized class system, although it did subjugate the warring *barangays* (kinship-based communities of the pre-Conquest era) under unified rule. This sense of community eventually suggested the possibility of nationhood.

United States Influence

Following the Spanish-American War, the Philippines was ceded to the United States on December 10, 1898, upon the ratification of the Spanish-American peace treaty in Paris. The abortive independent republic established by the Filipinos during the interim was short-lived. For the next forty-eight years, the country was to experience a different mode of colonial government, interrupted briefly by Japanese occupation —the American policy of "benevolent assimilation" (Taylor, 1964).

After the Philippines became an unincorporated territory of the United States at the turn of the century, the Americans approved a Bill of Rights for the Philippine Islands which was to parallel the American Constitution. There were two crucial deviations, however, whose significance was not well understood then although they were inserted specifically to suit traditions of Philippine society. The first is the greater centralization of power in the presidency in that control over the budget and local government is granted to that office. The second difference is that under the Philippine Constitution, "it is the good of the State, not the good of the individual that must prevail" (Taylor, 1964:70).

When the U.S. military government ended, the first nationwide census was conducted in 1903. In addition, concepts of due process of law, respect for private property, and public education in its rudimentary form were introduced, mostly by superimposing them on the Spanish legacy rather than by replacing it. Banking and insurance institutions, along with systems of communication (postal, telegraph, telephone, radio facilities, and printed material), were developed, with English as the medium of communication. Great improvements were made in public health and mass education, benefiting a sizable proportion of the populace for many years to come.

The Tydings-McDuffie Act, signed by President Franklin D. Roosevelt and accepted by the Philippine legislature in 1934, stipulated that complete independence would be granted to the country after the establishment of a ten-year transitional government called the Commonwealth. It allowed the United States to retain military bases in the archipelago and to cut off free trade with the Philippines after independence; it also restricted Filipino immigration into the United States, although American immigration to the Philippines was not similarly curtailed (Molina, 1960; Taylor, 1964).

When the Philippines celebrated its "independence" amidst the ruins of war in 1946, the country found itself politically free indeed, but still economically dependent on the United States as a result of the trade acts negotiated between the two countries.[4] The establishment of "free trade" with the United States beginning in 1909 had allowed the Philippines to export raw agricultural material without paying the U.S. tariffs normally levied against foreign goods, in exchange for U.S. manufactured and processed imports (McHale, 1952). Consequently, power production and manufacturing in the islands were retarded, since the U.S. decision to grant independence had stymied any long-term business investment interest that might otherwise have been shown in the Philippines.

The detrimental effects of such economic dependency on the United States are self-evident. From 1945 until 1969, Philippine imports surpassed exports, resulting in an unfavorable balance of trade.[5] On February 21, 1970, the government introduced the system of flexible exchange rates in an attempt to ameliorate the deteriorating balance-of-payments situation. The result was a devaluation of the peso by 60 percent (as of 1971). The exchange rate between the peso and the dollar in 1968 had averaged 3.90 pesos per dollar but it floated to about 6.25 pesos per dollar after the devaluation. By 1977 the currency exchange reached 7.50 pesos per dollar. Unfortunately, the system of flexible exchange rates did not really alter the import-oriented consumption patterns of the Philippines. An examination of the foreign trade data for every year from 1969 to 1974 (the most recent published data as of this writing) reveals that balance-of-trade deficits persist (NCSO, 1973a, 1973b, 1975c).

In short, except for the cash crops that were cultivated explicitly for export to the United States, agriculture and industry during the U.S. occupation remained basically as they were before the turn of the century. The three-tier economy of Spanish colonization was largely undisturbed. The legal restrictions the Spaniards imposed against the Chinese were lifted under the U.S. protectorate, and subsequent increases in the Chinese population—albeit insignificant in proportion to the total population increase of the country—only strengthened their role as middlemen.

Colonial Impact on the Social Structure

In addition to the religious, political, and economic impact of more than four hundred years of colonial experience, both Spanish and U.S. influence in the Philippines had distinct social-structural consequences as well. First of all, through its missionary zeal to spread the Christian faith, Spain introduced the *padrinazgo* (godparenthood) and *compadrazgo* (coparenthood) system which subsequently became entrenched and elaborated in its colonies. Historically, the ritual performed two functions: (1) it formally recruited new members into the Catholic community through the initiation rite of baptism, a sacrament designed to remove the stigma of original sin; (2) the rites after baptism (including confirmation) ensured that undesirable members of society were excluded from the religious community until they had proven their sincerity in becoming members of the church. The latter function was decidedly important in the early days of the spread of Christianity in order to protect the aboriginal converts from the "sinful" influence of pagans and heretics (Mintz and Wolf, 1950). However, in the Philippines as in Spain, the religious rite quickly became a multifaceted patronage system linking the participants vertically and horizontally in the existing social structure. Consequently, the individual is afforded a loaded "matrix" of costs and gains in social interaction and child-rearing, one in which the risks and probabilities would have been different if *compadrazgo* and *padrinazgo* had not existed, as will be seen in Chapter 11.

Second, both the Spanish theocratic government and the social patronage system displayed a hierarchical authority structure which was to leave lasting imprints in the Philippines. The preeminence of God over state, ruler over subjects, and family over individual remained unquestioned for several centuries. Order and harmony were (and still are) thus given absolute emphasis at both the political and the interpersonal levels.

Third, Catholic teachings and the presumptive right of the conquerors to partake in the spoils established a standard against which men and women were to structure their social and sexual relationships. Two logically dissonant concepts—premarital chastity for women and a virility complex for men—received colonial sanction, if not legal support. Furthermore, the supreme value placed on female sexual purity and the fact that marriage was an institution that linked two families rather than two individuals necessitated the adoption of chaperonage in order to "protect" the woman's and her family's reputation. The *querida* or mistress system evolved in the process as a "safety valve" to sustain the integrity of the family system and to maintain the double standard.

Fourth, by superimposing a modified version of the U.S. Constitution on an anachronistic Spanish legal structure, the system of government in the Philippines retained the form but not necessarily the substance of modern democracy. The concept of popular primary education introduced by the United States improved the odds of upward social mobility for the common *tao*. It also opened independent career opportunities for the unmarried woman who until then had been confined to domesticity by Spanish moral codes.

Fifth, the peculiar legal status of the Filipinos (who were defined as *nationals* but not citizens of the United States) and the widespread adoption of the English language generated an orientation toward "stateside" migration (cf. Keeley, 1973). This was originally for the purpose of obtaining a "liberal" education to implement democratic principles; subsequently it was used for economic betterment, political asylum, and professional enhancement. A small but steady stream of plantation workers and farm laborers migrating to Hawaii and the West Coast beginning in 1907 probably helped to ease the pressure of rapid population growth in selected areas at home. Moreover, the large postwar influx of ambitious and talented Filipinos into the United States for training in the health fields resulted in the direct transplantation of modern technical training and medical practices into the urban centers of the Philippines, but left the rural sector largely as it had been for centuries. This led to the existence of dual systems of health practices: the Western model for educated urbanites, and folk methods for the less privileged masses.

Lastly, in marriage and the family, the U.S. influence rendered public display of affection more acceptable and gave increasing respectability to the concept of unchaperoned dating, but only among the avant-garde members of the society living in metropolitan areas. However, it has gradually changed the role of the family elders in mate selection. The continuous importation of U.S. movies and other media materials spurs even greater consumption demand for foreign products and reinforces an orientation toward an "American" lifestyle as portrayed by Hollywood producers, thereby helping to accelerate the migratory flow to the United States. On return visits home, the *balikbayan*'s tales fan the strong wanderlust of townmates and cast doubt on the importance of adhering to traditional values and customs.

Filipino Culture and Society

In studying a society such as that in the Philippines, it is very easy to deduce from the protracted history of foreign domination that there is no distinctly Filipino culture. It is further tempting to conclude, on the basis of geographical fragmentation and ethnolinguistic insularity, that the country is a congeries of islands and nothing more. Nevertheless, a study of social-structural uniformities across regions, a look at the census statistics, an examination of earlier writings by the Spanish friars, and a reading of the more recent social scientific literature suggest that such swift generalizations should be regarded with skepticism. They ignore the stable cultural elements that reach far into the pre-Hispanic past and obscure the common threads of values and beliefs that a large number of Filipinos share.

Culturally, for instance, the Filipinos have been classified into three main groups since the Spanish era, mainly for administrative purposes: Negrillos, Indios, and Moros. While there are some inaccuracies in the Spainards' categorization of the Negrillos (they are made up of

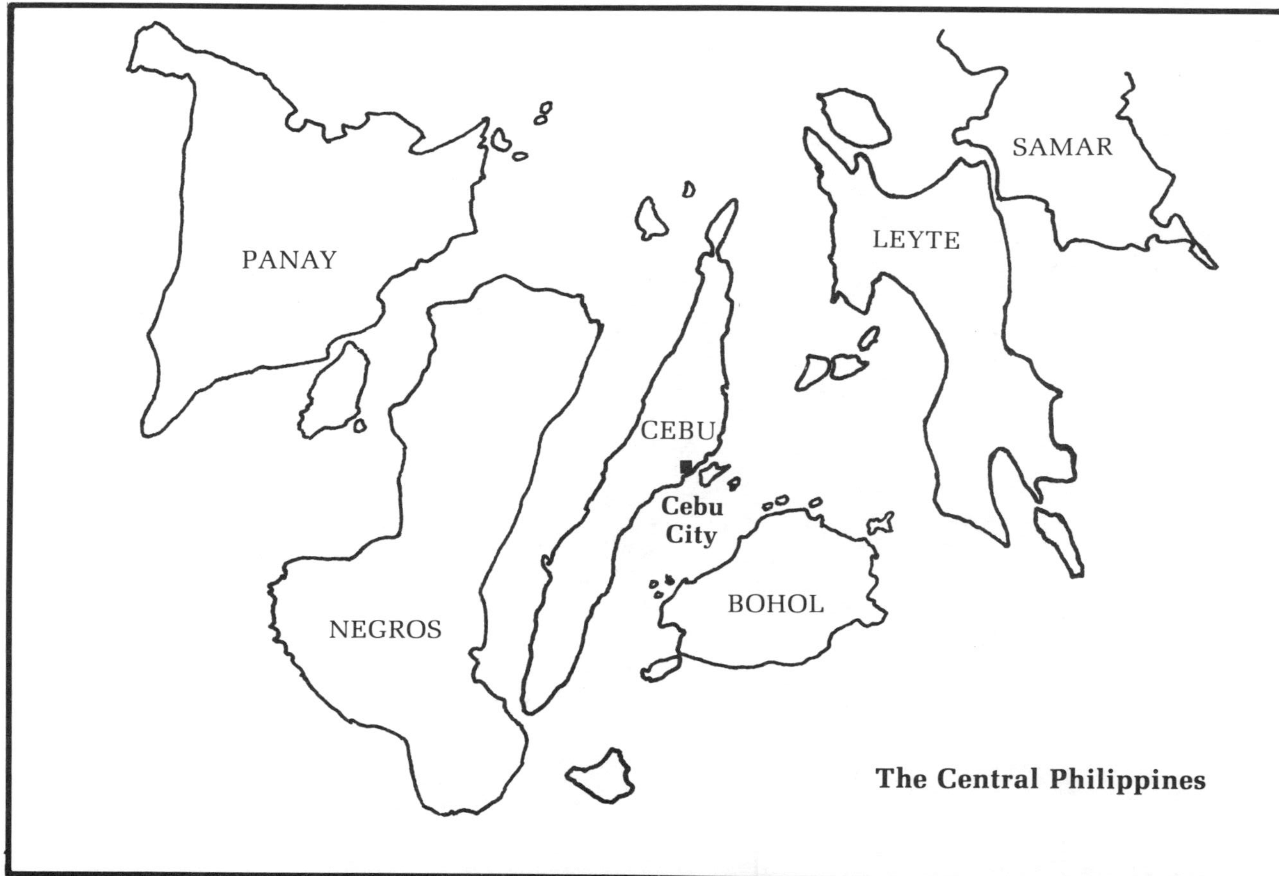

The Central Philippines

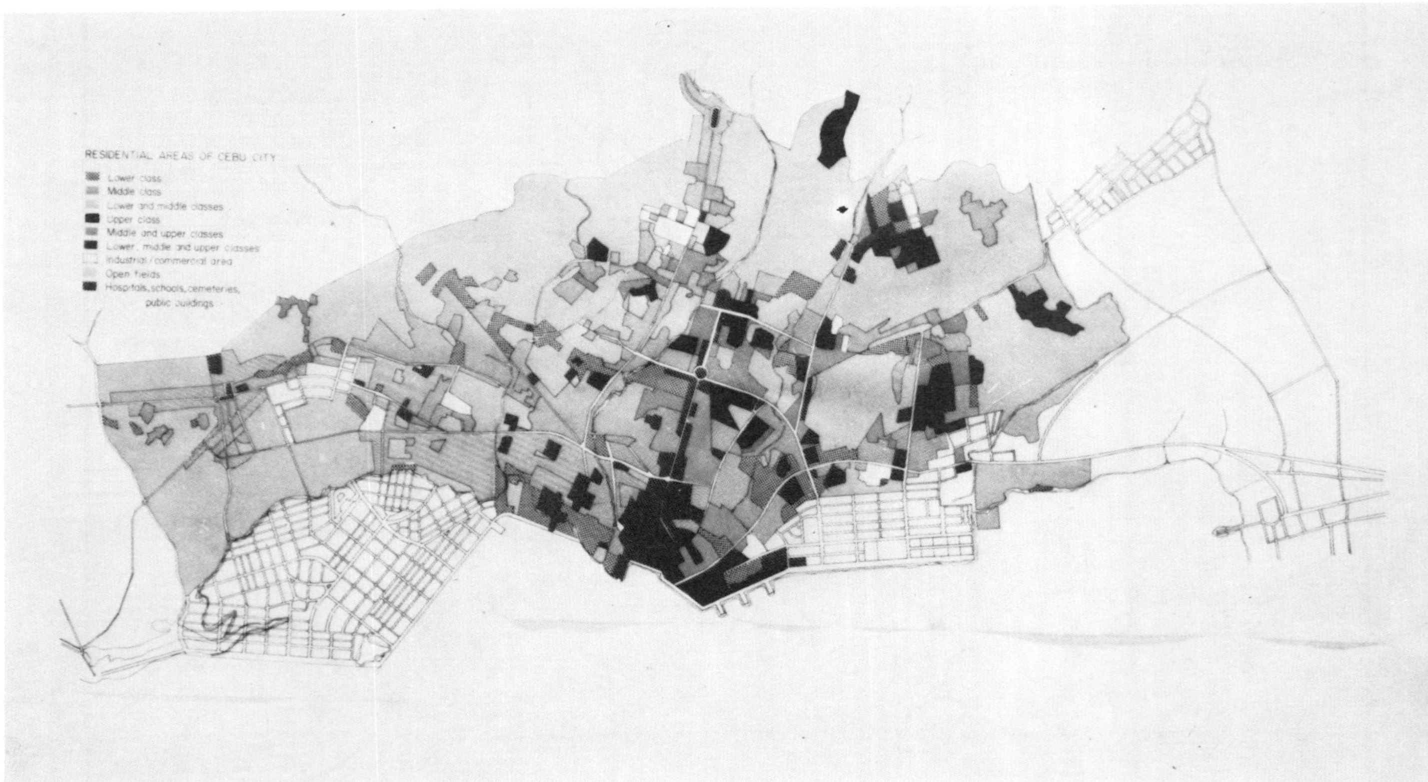

Residential Map of Cebu City

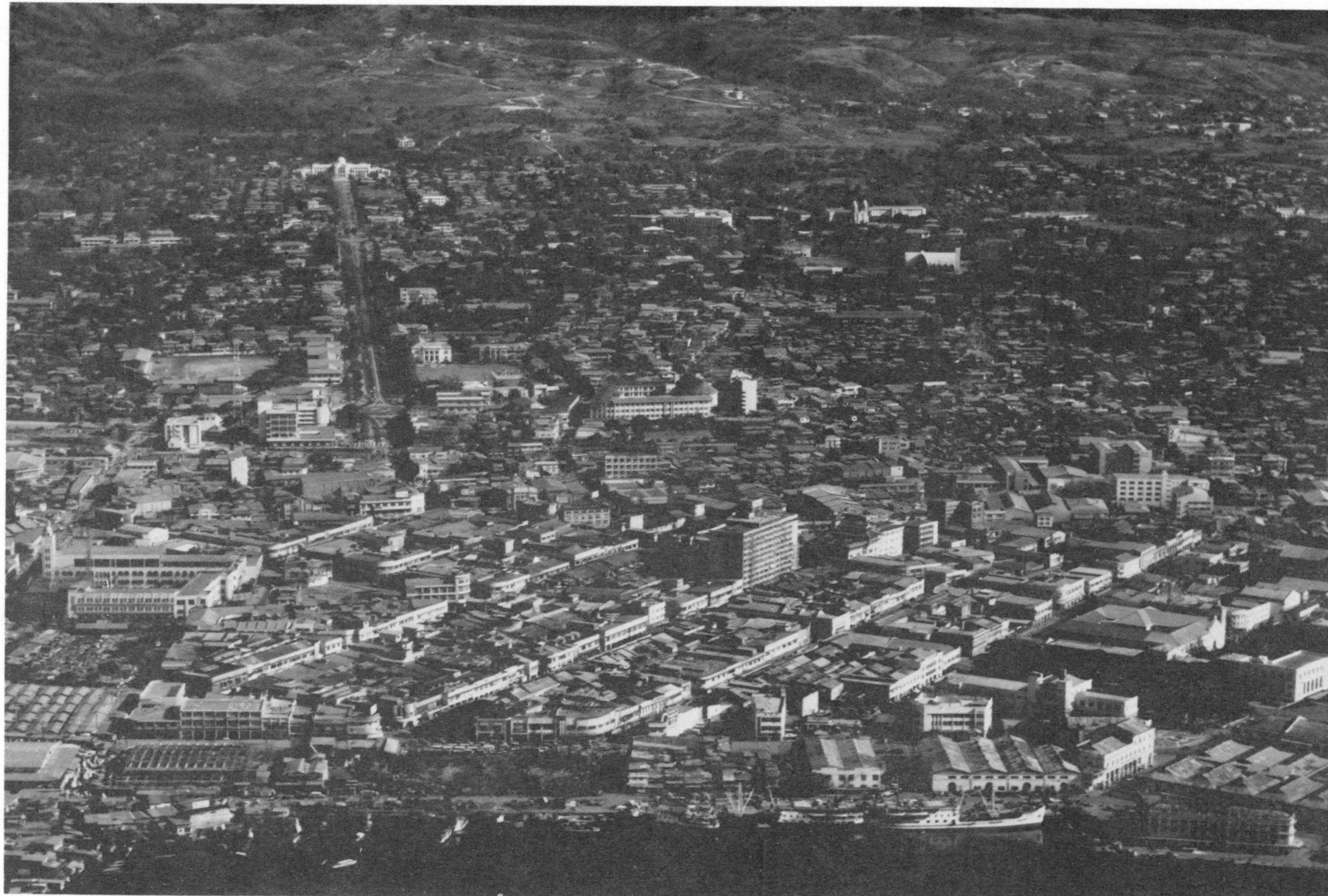

Aerial view of Cebu City.

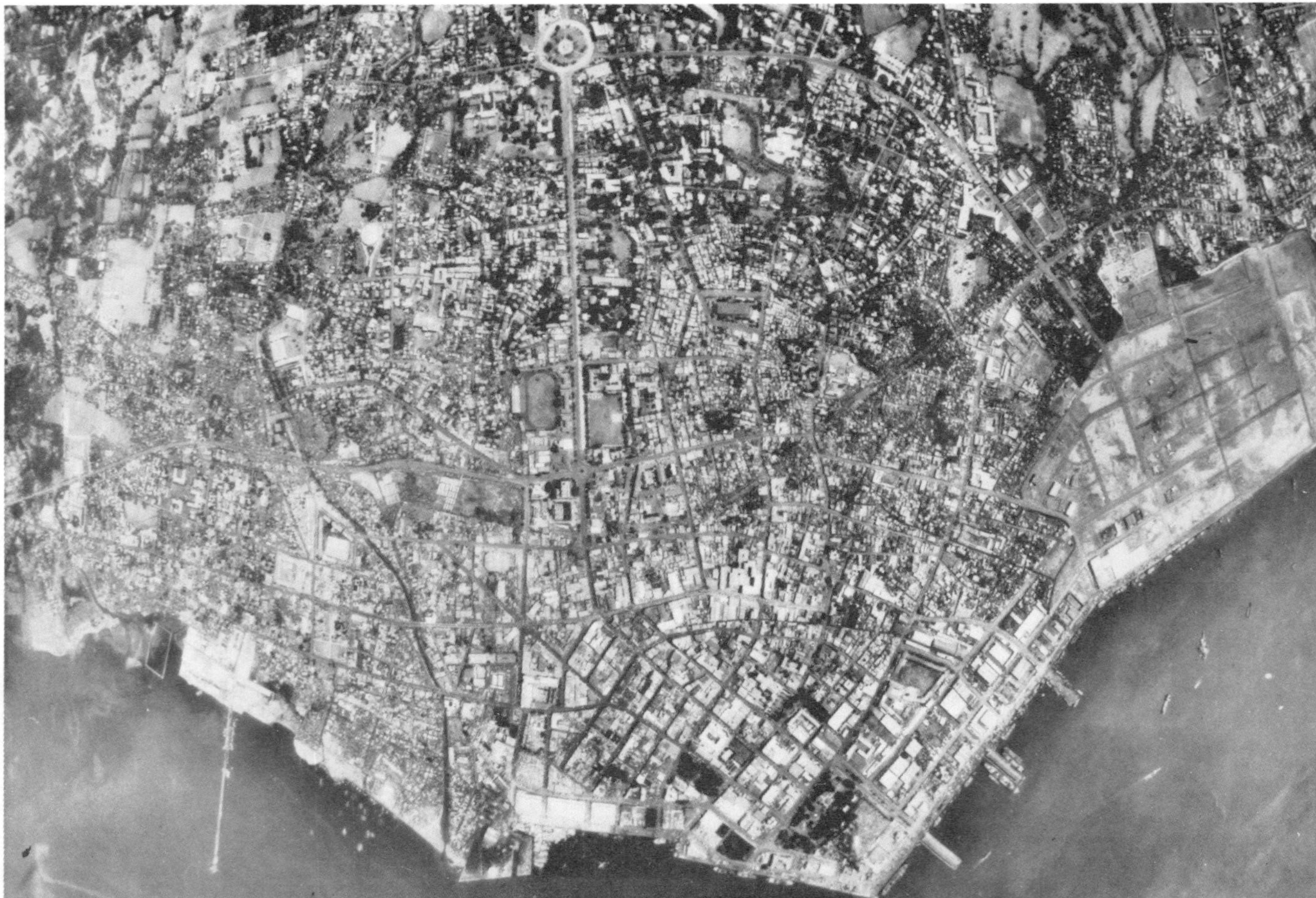

Aerial view of Cebu City.

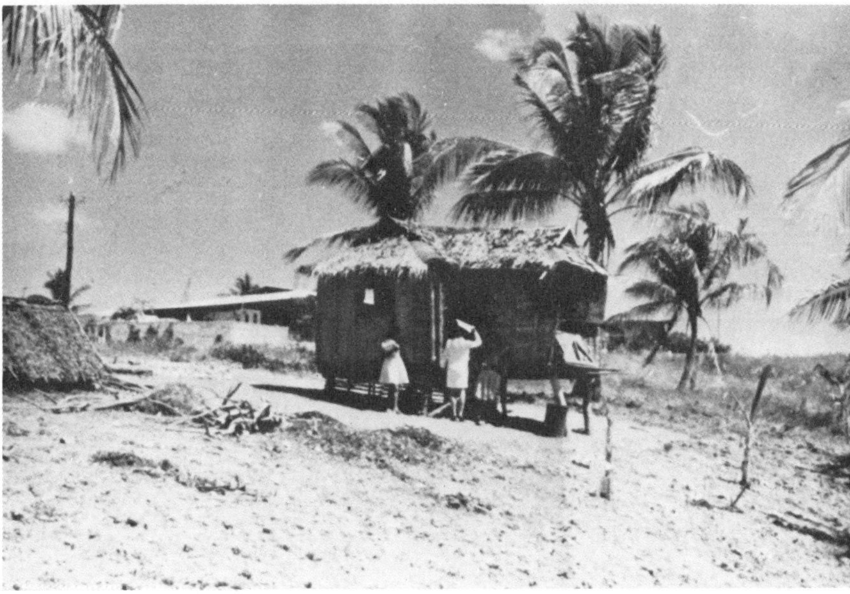

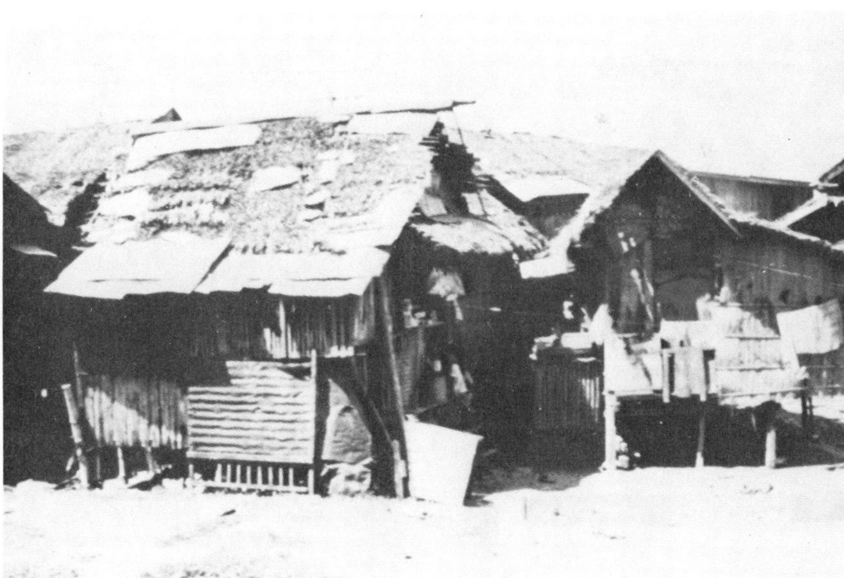

Lower-lower class houses.

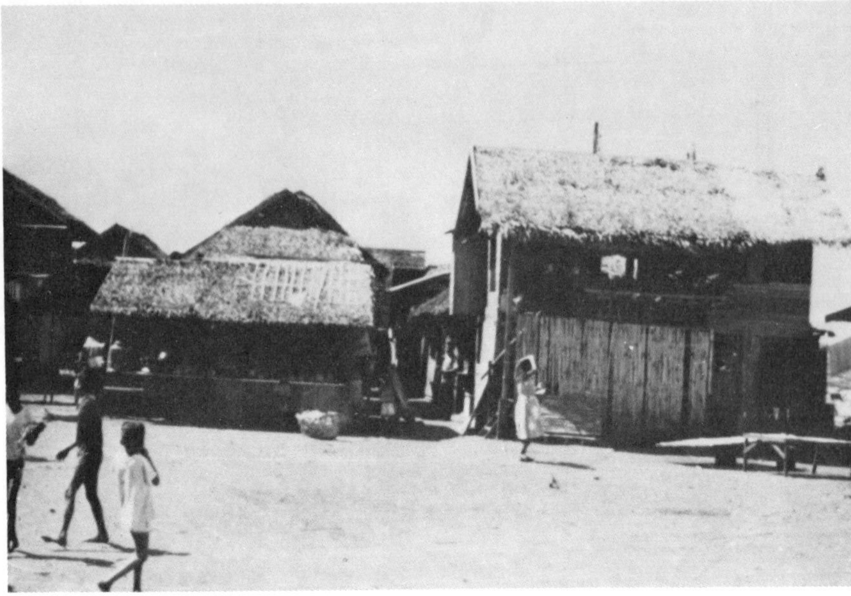

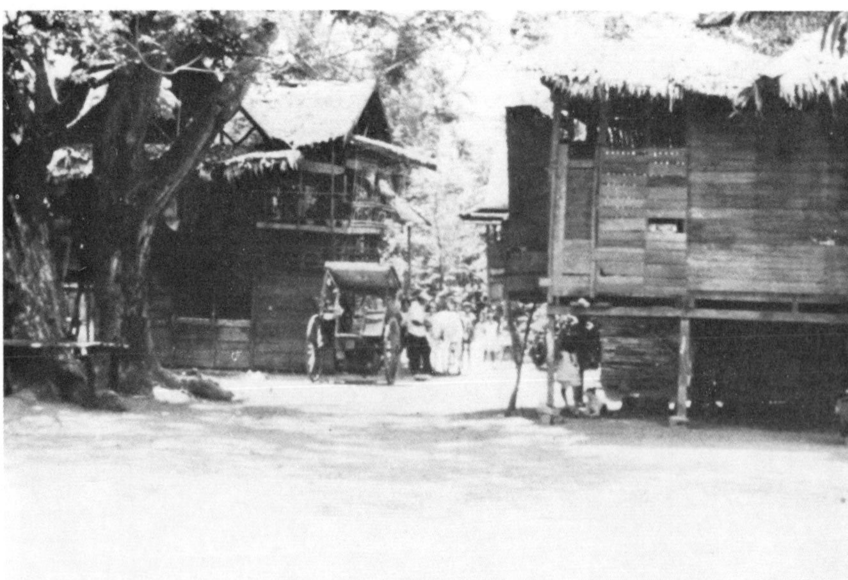

Upper-lower class houses.

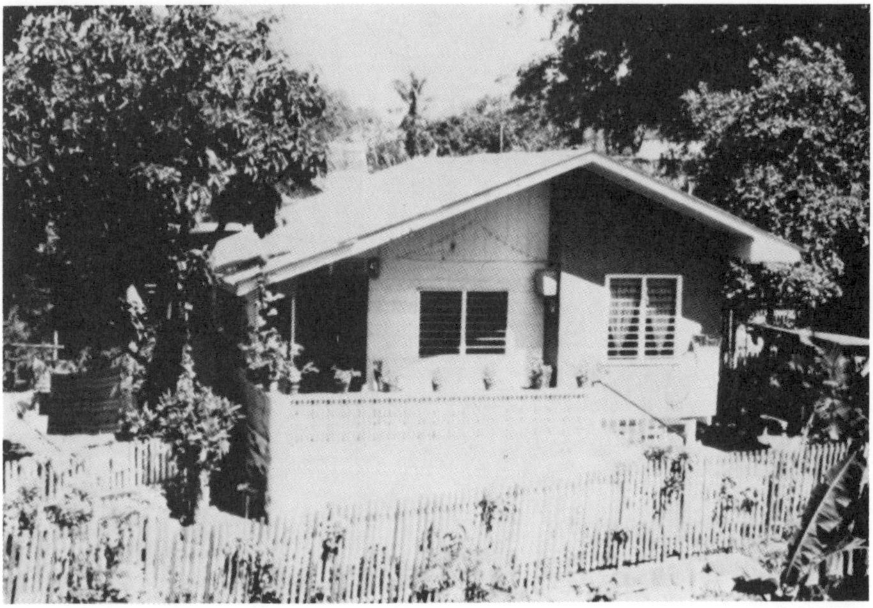

Lower-middle class house.

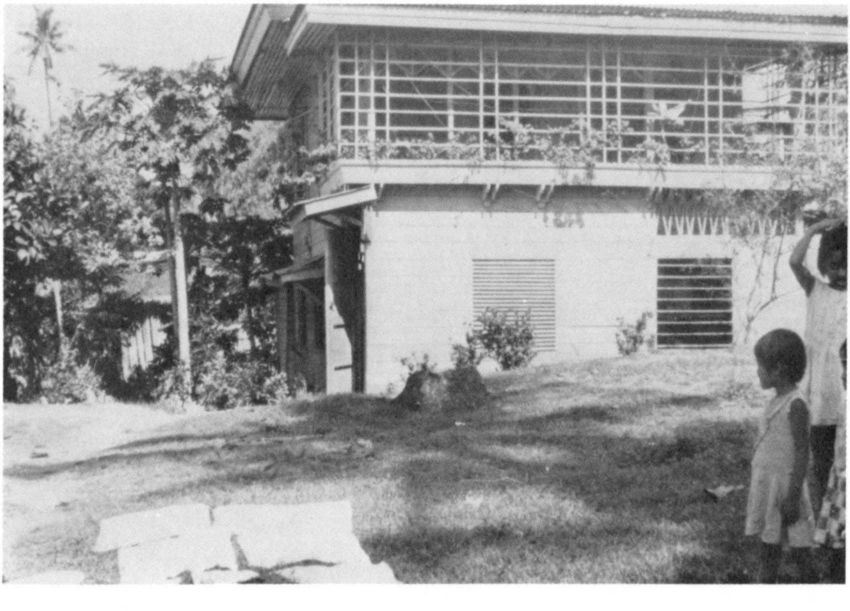

Upper-middle class house.

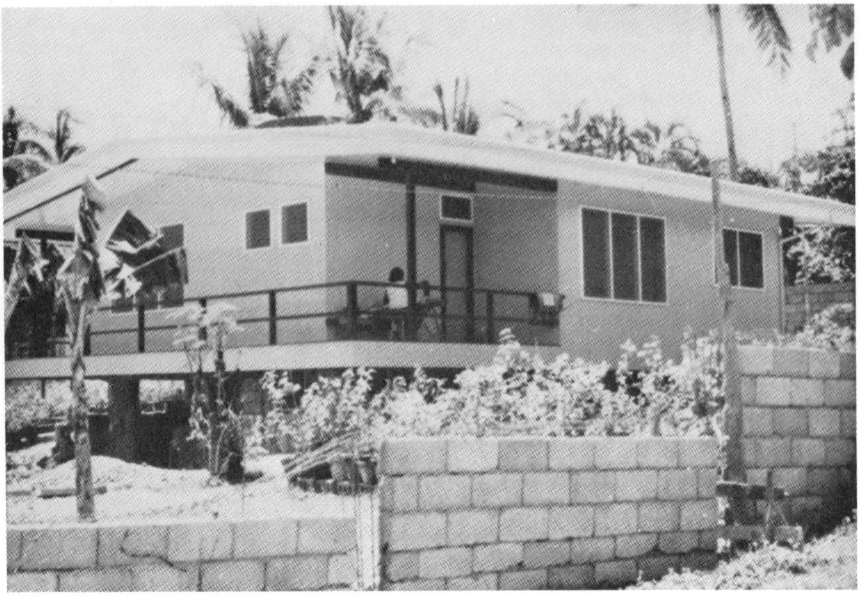

Lower-upper class house.

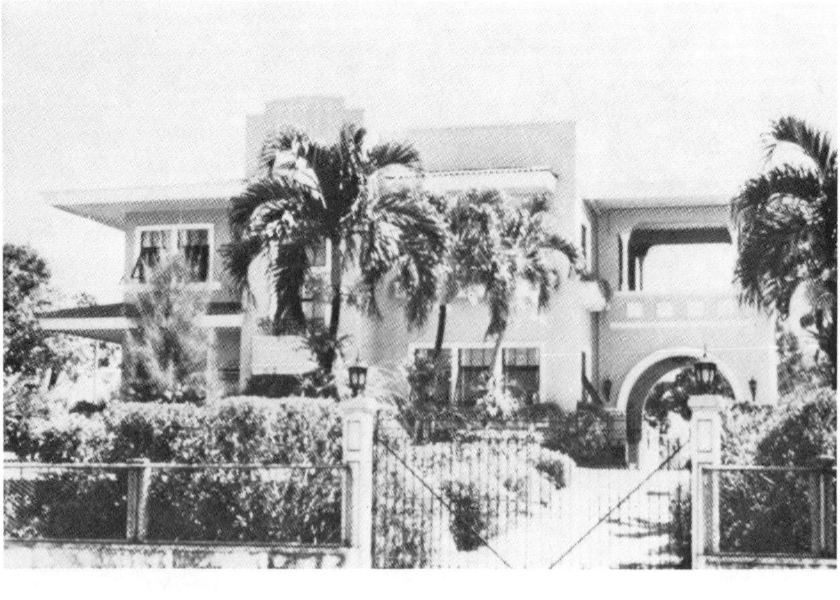

Upper-upper class house.

different tribes, exhibiting varying technological and subsistence levels), researchers in the Philippines have found the basic distinctions useful. Nowadays, the general delineations employed are "Mountain" people, Lowland Christians, and Moslems. The Mountain people include the Negritos, the Igorots, the Ifugaos, and other technologically simple tribes that are still found in Mountain Province, as well as in other isolated regions of the country (scattered in parts of Luzon, Mindanao, and Palawan). The Moslems are found predominantly in the south (Mindanao), and the coinage *Lowland Christians* is generally applied to those who are neither Mountain people nor Moslems.

It is often mistakenly thought that these three culturally distinct groups of Filipinos are so dissimilar that they share almost nothing beyond being confined within a geopolitical boundary. Yet, if one scrutinizes the basic institutional features of these contrasting groups, a uniquely Filipino social structure that antedates Spanish and U.S. contacts is evident. In Fox's words (1959:3–4):

> A fundamental and distinctive sameness is everywhere readily apparent—in the structure of the family and kin-group which reckons relationship *bilaterally*; in the organization of the society into horizontally distinct *generations*, supporting a powerful pattern of generational respect which shapes interpersonal relationship; in leadership based upon wealth, size of the supporting kinship group, personality qualities, and age; in the absence of effective and embracive political organization on the local level, except perhaps in the Muslim areas; in economic activities; traditional religious beliefs, and so forth.

Linguistically, it has been said that the Philippines is a Babel. In addition to Castilian Spanish, American English, and the Chinese Cantonese and Hokkien dialects, there are seventy-five Filipino dialects. Pilipino (or Tagalog), the national language, is the mother tongue of some 21 percent of the population,[6] but an earnest effort is made to teach it in primary and secondary schools across the country. However, English is used almost exclusively in college, by professional people, and in the business sector. The major newspapers and magazines are published in English. Hence, for all practical purposes, it is the *lingua franca*. However, to be able to speak Spanish remains a mark of distinction as it was during the Spanish Conquest when education was elitist.

While such ethnolinguistic pluralism may be construed as a divisive force, an inspection of the census material on the distribution of dialectal groups in the archipelago quickly dispels this belief. For despite the existence of seventy-five identifiable language groups, only eight are in fact major ethnolinguistic groups: Cebuano, Tagalog, Ilokano, Hiligaynon, Bikol, Waray, Pampangan, and Pangasinan (in that order).[7]

Vestiges of pre-Hispanic animistic beliefs have persisted over time as well. Phelan (1959), for example, cited some earlier documents that revealed the friars' recognition that the spread of Christianity had not supplanted the spirits that filled the Indio's pre-Conquest pagan religion. One problem that bothered the *padres* then and is still observable among some of the rural and less well-educated Filipinos from Cebu is that of asking permission from the spirits before doing things such as taking fruit from a tree or crossing a river (mentioned in Phelan, 1959: 80), or cutting an old tree (which we have observed and which Arens, 1959:38, also described in Samar and Leyte).

Historical stability is further evident in the practice of Cebuano sorcery and belief in witches. Lieban (1967:1), for instance, found a description of *barang*[8] in a manuscript dated 1578 and attributed to an early Spanish *encomendero* in Negros which bore a close resemblance to what his respondents supplied to him when he did his study on ethnomedicine in 1958 in two of the islands (Cebu and Negros) in the Bisayan region.[9] Similarly, Hart (1965:50) cites a study (Malay, 1957) which reported that in Obando *poblacion* (near Manila) in the early 1900s, expectant mothers were entreated not to venture out at night for fear of being spotted by the *aswang* (a type of witch believed to be capable of changing his human form into that of an animal, such as a dog, pig, bird, and the like, and who especially relishes fetuses). Among some Cebuanos such warnings are still given to expectant mothers. In addition, Demetria (1969) found that an indigenous method of induced abortion described in a sixteenth-century manuscript translated by Quirino and Garcia (1958:413) is in fact still in use among some inhabitants of Cebu.[10] Thus, centuries of external influence and evidence of regional variation notwithstanding, the Filipinos' beliefs in spirits and witches have persisted, especially among the rural segment of the population. Through their role as migrants and housemaids, these country folk have also shared their beliefs with some urban dwellers and city-bred youngsters.

At the risk of overgeneralization, the Filipinos as a whole can be said to share a number of common beliefs and values that cut across linguistic and religious cleavages. Among these are the norm of reciprocity or indebtedness (cf. Hollnsteiner, 1970), the image of the ideal child as one who is obedient and tractable (cf. Guthrie, 1966), the value placed on premarital chastity, the centrality of the family and kingroup, and the great emphasis on respect for the older generation. For better or for worse, they also share the common experience of being embroiled in a prolonged economic struggle to provide for an average of six children per family.

Ethnic Stratification

A grim reality in the Philippines is the existence of a stratification system that could almost be dichotomized into "have's" and "have-not's." The elite is extremely small, representing at the most 3 percent of the total population. It is composed of U.S. and European professionals, administrative technicians, and multinational corporate managers or shareholders; native-born Spanish-Mestizo politicians or landowners; native-born and naturalized Chinese importers and retailers; and well-to-do and foreign-educated Filipinos. According to one source (Yoshihara, 1971), two-thirds of the 254 manufacturing corporations with recorded sales of over 5 million pesos in 1968 were owned and managed by foreigners (Americans and Chinese, in that order). According to another source (Escultura, 1974), U.S. investments accounted for 77.62 percent of all foreign investments in the Philippines in 1970, and 91.62 percent of the total net profits. It was reported further that "of the 196 foreign top individual income tax payers in the Philippines, 117 are Americans and the rest are British, (Kuomintang) Chinese, Spanish and other nationalities. Of the top ten individual income tax payers in the country, five are Americans and five are Spanish. Of the top 20 taxpayers, only four Filipinos made the grade" (Escultura, 1974:64).

In the Philippines, therefore, ethnicity and social class for the foreigners mesh to produce a clearly defined ethnic stratification system. Although a Filipino upper class exists, the values they propound are often not manifestly different from those found among the colonial Spanish elite. They still treasure land ownership as the ultimate criterion of status, avoid manual labor, and support a class system that enhances the wide gulf between the rich and the poor (Fox, 1959:5; Madigan, 1959:17–18).[11]

At the bottom stratum of the social pyramid are masses and masses of mostly indigenous Malay and Mestizo Filipinos who are ill fed, ill clad, unlettered, and unemployed. In the precarious middle are the schooled, ambitious, but underemployed Filipino and Chinese sales agents, petty clerks, business and service workers, bureaucrats, teachers, and other poorly paid professionals. This system of ethnic stratification is a result of centuries of historical accidents, of course, and inertia.

Economic Conditions

The only source of systematic information we have to substantiate the economic conditions of the Filipinos is the Bureau of Census and

Statistics. Bearing in mind some of the criticisms scholars have made regarding their data-set, we may take note of some of their findings. For instance, their May 1966 survey of households indicates that the annual income of close to half (46 percent) of the estimated 5,126,000 families in 1965 was less than 1,500 pesos.[12] These same families received only 14.6 percent of the country's total family income for that same period. Finer breakdowns show that an estimated 11.6 percent (or 600 thousand) of all families had incomes of less than 500 pesos; another 17.7 percent (or 900 thousand families) reported incomes of between 500 and 1,000 pesos, and 16.7 percent were fortunate enough to have between 1,000 and 1,500 pesos to share with members of their family. By contrast, for families with income of 10,000 pesos or more, who made up only 2.6 percent of all families, the share of the total family income was 20.8 percent.[13] Using less than 2,500 pesos as their definition of the "low income" class, the BCSSH (1968) tabulated the data in Table 2.1 to give an overall picture of the socioeconomic condition of the families in the country. Table 2.1 suggests that in 1965 seven of every ten families (or 69.4 percent) belonged in the low-income range. And of the more than 3.5 million low-income families in the nation, 78.7 percent lived in the rural areas.

More recent conditions are difficult to determine with certainty since comparable published tabulations based on later surveys have not been located, although the data appear to be available. Nevertheless, a rough approximation may be obtained from a feature article in the *Journal of Philippine Statistics* (NCSO, 1975b) which shows the differential family income of employed versus unemployed persons during the May 1971 survey of households. The results reveal that of 12,018,000 employed persons in the country, over half (55 percent) reported a total family income of less than 3,000 pesos for the twelve months preceding the survey. The report further states that 29.5 percent of 3.1 million urban employed persons as opposed to 64.2 percent of the 8.8 million rural ones had to be content with this meager family income. Among *rural* employed persons, the farmers, farm laborers, fishermen, hunters, loggers, and related workers as a group comprise 6,043,000 persons (or 68.3 percent) and fare far worse than any other occupational group: 72.6 percent of them had a total family income of *less than* 3,000 pesos. To call this "subsistence" is a euphemism, for that amount had to be apportioned among family members and stretched over twelve months. Another 20.7 percent of this wretched occupation group had 3,000 to 5,999 pesos to share with their family members. Combining the two income classes, 93.3 percent had a total family income of less than 6,000 pesos.

The unemployment figure was more than six hundred thousand for

TABLE 2.1

DISTRIBUTION OF FAMILIES BY INCOME CLASS, 1965

Classification	*Income Range (pesos)*	*Philippines*	*Urban Total*	*Urban (metropolitan Manila)*	*Urban (outside metropolitan Manila)*	*Rural Total*
Total families (thousands)	—	5,126	1,520	458	1,062	3,606
Percentage	—	100.0%	100.0%	100.0%	100.0%	100.0%
Low income	under 2,500	69.4	47.4	29.4	55.2	78.7
Middle income	2,500–4,999	21.1	29.5	35.0	27.1	17.5
High income	5,000 & over	9.5	23.1	35.6	17.7	3.8

Source: *Journal of Philippine Statistics* 19 (April–June, 1968):x.

the same period under study (although according to Piron, 1972:339, the unemployment figure had reached one million in October 1968). Almost half (48.1 percent) of the officially reported unemployed were from families in the poorest income class (less than 3,000 pesos), of which more than half belonged to families with incomes of less than 2,000 pesos (see Table 2.2). Of the total unemployed persons, 31.3 percent had a family income of 3,000 to 5,999 pesos (pooled from the other working members in the family), while 13.7 percent belonged to families with incomes ranging from 6,000 to 9,999 pesos. The residual 6.9 percent of unemployed persons came from families with incomes of 10,000 pesos or more. In other words, nearly four out of five unemployed persons (79.4 percent) had a family income of less than 6,000 pesos for twelve months.

Table 2.2 also shows that of the total 636,000 unemployed persons as of 1971, a little over one-tenth (10.6 percent) did not even have an income earner in their family. If, therefore, they were to succeed in finding work, they would be the sole breadwinners of their families. More than two-fifths (41 percent) of the total unemployed came from families in which only one person was working for pay or profit. Less than half (48.4 percent) of those unemployed belonged to families with more than one working member. Furthermore, 353,000 of the total unemployed (55.5 percent) had no previous work experience. These data, obtained from official sources, give us an indication of the standard of living in the Philippines and serve as the basis for more detailed discussion in this volume on how the people cope with their economic exigencies.

Deeper insight into the plight of the unemployed masses is lucidly provided in Table 2.3, which is taken from the same study. The unem-

TABLE 2.2

UNEMPLOYED PERSONS DURING THE SURVEY WEEK; MAY 1971

*Number of Family Members Employed for Pay or Profit**	*Total*		*Family Income During the Past 12 Months (pesos)*					
	Number in thousands (with % of total)	*Percentage*	*Under 3,000*	*3,000–5,999*	*6,000–9,999*	*10,000–14,999*	*15,000–19,999*	*20,000 or over*
None	67 (10.6)	100.0	68.1	17.8	7.4	3.3	3.0	0.4
1 member	260 (41.0)	100.0	57.3	32.0	7.8	1.6	0.9	0.4
2 members	163 (25.6)	100.0	39.2	34.9	20.0	4.6	0.7	0.7
3 members	91 (14.3)	100.0	36.2	36.7	17.8	6.6	1.6	1.2
4 members	36 (5.7)	100.0	25.2	24.3	30.4	9.4	2.7	8.0
5 or more members	18 (2.8)	100.0	28.7	24.7	11.9	19.7	7.7	7.3
Philippines (total)	636 (100.0)	100.0	48.1	31.3	13.7	4.2	1.5	1.2

Source: *Journal of Philippine Statistics* 26, 1 (1975):xvi.

Note: Figures in thousands except percentages. Details may not add up to totals because of rounding.

*Does not include unpaid workers in family farms or enterprises.

TABLE 2.3

UNEMPLOYED PERSONS, BY INCOME CLASS AND SIZE OF FAMILY, MAY 1971

Family Income (pesos)	*Total (in thousands) (with percentage of total)*	*Number in Family*										
		1	*2*	*3*	*4*	*5*	*6*	*7*	*8*	*9*	*10 or more*[a]	
under 500	23 (3.6)	1	4	3	2	4	5	1	2	—	1	
500–999	47 (7.5)	1	2	4	9	4	6	5	9	3	5	
1,000–1,499	65 (10.2)	—	5	6	8	8	8	5	6	9	9	
1,500–1,999	48 (7.5)	—	2	3	3	6	7	6	11	1	8	1st
2,000–2,499	57 (9.0)	—	3	4	11	8	6	5	7	4	9	(101)
2,500–2,999	66 (10.4)	—	1	6	7	10	7	8	12	4	11	
3,000–3,999	85 (13.3)	—	1	4	9	11	11	7	12	8	22	2nd
4,000–4,999	69 (10.9)	—	[b]	4	8	8	12	11	5	5	16	(157)
5,000–5,999	45 (7.0)	—	[b]	—	5	3	5	6	6	6	13	3rd
6,000–7,999	56 (8.8)	—	1	1	3	6	8	5	4	8	20	(117)
8,000–9,999	31 (4.9)	—	—	1	5	2	2	4	6	2	8	
10,000–14,999	27 (4.2)	—	—	—	—	4	3	5	3	3	9	
15,000–19,999	9 (1.5)	—	—	—	1	—	—	[b]	3	2	3	
20,000 and over	8 (1.2)	—	—	1	—	1	1	[b]	1	1	3	
Philippines (total)	636 (100.0)	1	17	37	73	74	81	70	88	56	139	

Source: *Journal of Philippine Statistics* 26, 1 (1975):xv.
Note: Numbers are in thousands. Details may not equal totals because of rounding.
[a]Average size is 11 persons (11.1 to be more exact) for the Philippines, rural and urban.
[b]Less than 500.

ployed person's per capita share of the family income is calculated using finer income breakdowns of families and the midpoints of these breakdowns as bases for computations. The highest zig-zag line in Table 2.3 shows that an estimated 101,000 unemployed had to share only 200 pesos or less. If one uses 400 pesos per capita as the bare subsistence figure,[14] then 258,000 unemployed (families above the first and second zig-zag lines) fell into this bracket. When one divides the subsistence per capital income of 400 pesos by 365 days in one year, then, no words can convey the destitute situation of the unemployed, thousands of whom belong to families with even less than 400 pesos per capita to spare.[15]

In short, when the Cebu Family Health Project took place, the economy was plagued with many problems characteristic of former colonies. Many of the unemployed had never worked; many more never bothered to seek employment. However, the Philippines was not the only country in Southeast Asia with a serious economic development problem. With respect to literacy, for example, the country actually ranked among the better ones. Nevertheless, at least during the sixties and seventies, the Philippines experienced one of the highest population growth rates of all nations. It is against such adverse economic conditions that an average person must come to terms with his or her life demands, of which fertility expectations and behavior are merely one component.

3 / Methodology

The data for the more than two thousand women reported herein represent countless hours of planning and field work, of climbing hills and enduring heat, of dispelling suspicions and overcoming shyness, and of convincing reluctant respondents to participate. Social research of any type customarily must resolve methodological problems inherent in the adoption of a specific mode of data collection, but those which emerge from survey studies in a cross-cultural context are manifold, especially when the community has not been exposed to large-scale research. To most readers, the attendant field conditions are never really known, since the type of research adventures that do culminate in final reports, monographs, or other publications are "reconstructed logic" (Kaplan, 1964), devoid of vivid operational details. The authors' intention here is not to present irrelevant details, but rather to provide sufficient discussion to allow the reader an adequate insight into the field situation during the course of our research.

The Cebu study consisted of three phases of data collection, all directly supervised by William T. Liu, the project director. First, the *survey phase* was aimed at obtaining basic information on reproductive behavior from as nearly representative a sample as possible of Cebuano women. Second, the *kinship phase* focused on acquiring detailed case histories from a select group of women through unstructured, in-depth interviews. More specifically, these case histories were designed to reveal the structural effects of the family system on the interpersonal control of reproductive behavior. The third stage was implemented to explore Cebuano *husband-wife interaction patterns* through the use of the revealed difference method (Strodtbeck, 1951).[1]

Before the survey phase could begin, however, it became evident that the field work needed to be delayed to allow the investigators sufficient time for ethnographic inquiries into lifestyles, prenatal and postpartum care of infants and mothers, folk conceptions of pregnancies, the birth process, and mother-infant interaction. With the assistance of the Graduate Department of Anthropology at the University of San Carlos, which is staffed by German- and American-trained scholars and rated the best department in the Visayas region, we were able to recruit four research assistants who assisted us in conducting the ethnographic inquiries. They received training from us in reviewing fertility research literature and in making natural observations as well as unobtrusive interviews with expectant mothers, maternity ward workers, folk healers and midwives, and other individuals. As a result of this preliminary inquiry, a decision was made to conduct special studies on the *mananabangs* (folk midwives), neighborhood communication patterns, and Cebuano courtship and dating processes, each under the direction of one of the project staff. An effort was also made to gather other culturally pertinent information that we suspected might be related to Cebuano reproductive behavior.[2]

In order to collect reliable basic information on household composition, family structure, occupational profiles, income differentials, domestic relations, pregnancy histories, and network constellations of friends and relatives, the entire province of Cebu was designated as the sampling universe. In both urban and rural areas, a multi-stage, stratified, random sampling procedure was attempted. Each of these areas required somewhat different procedures because of ecological differentiations.

Preliminary Steps in Sampling Rural Barrios

Two types of barrios were delineated: urban and rural. An area was operationally defined as rural if, in our estimation, more than half of the gainfully employed persons were employed in agricultural or primary industries such as fishing, mining, or forestry. As a preliminary step in determining the barrios to be sampled, we obtained an accurate description of each barrio in the province. Urban barrios were set aside as a special category to be considered as part of the urban complex of Cebu City. To ensure that our rural sample would represent the broad spectrum of rural lifestyles, two defining characteristics of rural barrios were employed simultaneously:[3]

1. The nature of the economy, such as the production of
    a. sugar cane—coconut—corn
    b. coconut—corn—mango
    c. coconut—corn—abaca
    d. coconut—vegetables—rice
    e. fishing—coconut
    f. forestry—vegetables
2. The mode of transportation available
    a. has roads and regular truck service
    b. has roads but no truck service
    c. is accessible only by foot

With these two defining characteristics of rural barrios, a joint-description table was drawn to serve as our basis for rural sampling (see Table 3.1). Barrios that fell into each cell of the table were considered homogeneous units in a statistical sense and for our research purpose. In order to minimize costs and to maximize our manpower resources, clustered sampling was used, since systematic random sampling was infeasible.[4] More specifically, the procedure employed was as follows:

1. From 1 to *n* barrios were selected until all crops or types of economic life were represented.
2. If, within one municipality, more than one barrio grew a particular crop, a table of random numbers was used to select the barrio to be sampled.
3. Any barrio that could not be located on the map of the province was discarded.[5]

Following this procedure, a total of twenty-four rural barrios were selected[6] and an initial quota of 600 rural interviews was set. Specific subquotas for each barrio were determined proportionately to the particular type (economy and transportation) of the barrio.

Finding the Sampling Framework for Cebu City

Sampling in metropolitan Cebu and its urban barrios was more complicated, since we could not safely assume that urban barrios were a homogeneous unit. Census data did not provide barrio statistics on housing conditions, segregation patterns (in terms of age, sex, marital status, occupation, education), or other indices. There was, therefore, no foolproof method of ascertaining the degree of homogeneity of any two urban barrios. A crude way of solving this problem was to ignore jurisdictional barrio boundaries within the city in favor of the "natural areas," as human ecologists call them. (These are areas which have visible features reflecting lifestyles shared by their residents.)

To accomplish this, the research assistants were instructed to familiarize themselves thoroughly with the city of Cebu and to make rough divisions of what might be considered its natural areas. Industrial, business, warehouse, and waterfront areas were eliminated from the universe for sampling purposes. What remained was either the residential areas or a combination of residential and business areas. Finally, three classes were used to determine the social rank of an area: the upper (such as Beverly Hills), the middle (such as some areas in the Capitol Site section), and the lower classes (such as Pasil and Villagonzalo).

TABLE 3.1

TWO DEFINING CHARACTERISTICS OF RURAL BARRIOS

Modes of Transportation	*Modes of Economic Adaptation*			
	Corn-Rice	*Coconut*	*Fishing*	*Etc.*
Trucks				
Roads, no trucks				
No roads				
Miscellaneous				

This information was plotted on a map of Cebu City by designating each residential class with the use of different color codes.

After the map had been completed, the research assistants again canvassed the city and listed the household clusters in each block for all residential areas. Each group was assigned an identification number, and the number of structures per group was recorded. All blocks bearing the same color designation were assigned a number, and the total number of blocks of all colors was used to compute the fraction of particular blocks to be selected from the entire city.

The inaccuracy of the city map necessitated revision of streets and blocks with the aid of aerial photography. Arrangements were made for the U.S. Air Force in Mactan to fly a T-34 plane owned by the Philippine Air Force to take aerial photos of the city.

Next, the research assistants made a preliminary count of the number of homes clustered together in small groups within one city block (about the same size as a city block in an average city in Indiana). This laborious task was necessitated by the peculiar pattern of housing congestion so characteristic of urban centers in the Philippines, where wooden or bamboo shacks follow an unregulated use of available land space that often leaves no footpaths between two structures. It is also quite common for a group of such shacks to share only one narrow footpath. Another common sight was a shack in the middle of what seemed to be a pathway leading to a nearby street. Such housing congestion was frequent enough to occupy no fewer than fifty city blocks and made street or housing identification practically impossible.

For each city block the research assistants identified, all groups of shacks or houses structurally independent from one another but with no space wide enough for a footpath were given identification numbers, and for each group a count of the number of structures was recorded.

From this enumeration of areas, blocks, and groups of homes, a simple random, self-weighting sample was drawn by using all blocks bearing the same color as separate parameters and selecting specific groups of houses. Finally, the interviewers were assigned to take every fourth residential structure within the designated groups.[7] These procedures for selecting the sampling unit were employed for the middle-and lower-class areas but were inappropriate for the exclusively upper-class section because upper-class homes generally have much more space between them. Accordingly, the sampling unit for these sections was the block, rather than the group of residential structures.

Eligibility criteria were established to set the most inclusive parameters possible for the survey respondents, with the principal focus being on reproductive behavior. Accordingly, we required that the female respondent be between fifteen and forty-five years old, have at least one child, and, by her own definition, have been married at some time. Our research requirements did not demand that the respondent ever have been legally married or that her husband be living with her at the time of the interview. In addition, to exclude families who had recently moved to Cebu, the final eligibility requirement was that the respondent must have lived in the province for the preceding five years. In sum, these qualifications allowed a focus on women still in their childbearing years who had some experience with raising children, and who were relatively stable geographically within the province.

Selection of Households

In selecting specific households, we took the following steps: If the woman chosen from every fourth residential structure failed to satisfy the eligibility requirements and there was no qualified woman in the same designated household, the interviewer proceeded to the next preselected sample household. However, if more than one household was found in one residential structure, or more than one eligible respondent lived in a designated residence, the interviewer alternated the households or persons in terms of the ages of the women respondents. For example, if the first residential structure contained two households, one with a woman under thirty, another with a woman over thirty, the interviewer tossed a coin to determine who should be interviewed. If the woman she selected in this case was *under* thirty years of age, then in the next multihousehold structure she was required to select for interview a woman who was *over* thirty years of age. If the woman chosen by this method failed to meet the qualifications for a respondent (such as one who had never had a pregnancy), another woman of the same age group in the same household who was eligible was chosen as a replacement. If the originally chosen household did not contain eligible respondents, the interviewer was to go on to the next designated sample household. If a potential respondent was not at home at the time of the first contact, a maximum of three call-backs was made before considering this as a noninterview.

Social Class in Cebu City

Identifying the social classes in Cebu City presented several problems not generally encountered in North American cities. For one thing, there were no comparable residential districts cordoned off by zoning laws based on dwelling cost or median rental values. For another, owing to a widespread underreporting of income, there is a tendency for Filipinos to be reluctant to disclose their actual yearly earnings. Consequently, determining socioeconomic class solely by reported income or by residential address was deemed unreliable. Instead, the project developed a composite index based upon residence structure, material possessions, occupation, club membership, and estimated family budget which appeared most satisfactory for our research purpose.

During the first stage of social classification, the research team canvassed the residential areas of the city, making gross classifications by residence structure. Further refinements in classification were made by interviewing residents about education, income, and occupation as well as by observing material possessions within the home. Through this procedure, six social classes were discernible: lower-lower class, upper-lower class, lower-middle class, upper-middle class, lower-upper class, and upper-upper class.

To appraise the reliability of our classification, five or six investigators simultaneously classified homes; their agreement ranged from 80 to 90 percent. A description of the six social classes follows.

Lower-Lower Class

The lower-lower class includes the squatters who live on land either without rent or which rents for a very few pesos each month. Some squatters reside on government land such as the edge of the road or the dump and, although frequently evicted, they do not pay rent. Others living on private property are pressured by the owners to pay about two pesos monthly. In addition to squatters, the lower-lower class includes those families who are at a subsistence level of existence, earning about four pesos daily. (The figures for rentals and incomes indicated are those obtaining at the time of the survey.)

For livelihood, members of the lower-lower class scavenge the dumps and debris piles, sell raffle tickets, old newspapers, or broken bottles, and at times work at unskilled jobs or as rig drivers. Their dwellings are huts or tiny shacks constructed of discarded wood, paper, metal, and junk, mixed with nondurable wood such as bamboo and nipa. The area may be as small as ten by ten feet, and is usually only one story high. If it is elevated by four bamboo posts, the ground space oftentimes serves as a pigsty. The hut usually has only one room, which is used for all purposes—cooking, eating, and sleeping. Some of the larger huts may have a small, invisibly designated space for sleeping, leaving the rest of the area for cooking and eating. There are generally no beds. The occupants sleep either on the floor or on straw mats.

Only the barest number of cooking and eating utensils are found, such as an earthen pot or two, a kettle, an earthen water jar, and a few plates and spoons. Stoves are either fashioned from a tin can or improvised by resting a clay pot on three rocks. There are no tables, chairs, or any other furniture. A gas lamp is used for lighting. There is no toilet or running water. Generally water is fetched from a public artesian well, and bathing and toilet facilities are likewise public.

Although the government has declared that elementary education for all Filipinos is free and required, many families are still unable to send their children to school for lack of money to provide the barest necessities (such as shoes, clothes, pens, and paper). Also, for many of the lower-lower-class families, sending a child to school would reduce the help around the house and curtail possible earnings from doing menial tasks in the neighborhood such as shining shoes or collecting wastepaper. Thus, a great number of children from these families do not attend school. Their neighborhood is distinguished by school-age children congesting the street.

Upper-Lower Class

Upper-lower-class families are usually found near the lower-lower-class ones but are distinguished by slightly larger houses, generally elevated from the ground. They pay two to ten pesos in rent monthly for houses that are frequently found in the interior of a block at the back of other houses, or crowded together along the side of the road.

Like those in the lower-lower class, the upper-lower-class Cebuanos are unskilled laborers. However, their jobs are steadier or they are more successful jeepney[8] and taxi drivers with an average daily earning of seven pesos.

Their houses are small, enclosing about fifteen by fifteen feet, and subdivided into a *sala* (living room), which doubles as a sleeping room at night, and a kitchen-and-dining area, with the space between the elevated house and the ground serving as a pigsty. Construction materials are wood, bamboo, and nipa. Straw mats are spread on the floor for sleeping. There are cooking utensils, a few plates and other eating utensils, plus a gas lamp. Old, well-used furniture is at a minimum. Some of these houses have bamboo fences and a few flowerpots. There is no toilet, but sometimes public water is supplied for five pesos monthly. Generally, bathing and toilet facilities are public.

Although the upper-lower-class families exist at subsistence level, they are better able than the lower-lower class to send their children to school, since the mother may occasionally take in laundry or contribute in some other way toward increasing their meager family income (such as raising suckling pigs).

Lower-Middle Class

Members of this class are usually low-paid professionals such as school teachers, salaried businessmen, and less prominent doctors and lawyers, earning between 180 and 400 pesos monthly. Frequently, the husband's earnings are supplemented by the wife's efforts through part-time or full-time work, at home or outside. Among the people in this social stratum, it is a symbol of prestige (and a relief from humdrum household chores) to be able to afford a houseservant, usually an adolescent maid.

Their dwellings are more substantial than lower-class houses, even though they are not all that large. In most cases the ground floor is paved with cement, while wood is used for the second floor. Their houses are generally divided into bedrooms, *sala*, kitchen, and dining room areas. The dwellings may not be painted, but they are adorned with flowerpots and may have a small, well-kept garden. There are rattan beds, bedroom furniture, a *sala* set, electricity, and running water plus a toilet and bath. Ample cooking and eating utensils and pottery or glassware are available. Furnishings include lamps, radios, fans, and sometimes a used television set conspicuously displayed, along with other small electrical appliances. Glass windows adorned with curtains are common. Fences are generally found around these homes. Usually the family owns the lot and the house, and has lived in it for a number of years. If the family does not own the house, their monthly rent is generally about a hundred pesos.

Lower-middle-class children attend school, mostly tuition-free government schools, although some siblings may have to drop out after high school in order to supplement the family income or support themselves. Some may defer their college education for a few years. Others may attend school at night while working in the daytime.

Upper-Middle Class

Upper-middle-class families consist of professional people who either hold slightly better jobs than those of the lower-middle class or have family property or other assets. Their monthly income averages between 400 and 800 pesos. Frequently, both husband and wife work, and they may own a used car or a reconditioned jeep. They hire more than one housemaid to help around the house and to serve as *yayas* (nursemaids) for their children. Some of these maids may be remote kin from less fortunate families. They generally live with the family.

Upper-middle-class dwellings are made of more substantial construction materials than lower-class shacks. Their houses differ from those of the lower-middle class in that they cost a little more and are better painted and better kept. The house is clearly subdivided into bedrooms (with regular beds), kitchen, dining room, *sala*, bath, and toilet. Upper-middle-class families usually own their home, whose worth is estimated at 20,000 pesos. Furnishings are more expensive, but still well-worn. They possess more home appliances, in addition to better china and kitchen utensils.

Their children normally attend private schools in the city and have greater opportunities to complete college.

Lower-Upper Class

Members of the lower-upper class are well-paid professionals (such as doctors, lawyers, and managerial businessmen) who have been educated in the best schools in Cebu or Manila. A few may have studied abroad. In most cases, the wives are also well-educated professionals, some of whom work.

Lower-upper-class dwellings may be situated in neighborhoods where lower- and middle-class dwellings abound. However, there are some areas of the city, such as Capitol Site, some parts of Banawa, and sections of Lahug, which have become lower-upper-class housing subdivisions, primarily because they are less accessible from the center of the city and are a great distance from the usual means of livelihood for most lower-class Cebuanos.

Houses are large, consisting of two stories, and usually of modern architectural design built within the last ten years, with well-kept gardens, garages for two or more cars, and high fences of cement, steel, and/or other durable material. Many of these houses resemble the middle-class dwellings in warmer parts of the United States. The value of the houses, which are usually owned or being paid for, was estimated at between 20,000 and 50,000 pesos.

Electrical appliances, such as television sets, radios, refrigerators, gas or electric stoves, and hi-fis are common. There are usually more than one bathroom and quarters for several servants. Furniture is attractive and expensive.

Not only do lower-upper-class children attend the better schools in the country, but the opportunity to travel and study abroad is also within their reach, in part because they tend to be more fluent in English than the lower classes.

Upper-Upper-Class

From the standpoint of income and lifestyle, the uppermost stratum represents a highly distinctive class. For this reason, information about the upper-upper class was more difficult to obtain. For the sake of this study, we obtained the names of families who were considered the wealthiest and most influential in Cebu City from businessmen and other knowledgeable Cebuanos. There appeared to be some fifty to one hundred of these families, and there was general but not unanimous agreement as to who should be included in the list.

Briefly stated, the upper-upper class consists of families with landed wealth, and owners of substantial interlocking business interests including rice or corn milling and retailing, copra exports, foreign-goods imports, shipping, real estate, large department stores, and restaurant operations. Members of their extended families have diversified investments in numerous economic enterprises. The professionals within this class usually have incomes other than their fees and salaries, such as inheritances, land, dividends, and interest. Some of the wealthiest families (perhaps twenty of them) are Chinese. These are seemingly uninvolved in local politics but are said to be powerful behind the scenes. Their power stems primarily from their business acuity and interlocking financial holdings.

As a group, upper-upper-class families travel a good deal between islands and to other countries. Some of them are influential in international trade and national politics as well. Their children, as a rule, are not only educated in the exclusive, private schools of the country, but are also often sent abroad for their higher education.

The families own spacious homes with fish ponds, landscaped gardens, wooded acreages, and tall fences to keep curious onlookers out. Some of these homes are equipped with at least one swimming pool. Other families own cottages along the most beautiful beaches that stretch around the island. Still others have pooled their resources with other wealthy families and built an exclusive and jointly managed swimming pool and recreation facilities at one of the resort beaches near the city.

Despite their affluence, most upper-upper-class families have managed to keep the exteriors of their residences modest. Generally, there are two architectural styles: Western-Hollywood and Spanish-Filipino. The Western-style houses are usually more spacious than the Spanish ones. Each family owns two or more cars, one of which may be an expensive late-model European import, the other an American gas guzzler. Besides the chauffeur(s), there are numerous domestic helpers around the house, each specializing in one or only a few aspects of housekeeping and babysitting chores.

Recruitment and Training of Interviewers

Linguistic pluralism and the absence of a pool of research interviewers who are well trained in the social sciences were problems that we had to overcome in the early phase of the Cebu project. Since the qualifications needed to do interviewing inevitably excluded those who were not well educated, it also meant that those whom we considered to be qualified were likely to be gainfully employed. We decided to recruit as interviewers those who could work part time, in addition to those who were willing to work full time, provided that they were proficient in English and Cebuano (also called Visayan)[9] and would complete several weeks of interviewer training.

The project's affiliation with the University of San Carlos proved to be invaluable because it allowed us to draw upon their college students, advanced graduate students, and teaching staff. Through advertisements and by word of mouth, we were able to attract many applicants, of whom we selected twenty interviewers and kept ten more in reserve. All were fluent in Cebuano and English; many could speak Pilipino as well. Most of the interviewers had at least a college degree; those who did not were attending the university. All but six worked only part time. Four of the original recruits who could work full time were given special responsibilities besides interviewing, such as preparing field work organization, collecting basic information for sampling, and translating. They were given the title of research assistants. All four were in their early twenties.

For three months the four research assistants also pretested the preliminary version of the instrument, tabulated the data, and helped with the second and third revisions. By the end of the third month, all four had become proficient in the use of the survey questionnaire, knowledgeable about the field conditions, and familiar with the objectives of the first phase of the project. Then the interview training began, with the four research assistants serving as facilitators.

Two separate training sessions were held, one in the morning and the other in the afternoon, in order to accommodate the part-time trainees. Each session lasted for three hours daily, and the training went on five days a week for three consecutive weeks. It included an orientation program, a cursory explanation of the project, its theoretical foundations, sampling procedures, the interviewer's role, the sponsoring agencies, cooperating institutions, the background and interests of staff researchers, and administrative details (the procedures of reporting working hours, assignment, and methods of payment). In addition, seminars were conducted throughout the survey phase by the director and local professionals (anthropologists, physicians, and family planning experts) on a variety of topics directly related to reproductive behavior. This permitted a continual discussion and evaluation of new ideas and hypotheses that might be salient in subsequent analysis of the data.

During the interviewer training period, each interviewer was instructed on the nature of survey research, its strengths and limitations. Each was given an interviewer's manual (Katz, 1966) to read, which was accompanied by detailed, item-by-item specifications, explaining the intent of the questions and how probes should be made tactfully.

The group was broken into pairs so that each trainee could practice the art of interviewing and become familiar with the wording, style, and procedure of the interview schedule itself. After this initial role-playing, the correct techniques were demonstrated by the director and better interviewers. Specific problems that might arise in the field situations were discussed in detail. This exercise was supplemented with an actual demonstration of interviewing by one of the research assistants on an innocent subject in front of the group. The results were discussed and new suggestions were made by the group on certain wordings, problems of probing, and other points. A second demonstration followed; and similar discussions were held.

As soon as the English version of the interview schedule was completed, teams composed of the bilingual research staff and interviewers were assigned different sections of the interview schedule to translate. After one group completed the translation of an assigned section it was checked by one of the other groups until each section's translation had been independently approved by all of the groups. Upon its completion, the Cebuano version was given to an independent reader who had no prior knowledge of the original English version, who then translated it back into English. The back translation turned out to be exceptionally accurate, which obviated additional changes.[10]

Subsequently, each interviewer was told to interview an ordinary housewife—one who might be a potential respondent. Two such trials were administered: first to a cooperative mother, usually a friend or neighbor who met our eligibility requirements, and second to a total stranger. Every interviewer at this time had had a minimum of three weeks of training with an additional week of participation in the final revision and editing of the interview schedule.

Because techniques for securing the cooperation of the respondent are detailed in other texts, they will not be elaborated on here. As a general procedure, the interviewers were instructed to approach the potential respondent by saying:

> Good morning (afternoon, evening). My name is ______ and I am here representing the Cebu Family Health Project. This is one of the houses we have selected for the survey, which you may have heard about. Perhaps I can explain to you something about the project. A group of doctors have decided that they need to know all about Cebuano families. They want to know how many children Cebuano women have, and what children mean in the woman's relationship with her husband, and what kinds of problems parents have in taking care of their children. They need this information to give parents better advice when they ask for it. These doctors believe that only parents, especially the mother, can tell them what they need to know. So they have sent me, and several other Cebuano-speaking research assistants like myself, to ask some questions. This has nothing to do with the government.

If the woman consented to the interview, the interviewer proceeded with a set of screening questions to determine eligibility. When asked, the interviewer presented credentials consisting of an identification card and letters of introduction from the archbishop, the mayor, and other local government officials. In a country where modern contraceptive methods are still treated with some suspicion by the majority of the Catholic population, the letter of approval from the archbishop may have helped to convince some otherwise reluctant respondents. Regrettably, it was impossible to obtain information on the individuals who refused to participate, those who could not be located, or those who were not at home after three calls.

Methodological Obstacles

Some of the field problems we encountered have been noted previously, but a few others warrant elaboration, for although we were able to anticipate many of these problems—on the basis of reports of studies conducted in other developing countries—a number of methodological obstacles did not surface until the research was under way. Field conditions are, perhaps, minimally dependent upon the investigators' ability to adapt and their enthusiasm for field work, and maximally forged by the culture of the host community. Cebu was thus no different from any other field experience in that it presented particular problems related to the Cebuano culture. Some of the more outstanding problems are outlined here.

Generally, there were three types of problems: (1) those pertaining to the technological aspects of the cultural setting; (2) those pertaining to the interpersonal aspects of survey interviews; and (3) those pertaining to the recall of dates and facts.

With regard to technological problems, the time-consuming task of simply locating the sample households has already been described. Even with hand-drawn maps especially constructed by the project staff, locating the houses proved to be a major challenge. In the urban areas the interviewers were taken as far as possible by the project vehicles or by jeepneys. Still, in many sections they had to walk some distance into the interior of an area before finding the appropriate group of households to be sampled. Since telephone contact was all but impossible for the majority of the respondents, the interviewers were forced to rely upon repeated visits to try and obtain the cooperation of the selected respondent.

In many of the rural areas where the houses were far apart and often inaccessible by local transportation, the difficulty of locating respondents was compounded. To minimize the time spent in any one barrio, the interviewers went out in teams, accompanied by the field supervisor and a driver. The teams remained up to five nights in some of the rural barrios before the interviewing could be completed. This was necessary because news of strangers in the area spread with astonishing swiftness and it was imperative to minimize communication between neighbors about the contents of the survey. On most occasions, the onlookers' interference was minimal and could easily be avoided, but occasionally a problem did arise, as suggested by the following report from one of the field supervisors:

> An unfortunate incident occurred when a woman refused to be interviewed by Mrs. ______. Further efforts to get her cooperation were only met by

scandalous language thrown at the interviewer by the woman. A small crowd that was around laughed and jeered in agreement with the woman's "So what do you care if I enjoy the sex act! [A clear misunderstanding of the intention of the research.] What is it to you! You enjoy it too, don't you! I enjoy it, and it's none of your business!"

At 10:15 that same morning, about twenty houses away, this woman happened to be around when L_____ (another interviewer) was about to start an interview. It was with some effort that this woman was made to understand that the interview was best done if the respondent was alone. The woman had said, "Oh, it's all right. I know what it's all about. You are going to ask her how many times she makes sex. Ha! Ha! I have a husband, too! It's all right, go ahead and interview her."

Interviewer: A third person's presence will somehow affect the answers given. If I were interviewed, I might not give the same answers as I would if I were alone, as when somebody else is around. If you don't mind . . . ?

Woman: She won't be ashamed. We all do the same things. . . .

Interviewer: I really am sorry. Perhaps it's better if I wait until you're through with her.

The woman finally left, laughing to herself.

In many areas of Cebu, both rural and urban, the concept of privacy is quite different from the American middle-class notion. Given the very crowded living conditions, with the consequent opportunity for close communication between neighbors, privacy is not insisted upon as strongly as it might be under different circumstances. Therefore, the lack of privacy occasionally resulted in a predicament. The interviewer is, after all, an intruder into the routines of the neighborhood and cannot risk antagonizing a neighbor to gain privacy for the interview. At most, the interviewer can explain to the respondent and third party that privacy is essential, but little else can be done.

While the crowded conditions in some of the urban areas presented methodological problems, in the rural areas, where many houses were spaced far apart, a different problem arose. In these areas the interviewers often had to walk several kilometers to reach the designated household, often over hills and during the hottest part of the day. This expenditure of time and energy proved worthwhile when the respondent was home and agreed to be interviewed, but it severely taxed an interviewer's morale to walk several kilometers only to be refused. Consequently, in some of the rural areas where the homes were a considerable distance apart, clustered sampling was utilized to minimize the time wasted on nonproductive sojourns into the countryside. The following notes written out by one of the field supervisors after a trip to a rural barrio should give the reader a glimpse of the field situations that confronted our interviewers:

April 29

8:00 A.M.—Team of five female interviewers, two male interviewers, a driver, and a research assistant left for Borbon, the first far municipality. . . .

11:00 A.M.—At point on highway (Barrio Sagay) where one finally turned right to Borbon town, we had our first power failure. Van simply stopped. Alex [the driver] and the interviewers had to get out and push. Once started again, group proceeded to place in Barrio Sagay prearranged for lodging quarters. This turned out too long a walking distance from the street where van had to be parked for the night, since the only way to the house was a long trail. House owner gave us key to their old house in Borbon *población*. The ride to town turned out to be seven kilometers of dangerously narrow winding mountain roads. Group decided against traveling this way daily. Fresh provisions were cooked and preserved by the team at the town's home economics building with the help of home economics teachers at the request of the mayor.

2:00 P.M.—With van piled high with provisions, team left for work with police guide. While interviewers proceeded to do parts of La-aw along the highway and 2–3 kilometers to the interior, research assistant made arrangements for group to stay at a Mr. ______'s cottage in Sagay which is a good riding distance to point on highway where interviewers could start hike to interior *sitios*.

Next, barrio captain described locations of dwellings in his barrio. This turned out to be miscommunicated. For instance the cluster of houses indicated as "back of the school house" turned out to be 2 kilometers from back of school house and the "clusters" of houses were 5–10 tobacco and corn fields apart.

Interviewing ended at 6:00 P.M. with eleven interviews completed. Team decided long hikes would leave group too fatigued to attend to cooking. A cook was hired at one peso per day.

A missing item discovered—rubbing alcohol. Sore muscles were not anticipated.

April 30

After a public bath (only bathing facility available), team left to proceed to B. La-aw. *Sitios* were 1½–3 kilometers apart; houses were 5–10 fields apart; area mountainous. Where mountains gave way for a little breathing space, foot paths circled round rocks huge as large city homes. At two *sitios* some homes tended to cluster but at each of these, only one or two respondents could be had. Half the women were out to help in a harvest. The rest turned out to be old women. At two huts visited not too far from the highway, two women who had heard about the interview questions refused to be interviewed. They said they had to ask the barrio captain's permission. Barrio captain's house was too far into the interior, and the women were not too eager to go with interviewer in search of the captain at the moment, and so the attempt to interview was given up.

An interview with a wife, in the same area where interview questions were heard about from previous day's work, was met with a refusal by the husband when it [interview] was about half done. Woman could not be taken aside to be interviewed alone. Husband wanted to listen in. Questions husband particularly objected to: "What methods have you heard about," "Do you want more children than you now have?"

Twenty-one schedules were completed the second day. Work ended at 6:00 P.M.

May 1

While team packed lunches and snacks, van was brought to local vulcanizing shop. Battery seemed to be very weak. Nearest battery-charging station was two municipalities away. . . .

At 6:00 A.M. van drove team to B. Cajel part of the way. A kilometer and a half was hiked to reach Cajel proper. Other *sitios* were 1½–5 kilometers apart and houses were rolling hills and bare, sandy fields apart. A group with one male interviewer took *sitio* Cajel and Katugasan. A second group took toward *sitio* Dapdap and Yate. After an hour for lunch break the search for respondents resumed with the team which left for *sitios* Katagusan where trees could still be found. At Dapdap, which was bare of trees and shrubs, interviewers who ventured under the noon sun had to turn back [because of the scorching heat].

The barrio captain's home was situated at a point where foot paths led to and from three other *sitios*. Mothers who passed by from the fields were called in by the barrio captain. These women were interviewed at the captain's home. Toward midafternoon when it was not too hot, interviewers went toward *sitio* Yate.

Work ended at 7:00 P.M. with thirty-four interviews completed.

This report illustrates the kinds of difficulties our interviewers encountered. It does not, by any means, exhaust the range of problems we had to resolve.

Second, interpersonal problems in the field stem from the so-called cultural traits of the Filipinos, most of whom are relatively shy, humble, and often deferential. It is considered presumptuous to take the initiative in a discussion or interview. Hence, in general verbal exchange, the Cebuanos often volunteer only the minimum amount of information necessary to answer a question, sometimes without even saying a word, but merely by gesturing with their eyebrows. Although to an American observer men manifest shyness and deference to an obvious degree, women are even more shy, hesitant, and subservient. These behavioral attributes are definitely changing among the younger generation, particularly in the urban areas, but for the majority of the rural respondents, such a personality configuration may still be readily observed.

In order to obtain the family history information demanded by the study, certain intimate inquiries had to be made concerning the woman's pregnancy history and family planning data, if any. Owing to this culturally prescribed shyness, gathering information on sex and pregnancy involved an even more delicate situation. Using married female interviewers was one step in mitigating this problem, as was carefully preparing the interviewers to expect a certain reluctance and shyness.

Perhaps the most embarrassing situation for all respondents was discussing the frequency of intercourse. This involved only two questions: the first, the number of times per month for the first year of marriage, and the second, the number of times per month after the first child. This topic, which is embarrassing in most cultures, was made more complicated in Cebu because the Cebuano language contains no culturally acceptable word for sexual intercourse. The words *kayat* and *iyot*, usually used by men, are vulgar and unacceptable to use when speaking with women. Although the English language allows many euphemisms for sexual intercourse, such as "marital relations," "sleeping with," "being intimate with," and so on, in Cebuano the synonyms are considerably limited. After a great deal of search and consultation, two words were eventually chosen: *gamit*, meaning "to use," and *du-ol*, meaning "to come close." Since many Filipinos know some English, the interviewers were encouraged to use the words *sexual intercourse* as a supplementary phrase after using *gamit* or *du-ol*. Despite these precautions, it must be assumed that some respondents misunderstood the question, because a few of them reported a frequency for sexual intercourse in excess of two hundred times per month for the first year of marriage! (It appears that instead of the number of sexual acts, the respondents had given us the number of thrusts.)

Another problem that occasionally arose was the reluctance of people to be interviewed because of apprehension that the interview data were being collected by the government for tax purposes or other reasons. This may help to explain the higher refusal rate among the middle and upper classes than for the lower class; the former would have more to hide (about their actual earnings or other related information) and, ultimately, more to lose than the latter. We were informed that a sizable number of people in the Philippines do not report their earnings to the Bureau of Internal Revenue (as required by law), and that those who do frequently understate the reports. For similar reasons, people will often refrain from constructing ostentatious homes lest they attract too much attention. There are notable exceptions, of course, principally in the homogeneously upper-class area of the city appropriately named Beverly Hills.

Third, the difficulty in remembering dates and facts deserves mention. The war years in the early forties disrupted the routine of the lives of most Filipinos, and interrupted their normal patterns of reproductive behavior. While this is difficult to demonstrate because of the lack of reliable data, the loss of records (such as birth certificates) and failing memories among many of the respondents proved to be very real. Experience indicated that for older mothers or families living in remote barrios, time is more relative and thus fertility information contingent upon dates was not readily obtainable. Interviewers were taught to help mothers remember dates or, at a minimum, to narrow the time period. For example, an older mother who did not remember her marriage date was asked whether it was before, during, or after the war. If she was married during the war, she was asked whether it was during or after the bombing. A younger mother might be asked to recall the name of the mayor or governor who was in office at the time of her marriage. At times, older children remembered the birth dates of their siblings. Although these techniques were definitely not foolproof, under certain circumstances they did facilitate the interview.

To sum up, since survey research was unprecedented in Cebu when we began our study, there were very few people with prior interviewing experience, or with knowledge of what social research was all about. Thus, it was necessary not only to implement a training program for prospective interviewers, but also to adapt to the realities of the field situation. Many of the methodological procedures we employed were, therefore, made in response to local field conditions which, although probably similar to those in other developing countries, were quite disparate from those found in the more urbanized areas of the United States.

4 / Cebuano Reproduction and Courtship

Cebu is the oldest city in the Philippines, having been established by the Spaniards in 1565. Because of its natural harbor and central location, it has since served as an entrepôt not only for interisland shipping, but also for international trade. Moreover, it is the second largest educational and cultural center, surpassed only by Manila, the "prime" city of the Republic. Its dialect, Cebuano (also called Visayan or Bisayan), is widely spoken in many parts of the central and southern Philippines. In fact, according to the latest census figures, Cebuano is spoken by 24 percent of the Filipinos whereas the country's national language, Tagalog (also called Pilipino), is spoken by only 21 percent of the total population.[1] Far more significant is Cebu's status as the second most densely populated province in the country, topped only by Rizal.[2] As of 1970, its population was estimated to be 1,634,182. The fact that outmigration from Cebu has been evident for decades does not obscure its accelerating population growth. This, along with the fact that at least two prominent politicians' families hail from Cebu, makes it an important locus for politics as well.

In this chapter, we shall concern ourselves with patterns of Cebuano reproductive behavior and with some of the institutional forces that contribute to the regularities of these patterns. The data presented here come from twenty-two unstructured, intensive interviews and a total of more than two thousand cases obtained through sample surveys conducted in the city and in the barrios. Of the total, 1,521 cases were from the metropolitan area of Cebu City.[3]

Cebuano Natality Profile

As a start, it is useful to consider the age at marriage among our respondents. Under Philippine law, the minimum marriage age for men is sixteen years and that for women is fourteen years. However, men who are under twenty and women who are not yet eighteen are required to obtain written consent from at least one parent or guardian before applying for a marriage license at the local civil registrar. Vital statistics data obtained from the National Census and Statistics Office indicate that from 1961 to 1965 the median age at first marriage for grooms was twenty-three years old, consistently. It went up by a few months in 1969 and stood at 23.6 in 1973. The median age at marriage for brides was twenty years old from 1961 to 1963. As of 1973, it stood at twenty-one years of age.

In examining our data, we found that the figures we obtained did not deviate significantly from the national average. Table 4.1 shows the median age at first marriage in our total sample, broken down by social class, sex, and urban or rural background. The small increase in median age at first marriage as one moves up the social ladder is consistent for both sexes. The figures for rural women do not differ significantly from those for urban wives. On the whole, the median age at first marriage between subsamples is fairly close, with the greatest age gap occurring between rural lower-class wives and urban upper-class husbands.

At the time of the interview, the respondents had been married for an average of between 10.5 and 12.7 years, depending on their social class and urban or rural background (Table 4.2). The rural lower-class and the urban upper-class respondents had each been married for 12 or more years, while the rest had been married for slightly shorter periods.

Urban-rural differences in fertility ratio are shown in Table 4.3. Here the number of births per thousand women in each group is consistently higher for the rural sample.

Cohort breakdown reveals that within the first two younger age cohorts, the number of children ever born to urban women is slightly greater among middle-class respondents than among those of the lower class (Table 4.4). This difference begins to reverse among the cohorts of women twenty-five years or older: the lower class consistently reported the largest number of children ever born, followed by the middle class, with the upper class reporting the smallest corresponding figures. A

TABLE 4.1

MEDIAN AGE AT FIRST MARRIAGE, N = 2,094

	Urban		*Rural*	
Social Class	*Husband*	*Wife*	*Husband*	*Wife*
Upper	26.1	23.2	—	—
Middle	24.1	21.3	23.2	21.0
Lower	23.0	19.9	22.1	19.5

TABLE 4.2

YEARS OF MARRIAGE AT TIME OF INTERVIEW

	Urban			*Rural*		
Social Class	*Mean*	*Median*	*N*	*Mean*	*Median*	*N*
Upper	12.7	13.4	101	—	—	—
Middle	11.6	10.9	720	10.5	11.6	170
Lower	11.6	11.1	700	12.0	9.8	403

TABLE 4.3

NUMBER OF BIRTHS PER THOUSAND WOMEN

Age Cohort	*Postmarital Place of Residence*	*Number of Children*	*Number of Cases*	*Per 1,000 Women*
Under 19	urban	46	23	2,000
	rural	12	7	*
20–24	urban	492	205	2,400
	rural	150	63	2,540
25–29	urban	1,174	354	3,316
	rural	421	120	3,508
30–34	urban	1,948	414	4,708
	rural	542	112	4,839
35–39	urban	2,143	345	6,212
	rural	510	78	6,538
40–44	urban	1,530	227	6,740
	rural	426	59	7,220
45 and over	urban	323	57	5,670
	rural	139	17	8,176

*Number too small to report.

TABLE 4.4

NUMBER OF CHILDREN EVER BORN

Selected Characteristics	Urban			Rural	
	Upper	*Middle*	*Lower*	*Middle*	*Lower*
Age cohorts					
Under 19	*	2.90	2.25	*	1.86
20–24	*	3.15	2.72	2.61	2.80
25–29	2.30	3.78	4.00	4.15	4.11
30–34	4.77	4.99	5.52	5.10	6.70
35–39	6.29	6.64	7.37	5.91	7.18
40–44	6.41	6.61	*	*	7.72
45 or over	*	6.75	7.37	*	10.21

*Number of cases too small to report.

class differential is also discernible in the rural sample. Except for the cohort of twenty-five to twenty-nine years old, the middle class had fewer children ever born than the lower class.

Taking age at marriage into account, Table 4.5 shows that for those who married at less than twenty years of age, the urban upper class has the largest number of children, followed very closely by the rural lower class. The range narrowed among those who married between the ages of twenty and twenty-five, where variation in number of births is slight. Finally, marriage after age twenty-five lowered considerably the number of children ever born.

The question of whether the educational attainment of our respondents influences fertility is addressed in Tables 4.6 and 4.7. Among married women under twenty years of age, those whose husbands had a college education reported more births (Table 4.6). But in the cohorts of women aged thirty or older, those with college-educated husbands reported the smallest number of children ever born.

When the wife's educational attainment is used instead (see Table 4.7), the picture comes into much sharper focus. In every age cohort, women with a college education reported fewer births than the rest of our respondents. Among women under the age of twenty-five, those with a high school education reported the largest number of births. For the next two age cohorts, twenty-five to twenty-nine and thirty to thirty-four, those with no education had the highest number of births, and we see the variation by educational levels beginning to take shape. It is among the respondents aged thirty-five or older that the relationship between educational differences and the number of births is most pro-

TABLE 4.5

AGE AT MARRIAGE
AND NUMBER OF CHILDREN EVER BORN

Age at Marriage	*Urban*			*Rural*	
	Upper	*Middle*	*Lower*	*Middle*	*Lower*
Under 20	6.00	5.08	5.22	4.85	5.67
20–25	4.39	4.62	4.60	4.67	4.55
26–30	4.00	3.53	3.69	3.176	3.63
30 and over	[a]	[a]	3.43[b]	[a]	[a]

[a]Number of cases is too small to report.
[b]Subject to error, based on less than ten cases.

TABLE 4.6

NUMBER OF BIRTHS,
BY HUSBAND'S EDUCATIONAL ATTAINMENT

Age Cohort of Woman	*Educational Attainment of Husband*			
	No School	*Grade School*	*High School*	*College*
Under 19	*	1.73	1.95	2.20
20–24	1.73	2.40	2.73	2.31
25–29	2.83	3.68	3.46	2.94
30–34	4.45	4.85	4.99	4.41
35–39	6.15	6.59	6.17	5.71
40–44	5.91	6.88	6.67	5.76
45 and over	6.42	7.15	6.27	5.68

*Number of cases is too small to report.

TABLE 4.7

NUMBER OF BIRTHS,
BY WIFE'S EDUCATIONAL ATTAINMENT

	Educational Attainment of Wife			
Age Cohort	*No School*	*Grade School*	*High School*	*College*
Under 19	—	1.72	2.33	—
20–24	2.55	2.33	2.74	2.19
25–29	3.90	3.58	3.51	2.54
30–34	5.50	4.93	5.13	3.74
35–39	6.59	6.79	5.96	5.20
40–44	6.76	7.33	6.43	4.74
45 and over	7.00	7.43	6.18	5.06

nounced, with grade school education or less dividing the relatively "high" from the "low" natality groups.

Cross-tabulation by husband's occupation (Table 4.8) shows that, except for the cohort of women younger than twenty-five, those in the "high-status" occupational group have fewer children than others, and, starting from the cohort of women aged thirty or older, those whose husbands are in blue-collar or other low-status jobs generally report the largest number of children. By the time their fertility is completed, the natality difference between women whose husbands are in professional or administrative occupations and those whose husbands are in blue-collar or other jobs is 2.2 children.

Taking all these tables into account, the Cebu data suggest that women of the lower class and from rural backgrounds commonly married young, continued to have children for a longer time than the other respondents and, as a result, had a higher natality than the other groups of respondents. The tables also suggest that class differences in natality are more subdued than urban-rural differences. By the time Cebuano women have completed their reproduction (aged forty-five or older), urban lower-class respondents had as many as 7.37 children compared to 10.21 children among the rural lower-class respondents. The uneven number of cases that result from finer breakdowns of social class and urban or rural background renders a more definitive conclusion difficult since, in some cells, the number is too small for analysis.

Timing of the First Child

An examination of the time lapse between the respondents' reported marriage dates and the births of their first children shows the

TABLE 4.8

NUMBER OF BIRTHS,
BY HUSBAND'S OCCUPATION

	Occupation of Husband		
Age Cohort	*Professional, Administrative*	*White-Collar*	*Blue-Collar*
20–24	2.66	2.35	2.53
25–29	2.65	3.45	3.27
30–34	4.15	4.35	4.97
35–39	5.36	5.89	6.48
40–44	5.10	6.82	6.87
45 and over	4.31	6.30	6.55

rapid fire of successful births that befall Cebuano women. Table 4.9 presents the average number of months elapsed between marriage and each consecutive live birth for women of three different age cohorts in our total sample. In calculating these averages, only women with live births in each of the parities were used. Those who had a miscarriage, an abortion, or a stillbirth in any parity were excluded from the computation of that particular parity. Women who might be subfecund are not excluded from the total sample, because such a factor is practically impossible to single out unless data on the precise use of contraceptives between successive births are reliable. (As we shall see in Chapter 5, our data on contraception were based on self-reports by women whose knowledge about birth control was often mixed with folk knowledge about reproduction and childbirth. Therefore, any attempt to employ such analyses introduces further errors.)

In reading Table 4.9 across the row, for instance, one notices that for those women born before 1935, the average length of time that elapsed between marriage and birth of the first child is 14 months, or just two months after the first wedding anniversary. Between the first and second parities, there was a gap of 25.3 months. This gap varied only slightly for all subsequent births.

Reading down the columns, one realizes that for, say, the first parity, younger women (those born after 1935) had an even shorter time gap between reported marriage date and birth of the first child. Thus, those born between 1935 and 1940 had a mean gap of 13.5 months, while those born in 1945 or later had a gap of 12.9 months.

Table 4.10 gives a different perspective on the same phenomenon. Here, we have limited ourselves to those couples who have had their first child (for convenience, we shall call these couples "fecund"), and

TABLE 4.9

MEAN TIME BETWEEN MARRIAGE AND SUBSEQUENT BIRTHS, IN MONTHS

Parity	1		2		3		4		5		6		7	
Women Born	*N*	*Mean*	*N*	*Mean*	*N*	*Mean*	*N*	*Mean*	*N*	*Mean*	*N*	*Mean*	*N*	*Mean*
Before 1935	(781)	14.0	(755)	25.3	(720)	26.5	(656)	27.0	(572)	27.5	(484)	27.8	(383)	25.9
1935–1944	(1003)	13.5	(925)	23.8	(764)	24.6	(582)	24.2	(388)	24.0	(234)	24.8	(121)	24.3
1945 or later	(310)	12.9	(236)	21.8	(118)	22.4	(43)	22.3	(14)	25.4	(9)	27.8	(4)	—
Total women who had live births	(2094)	13.6	(1916)	24.2	(1602)	25.3	(1281)	25.6	(974)	26.0	(727)	26.8	(508)	25.5

Note: The total number of women decreases as one reads across the row, indicating that at each parity, the number of women is different, depending on the total live births the woman had. These figures do not include pregnancies resulting in miscarriages, abortions, or stillbirths.

TABLE 4.10

TIME BETWEEN MARRIAGE AND FIRST CHILD, N = 2,094

Social Class	*Time Between Marriage and First Child*				
	1 year	*2 years*	*3 years*	*4 years*	*5 years*
Urban					
Upper	82.7%	13.3%	2.0%	1.0%	1.0%
Middle	81.2	14.5	3.1	0.6	0.3
Lower	77.0	15.6	4.8	1.2	1.0
Rural					
Middle	80.4	11.9	4.2	3.0	0.0
Lower	78.8	14.9	4.3	1.8	0.3

tabulated the latency period between marriage and the birth of that child. Table 4.10 shows the near universality of the short time lapse between marriage and the first child. In all subgroups, urban and rural, more than three-quarters of these fecund couples had had their first child by their first anniversary. As a matter of fact, the higher the social class, the greater the percentage of women who had had their first child by the end of their first year of marriage. Furthermore, by their third anniversary, 98 percent of all couples had had their first child.

We also collected further data that only served to emphasize the consistent pattern of early childbirth these tables represent. We had wondered whether there might be a connection between the timing of the birth of the first child and variations in the kind of living arrangements couples made after their marriage. We found there was no apparent connection: whether the couple lived alone or with some or another set of relatives, their first child came predictably—in most cases —shortly after their first wedding anniversary. At the same time, we did find that regardless of their social class or rural-urban background, over half of all young married couples lived with or very close to their immediate relatives. As many as 56 percent of the urban upper and middle classes and 77 percent of the rural lower class respondents had lived with the husband's parents, either in the same house or in the same *sitio*. Likewise, about 47 percent of the urban upper and middle classes and 65 percent of the rural lower class had either shared a house with or lived in close proximity to the wife's parents. In addition, close to 50 percent of all respondents had lived with or near to the husband's married siblings, while about 40 percent had resided with or near to the wife's married siblings. Such arrangements could be taken to be matters of necessity for the poor, who are often forced to live where they can find room to live, moving as many times as necessary from one relative to the next. But the fact that many well-to-do couples also lived with or near their relatives, when they presumably could be on their own, suggests that the Cebuano's patterns of postmarital residence are indicative of preferences that are based on more than considerations of financial means. In a sense, then, there *is* a connection between the consistency of the timing of the first child and the preference shown by newly married couples for living with or near their immediate relatives. Both are manifestations of the centrality of the family for social identity as well as for economic survival, and there is between them a strong current of *cultural* patterning that creates a situation of mutual reinforcement: the family encourages the young couple to have children quickly, and the sooner and more frequently the couple does have children, the more tightly they are bound to the support and the expectations of the family.

Indeed, pregnancy in the year following marriage has a symbolic meaning that cannot be extricated from the web of kinship obligations or from the cultural norms of Cebuano society. Because family and kin are essential both for economic survival and social identity, kinship and family pressures encourage early pregnancy and a subsequent rapid succession of births. As we shall see more fully in chapter 10, such pressures may be not at all subtle.

In the rest of this chapter, we wish to examine the way in which young unmarried people meet each other, become engaged, and enter into the web of kinship supports and obligations that come with marriage. In doing so we shall see that the peculiar pattern of Cebuano courtship and the norm of premarital chastity also play important parts in contributing to the rapidity and frequency with which married couples have children.

Courtship and Premarital Chastity

In the Cebuano language, the terms *dalaga* (young lady) and *ulitawo* (young man) are used to indicate the social recognition of adolescence, which often coincides with the onset of puberty. These words stand in contradistinction to *bata*, meaning "child." Public initiation rites marking the process of growing up are unheard of. For the girl, however, the unexpected discovery of blood spottings on her underwear is usually followed by a private mother-daughter ritual, a practice more closely observed among rural folk and the urban lower and middle classes than among the well-to-do. The following account is typical. (Unless otherwise specified, throughout this book, *M* denotes a middle-class respondent while *L* stands for lower-class.)

> *M:* I remember that . . . it happened in the classroom. While the lessons were going on I felt that I was getting wet and uncomfortable. I excused myself to go to the bathroom and found out that I had blood on my pants. Without going back to my class and without asking permission, I rushed home. My mother was surprised to see me and when she knew, she told me right away to go to the bathroom and take off my clothes. She then poured one can of water on my head, and another two on my shoulders. I knew what this was for because it was also done to my other sisters. After the "bath," I jumped three steps of our stairs and as I was doing it my classmates approached our house; they began to tease me. The next morning I refused to go to school for fear that the two classmates who had come to the house—they were asked by the teacher to inquire about what had happened to me—would tell the others and for sure I would be teased by everybody. [Did your mother ever give you any sex education, either before or after you had your first period?] I never dared to ask questions regarding matters about sex, for our parents never allowed us to talk about it.

That this ritual is still being practiced nowadays is evident among some of our respondents who reported having performed it on their daughters as well. Their descriptions did not differ substantially from those of a generation ago:

> *L:* When my oldest daughter had her menstruation, she became afraid because she thought something was wrong with her. [Probe.] I explained to her, and we had to do the pouring of three cans of water, one on the head, one on each shoulder . . . to ensure that she won't have too many days of menstruation. Then, also, she was made to jump three steps of the stairs for the same purpose. And her panty which had the first spots of blood was used to wipe her face. This is to have a good complexion; to prevent pimples from coming out in great number. [Probe.] Yes, my mother did that to me, too. . . . I was forbidden by my parents to talk about sex. In school, whenever I heard somebody mention something about it, I felt ashamed and would shout "*bastos!*" [That's base, gross, indecent!] [Probe.] I forbid my children to talk about it literally. I never tolerate them to say things like, for example, the dialect for the sexual organs. . . . I invented another name for it: "flower" for the girl's, and "tin-tin" for the boy's.

For a great number of Cebuano *dalaga*, the lack of sex education that accompanies their initiation into young adulthood is striking. In some cases, this fosters the conception that sex is *hilas* (embarrassing because it is bawdy). As one middle-class respondent put it, "Even when I was already in college, *hilasan ko* [I got embarrassed] when our zoology instructor discussed the subject of sex. . . . I did not want to listen." It comes as no surprise, then, that in some families, the woman is sexually unprepared even as she enters into a marriage:

> *M:* No such thing [sex] was ever discussed in our home, because our father was a very conservative man. We were even forbidden to swear or say bad words, how much more sex and anything like it. My mother never told us anything, even when we were about to marry. So we plunged into marriage

ignorant of everything. I did not even know what it would really be like, until I myself got married. It was Berting [husband] I should say who taught me every single thing about sex. While we did it, he would at the same time explain things to me, like how to respond to him.

Not all married women are as well informed about sex as this respondent. Of the women we interviewed intensively, only one reported that she had received informal sex education from her parents:

M: When we became *dalaga*, my father gave us sort of a lecture. We enjoyed these sessions especially when he inserted some jokes. . . . The lectures were about the difference between a boy and a girl; how human beings were created, *the danger of giving in to a boy* [emphasis added], and so on and so forth. Before this, we thought children were created by the magic hands of God, just as they say so in the Bible. [What did your father tell you?] *It was not the real thing* [emphasis added]. It was just to make us understand that sex is healthy and not a bad thing for us children to know. Besides we read articles and books about it. The *True Confessions* magazines which other parents prevented their children from reading were nothing to us. We read it and in my opinion there is nothing dirty about the stories. . . . Of course, in our early teens . . . we also had some misconceptions like, when you let a boy kiss you, you will get pregnant. But they weren't really grave [ignorance], for as I said, our father would once in a while explain things to us.

These remarks give the impression that the parent's principal objective in providing sex education is not to inform the *dalaga* of the facts, but to caution her about "the danger of giving in to a boy"—an objective the other parents probably hoped to accomplish simply by avoiding the discussion or by withholding sexual information.

Not to give in to a boy's persistent requests for intimacy is critical, for in the Cebuano culture, and in the larger Philippine society as well, premarital chastity is not an anachronous virtue but the ideal norm. Sexual naïveté in women is highly valued and regarded as a reflection of virginal innocence. However, with few exceptions, an *ulitawo* is expected to desire sexual adventures. It is considered "natural" for him not to pass up an opportunity when it is available; to refuse it implies a weakness in his manhood (*pagkalalaki*). His ability to be persuasive with women is part of his male role. It is the woman's responsibility to halt his advances, to "guard her honor," and "to keep her family's reputation"; should it be threatened or violated, she must do everything she can to restore respect to herself and her family. [See Jocano (1969) for a description of similar values in another Philippine province.]

The onset of puberty intensifies traditional sex-role socialization. The *dalaga* is taught to act in a ladylike manner and to learn housekeeping skills more seriously, now that she is grown up. She is admonished against playing with boys or mixing with them too often in school. She should certainly not be seen alone with them. She is told always to have somebody go with her wherever she goes; her social life is closely monitored by her parents and other members of the family. Only the girl who for one reason or another is not living in her parents' household can escape the watchful eyes of her elders. Even when she leaves home for college her social life is group-oriented. Unchaperoned dating is not so common in the Cebuano culture as it is in North America. A young girl who dares to break these codes risks being called the most damning of all names—*biga-on*, an adjective derived from the verb describing dogs in estrus. Under such conditions social mixing, courtship, and marriage take on a unique pattern.

It is regrettable that despite the rich folklore regarding the Cebuano proclivity for gallantry and romance, social scientists have not systematically studied their courtship behavior. For this reason, we had to rely upon our project staff to collect the relevant material. From the ethnomethodological accounts of courtships provided by our Cebuano research assistants,[4] we have the following distillation of firsthand and vicarious experiences in Cebuano courtship.

Conceptually, courtship begins at the *magka-ila* or "acquaintance" stage, where the *ulitawo* "spots" the girl he likes. Occasions for group activities provide the most common opportunities for boys to meet girls. Since both the boy and the girl are likely to have their individual peer groups (called *barkada*) as constant companions, the latter can inquire about or transmit any affective intentions between two potential lovers without causing undue embarrassment to either party. The *barkada* is thus an indispensable go-between during courtship. In most cases, heterosexual friendship proceeds cautiously and sometimes casually. In the rural areas, the boy (and his companions) may try to meet the girl (with her companions) at the well or by the river where she usually does her laundry. In the city and in school, he may try to find excuses to borrow her notes or phone her on the pretext of inquiring about their assignments. If the boy wishes to hint at his "special" feelings for her, he and his friends may trail behind her in school, sit at a nearby table in the cafeteria, or get into the same jeepney with her after class. The girl makes efforts to deny that she is aware of his interest, although her friends tease her incessantly about it. The boy is also teased by his friends especially in his first few tries to talk to the girl alone. Among male adolescents, trying to sneak a few private moments with the girl alone is called "chancing-chancing," or taking chances.

The second stage, *nang-ulitawo* or courting, involves more open interaction between the boy and the girl. When teased about it, each would insist that they are just *amigo* or friends. At this stage, the boy normally asks for a few private moments with the girl. The more persistent he is, the more genuine his feelings supposedly are. The girl, in turn, is expected to test his sincerity by saying no to the first—if not the first few—invitations. Depending upon the boy's persuasive power and the girl's eventual response, *amigo* relationships may or may not blossom into the more advanced stage of *managtrato* or "going steady." The *ulitawo* finally musters enough courage to visit the *dalaga* at her home. (In rural areas the boy, accompanied by a friend or his peer group, may serenade the girl.) If her family likes the young suitor, he may be invited into their home, but the girl is rarely left alone with him. A younger sibling or a grandparent is usually within hearing distance. Theoretically, there is no hand-holding or kissing in public, and if they attend parties or go to a movie the girl's family normally insists that she be chaperoned. Affection is communicated in public through gestures rather than vocally, and a sense of exclusiveness envelops the young couple. It is also a sign for other interested males to "stay away" from the *dalaga*.

In practice, however, "going steady" behavior varies a great deal between the sexes, for this is the stage of courtship where men try to persuade women to submit to coitus, while the latter must weigh the advantages and disadvantages accruing from such a concession. The layman's suspicion that sexual intimacy for men does not necessarily mean that marriage for the woman is within reach is given credence by one of our staff's findings on a sample of more than one thousand Cebuano college students (Pinard, 1971). He found that 43 percent of the men who responded to his questionnaire had had coital experience, as compared to only 3 percent of the women. Furthermore, for two-thirds of the women, the first petting experience occurred in the going-steady stage of courtship. For the other one-third, petting was experienced much later, during the engagement stage. The data collected from the men who have had coital experience are striking. Fully 65 percent of these men's first sexual partners were someone other than the person they were going steady with or engaged to. In 30 percent of the cases, the woman they were sexually intimate with was an unmarried stranger. In 17 percent of the cases, she was an unmarried casual acquaintance, and in still another 17 percent of the cases, she was an unmarried friend but not a "steady." Given that the sample as a whole does not approve of sexual intimacy for women, but that men do in fact acquire such experience with someone other than their "steady" or fiancée, it must be inferred that a strong double standard exists. A substantial number of men probably try to promise marriage in order to obtain sexual favors. Hence the wisdom in the advice that every woman must be wary of men promising marriage.

In cases where the man's sincerity has been tested and his marriage intentions are considered "serious" (genuine), the courtship then progresses into the *pamalaye* stage. This is when the boy's parents make their son's intentions known to the girl's parents. It is either done by the father himself or delegated to an articulate person, usually a relative, called the *mamamaye*. Wedding details and brideprice or gifts are discussed. The couple is now called *kaslunon*, "to be married." They can each freely admit their feelings, and no *ulaw* (shame) is involved anymore, even if they are teased by friends. Relatives and neighbors are generally informed and a wedding invitation is soon anticipated. In spite of the relaxation of restrictions at this stage, many a woman who considers herself properly brought up would avoid holding hands or kissing in public for fear of being considered "easy" by others and losing her fiancé's respect.

According to Pinard's findings, there is a discrepancy between the ideal and the actual time intervals for the different stages of courtship. Ideally, both sexes maintain that each progression (from going steady to engagement, and from engagement to marriage) should last about 11 months. But actually, the time span is much shorter. Boys reported knowing their girlfriends for only 2.1 months before they went steady. On the average, engagement followed after 7.8 months, and marriage after 20 months.

These figures are merely averages. In reality, the entire period from first acquaintance to marriage may range from as short as one month to as long as eight years, depending on the situation. The following (taken from our unstructured in-depth interviews) is an example:

> M: We met when we were both students at the University of San Carlos. Our courtship lasted a year and was characterized—during the later part when I finished my degree and returned to my hometown while he stayed in the city to finish up—by visits and letters. We wrote each other at least five times a week; we saw each other at least once a month. He visited me in my home town . . . or at my aunt's house whenever I came to the city. [When] I was a boarder at Sto. Rosario [a dormitory run by nuns] . . . the boarders did not talk about sex. . . . Boarders talked about clothes, college activities. Boyfriends visited but [we] did not go out [alone]. During that time, we stayed home on week-ends. All that time, *we never went out on dates. Once a boy and a girl are seen together people start talking so even if the girl has not really decided to marry the man, she will* [have to] *say yes because she is ashamed* [emphasis added]. In those days we [groups of friends] went out to parties together from the dormitory. . . . I never saw anyone kissing so it was farthest from my mind that things like that happen on dates. It was not until I was married and saw people kissing in movies that I realized that moviehouses are also places for lovemaking. This is why I don't allow my children to go by themselves.

Not all Cebuanos observe the strict rule of no single dating, as evidenced in the following:

M: I met my husband at a friend's birthday party. At first, I did not like Virgilio* as he had the air of a *palikero* [playboy]. Right that evening, he asked me to go with him to Yarrow [a night spot in Talisay] for dancing. I refused, because besides being brought up strictly by my father, I did not like his attitude and I had also told my father that I would be home before ten o'clock. Three days later, I received a phone call from Virgilio asking to meet me at one of the downtown restaurants for a snack and to "talk." I went. It was on that occasion that he asked me to go with him to see a movie that following Saturday. *I accepted on the condition that I would be bringing somebody along* [emphasis added]. . . . He began coming regularly to the house, fetching me from the office and escorting me on some engagements. . . . Then, just one afternoon, he called me up in the office where I was working, asking me a very funny question—"Would you get married if somebody were to ask you?" I responded that I would if I liked the man. The next thing I knew he asked me to marry him. *This was four weeks after knowing each other* [emphasis added]. I was not able to give him an answer right then, but asked him to give me time to think it over. After office hours on the same day, when we met at our particular rendezvous, he asked to meet my father. But he was not in town then, as he was busy going with the [political] campaign of a relative. So I suggested that . . . why not meet my older sister Juanita? I brought him over to see Juanita that Sunday and they clicked with each other, as Juanita also drinks a little. . . . The next Saturday after meeting Juanita, I brought him over to Opon to see my Aunt Dolores. Dolores liked Virgilio, as he is really a gentleman, so she gave me her opinion . . . of approval. . . . When he [father] came home, he got angry and disappointed, as he was [supposed to be] the first one to be told. I told him it was not my fault that he was not home. [Probe.] When he met Virgilio, he gave his blessings. The Sunday after this meeting, Virgilio came with his mother, father, and uncle and asked for my hand in marriage. They were given consent and the wedding was scheduled for the fourth Sunday after that meeting. They agreed on the terms of expenses and preparations, where the wedding was supposed to be held, and the kind of reception needed.

L: We had been sweethearts [*trato*] for eight years. . . . We had agreed beforehand to get married as soon as he finished his studies without necessarily [waiting for him to take] the board exam [for C.P.A.]. To this, his mother objected. Sensing that she might use this as a delaying tactic to prevent our marriage, I gave my husband an ultimatum, either we elope or we separate. He was already employed in a shipping company and he just asked me to accompany him on that trip. I went but not without leaving a sentimental note to my parents telling them of my decision. We came back after two weeks. He took a leave of absence and we got married.

In the last example, the lower-class respondent's aggressive ultimatum must be understood in the context of Cebuano culture. Being sweethearts for such a great length of time and not to be married afterwards would have meant a considerable loss of honor and self-respect for the woman, since at that stage of their courtship it is unlikely that their relationship could be kept out of public view. Hence, the woman must de-

*All names have been changed to ensure the respondents' anonymity.

fend her reputation, and defend it she did! Note, however, that she achieved this by compromising the ideal norm of premarital chastity, and neither in this particular session nor in subsequent interviews did she express regret over their infraction.

Not all courtships take the normatively prescribed path, as evidenced by the following lower-lower-class respondent, the daughter of a poor farmer in Leyte:

> *L:* I always wanted to come to the city [of Cebu]. So when my two cousins were planning to come here in 1958 to work as housemaids, they encouraged me to come along. [Probe.] They offered to pay for the boat fare of six pesos. I grabbed the opportunity and left with my parents' permission. [Probe.] I was fourteen years old then; had no thoughts of how I would earn a living nor how I could return home [to Leyte]. . . . [I was] forced to work as a maid for a Tagalog family. Unable to understand them, I left after two weeks and went to live with my aunt [father's cousin]. I could not go back to Leyte because I did not save enough for fare. The following day, a neighbor introduced me to Julio [husband, nine years her senior], who brought me to his married brother's house. I went with the impression that I was to work as a housemaid. To my surprise, I was told by the married brother that my marriage to Julio would be fixed soon. That night, we all slept in their one-room shack. [Probe.] No, *oy!* He never touched me. He came home every night and brought me food or little gifts. Occasionally, he brought me to the movies. *Every week he gave me his earnings, but he never proposed to me or mentioned that he loved me.* He only inquired if I had a boyfriend. Our relationship remained like this for a month. [Probe.] I had nowhere else to go. I was also too ashamed to ask questions or demand explanations. [Probe.] Gradually, I developed *feelings of pity* [emphasis added] toward him. Among his friends and relatives, it was understood that I was his woman. [Probe.] After a month's stay with Carlos [Julio's brother], we transferred to Tining's house [HuSi] because there was no more space; Julio's married sister came to live with Carlos. At Tining's house, we were given a separate room [from them] together with Tining's five children. We had to wait until all the children were asleep before we could sleep together. This was the first time we had sexual intercourse. It was only then that he told me he wanted to marry me.

Such a courtship pattern is undoubtedly unique. But even when the couple was initially able to become *magka-ila* or acquaintances, and a marriage proposal was articulated, the extent to which "feelings of pity" form the initial basis of a husband-wife relationship is not entirely rare, particularly among the lower-class respondents. The following is another example:

> *L:* I came from Argao [a coastal town sixty-seven kilometers south of Cebu City]. I used to come to the city regularly to peddle fruits and vegetables and stayed overnight in Villagonzalo 2 [a slum section of the city where her aunt lives]. This is where I met him [husband]. [Probe.] When he had a chance to work on a government project in Argao, he came to see me regularly . . . asked my parents' permission to marry me. [Probe.] He was eighteen; I was

twenty-two. [Probe.] I really did not plan to marry him. I did not like him because he was too small. When I said yes to him, it was only like play [*ti-aw ti-aw*]. We did not even go dating—*not even once*. I did not know he would take me seriously. When he told me that he was going to ask my parents' permission to marry, I answered him in jest, "Well, if you are ready and prepared to spend for the banquet, I won't object." He was always at our house because he was working with the Magsaysay Community Project. When I was washing clothes, he was there to fetch the water. When I weeded the fields, he was also there. I secretly planned to run away, but my mother caught me while I was packing my clothes; she cried. She advised me about the old saying, "*Mahaplato, mahabagol.*" [To eat decently from a plate or to eat in shame from a coconut shell.] And then she called my aunts and uncles and grandparents to the house. They all pressed me to accept the proposal so that I had to give in. [Probe.] He also threatened his parents with suicide if he could not marry me.

[How was it during the first month of your marriage?] I hated him and I had no affection for him at all. I used to sleep between the floor and the mat so that he would not find me; I would hear him asking his mother where I was. [Probe.] *I started to pity [lu-oy] him only after [first child] was born* [emphasis added]. The child looked like him, so when I looked at my baby, I see my husband and that's when I started to pity him.

Consequences of the Double Standard

In the Cebuano culture, the fact that girls are socialized to be sexually naive and socially sheltered makes them most vulnerable in any heterosexual encounters, a situation not too different from that of Jamaican girls as described by Blake (1961). Because of overzealous parental supervision and the severe punishment meted out to the budding girl if she is seen with a man the parents do not know or approve of, the circumstances that precipitate courtship and culminate in marriage are not always separable from her fear of censure or her motivation to be free from parental control. The following respondents' revelations as to how they reached the decision to get married are illuminating:

M: When I was still young I had many suitors who were determined [*desidido*] to marry me. One of them was Pedro, a man who was "evil" in thought and action . . . he tried to kidnap me three times. But all was a failure because one of my brothers would come to know of it. . . . There was also an accident when this man wounded another suitor. . . . Since then, Pedro would watch over our house with a shotgun on his shoulders. My family was not able to do anything about it, as he was a nephew of the Mayor of Dapitan [Zamboanga] and besides, he is feared by the others. [Probe.]

One February morning, Rodolfo [husband] came to Dapitan together with some Cebuano politicians, Mayor ______ and Judge ______. He acted as their bodyguard. I was attracted by his good looks, and he was [attracted to me], too. It was "love at first sight." Three days later, I was in the school canteen with some friends waiting for our P.E. teacher. Again met Rodolfo who invited us to some snacks. Then suddenly Pedro appeared outside with a gun. Because I was afraid of what might happen, I suggested to Rodolfo and another friend, a boy, to help me escape through the back door. [Probe.] I knew from a friend that Pedro planned to get me that day, "by hook or by crook." It was already six o'clock in the evening when we left the canteen and just by walking, we reached Calamba, another town, at four o'clock dawn, where I was seen by a relative who was delivering bread to the community, as they own a bakery. It was she who told me that my mother had gone mad looking for me, and it was she also who told my mother that she saw me with my [male] companion. *My fear grew more, as my mother is very strict. So I decided there and then to go ahead and escaped with Rodolfo, not caring for the consequences anymore.*

We then took a bus . . . so that we can take a boat for Cebu. But we were so unfortunate, as all boats were notified about us and that in case we would be on board, it was all right for the police to arrest us. So it took us a week to wait for the chance, until finally a captain friend of Rodolfo hid us in his cabin. After we arrived in Cebu, we took a launch for ______ [a neighboring island], where we stayed over in a friend's house. Rodolfo's friend. A few days later, our whereabouts were again known by my mother. A warrant of arrest was posted . . . we were then arrested, but I was placed under the custody of Mayor ______ [the same mayor mentioned earlier] and Rodolfo was under the custody of a police sergeant who was also a cousin of the mayor. Since my mother was really interested in having Rodolfo in jail for kidnaping a minor, Mayor ______ out of pity advised both of us to escape until all will be settled between our parents. . . . The mayor further advised me that I should stand for Rodolfo no matter what will happen so that Rodolfo would not suffer the catastrophic consequence. So again, we were able to escape with the use of a bicycle which was outside the *carenderia*, not knowing who the owner was. . . . [lengthy details of complicated escape routes deleted] . . . where we stayed at Judge ______'s [the same judge mentioned earlier] house. Then, the mayor, Judge ______, and the father of Rodolfo went to Dapitan, to ask for my hand. My mother was angry . . . [but] it was then agreed that *the only way my honor could be saved was for me to marry Rodolfo* [emphasis added].

L: My relatives objected to Eusebio. They had hoped I would marry a more educated man with better family background and who had a permanent job to speak of. My mother never stopped reminding me how they took pains to educate me [as far as high school] so that I would have more chances and better opportunity to meet the right man. *Knowing that we would not be allowed to marry, we decided to elope* [emphasis added]. After three days and knowing that we would eventually have to go back anyway, without having enough money, we went straight to my Ninang Lourdes (mother's cousin), because we were afraid that if we went straight to my parents, Eusebio might be shot by my father. While Lourdes did not either particularly like Eusebio, her main concern was that *after all we had indulged in the marital act already*, besides Lourdes was worried over what neighbors and friends would be saying especially if I became pregnant without the benefit of marriage. She reprimanded us heavily but also sent for my parents who were then residing in Toledo. My parents expressed the same anger but felt helpless [about what we had done]. . . . Their main objective was to finish everything [arrange the marriage] in a hurry.

M: Our marriage ended one of the most turbulent chapters of my life. I cannot now say whether this was a stroke of good or bad luck. *What I am sure of is that I did not love Opao then* [emphasis added]. He had been separated from his wife for eight years already when he started courting me. His children then were living with his older sister. . . . Early evenings, he would come to the sidewalk *sari-sari* store that I tended. One thing I can say about him is that he was most persistent. I hated him because of his looks. My friends often teased me by saying "the more you hate, the more you love." I completely agreed with my relatives when they stated their objections to this man. We all knew him to be married with two children and he did not have much to offer. He was no longer young and I faced the prospect of going to jail for bigamy.[5] Several times Opao wanted to walk me home. I always refused not only because I did not love him, but also because I was ashamed to be seen with him. You see, he was already bald then. But he would insist, and even though he could not walk me home, *he would follow me very closely all the way.* My older sisters noticed this and *they would punish me for it* [emphasis added]. They never believed me when I told them we were not sweethearts. I was hoping they would find out the truth later on, but somehow their hatred for the man knew no bounds. *With each passing day, their punishment [for me] became more severe. They would hit me, pull my hair, slap my face and inflict other indignities on my body* [emphasis added]. One day, I got so fed up. I was young, inexperienced, and very disgusted, and *I was just trying to free myself from the situation. I dared Opao to take me away* [emphasis added]. At this point, I also discovered the sincerity of his intentions. He did not agree to an elopement. Instead, he made all the legal preparations to have his wife—whom he had not heard from for seven years—[declared] legally dead. . . . For six months, we waited while the court deliberated on the case. My relatives eventually heard about this and they began to change their attitude toward Opao. It is at this point that they stopped beating me, but *they still refused to allow me to go out with Opao* [emphasis added]. So I had to find an alibi, and [I] used [the excuse of visiting] Basio [married brother].

From the North American perspective, the girl's decision to enter into marriage in each of these cases is characterized by a high degree of impetuosity. Strict confinement, sexual naïveté, social inexperience, and severe disapproval make a romantic escapade a most attractive solution to an unbearable situation. Elopement thus becomes an effective means of weakening parental blockage. Under such conditions, observance of the premarital chastity code hinges not so much on the daughter's internalizing the norm and developing "inner controls" as on the family's ability to provide the most punctilious surveillance of her activities. Yet the very fact that the operation of a double standard directs such scrutiny almost exclusively on daughters rather than on sons as well creates not only tensions from within but pressures from without, for the men must find suggestible females in order to realize their sexual adventures. Furthermore, the strict premarital code for women makes one single infraction, whether imagined or real, a sufficient and facile ground for forcing parental consent and speeding up conjugal union, the legal restrictions on minimum marriage age notwithstanding. One mother expressed such apprehension poignantly when she explained why she wanted to hasten her daughter's wedding when she was only sixteen years old: "*Simbako magbinu-ang ang lalaki! Desgrasyahan unya ang atong anak. Wala'y round ming ginikanan.*" (Just in case—God forbid—that the boy makes foolishness, our daughter would fall into disgrace. We parents would have no fighting chance!)

These respondents, of course, are women of childbearing age. It could be argued that in the face of urbanization and modernization, some changes may have taken place. The question of how widespread these attitudes are nowadays throughout the country or even in Cebu Province awaits further study. But based on two sets of questionnaires administered to two groups of college students in Cebu City, Pinard (1971) found that, expectations of modernization notwithstanding, the double sexual standard—as measured by his CATS instrument—was very much in evidence. By every measure, proportionally more men than women have gone out on dates without a chaperone and without informing their parents; more men than women also reported having petted, necked, and engaged in sexual intercourse either with strangers or with someone they knew at various stages of courtship. Furthermore, both male and female students appeared to uphold this double standard in that almost the same percentage of each sex (94 percent of 369 males and 90 percent of 298 females) favored the man marrying a virgin. Table 4.11 provides a good summary of the discrepancy in the latitude that males have over females in dating activities, and the extent of perceived parental approval for these activities.

Group dating, going on outings, and going to parties are activities most men and women have engaged in and which many of their parents approved. However, more men than women have gone to a beach or nightclub with their steadies, and even with nonsteadies. Neither of these places is considered exactly a "wholesome" playground in the Cebuano culture. Sex differences in parental approval are even more striking. While only 11 percent of the females felt that their parents would approve of their going to the beach with a steady, almost four times as many (40 percent) of the men reported that their parents approved. Similarly, 4 percent of the females versus more than five times that many males (22 percent) claimed to have parental approval for going to a nightclub with their steady.

On the whole, one can hazard a guess that even among the younger generation nowadays, courtship and the premarital chastity code still mirror the traditional double standard, although some women in Pinard's samples admitted to having deviated from a few of the traditional

TABLE 4.11

STUDENT DATING ACTIVITIES AND PARENTAL APPROVAL

	Male (N = *369*)			*Female* (N = 298)		
	Have Done	*Parents Approve*	*Don't Know*	*Have Done*	*Parents Approve*	*Don't Know*
Going to parties with steady	65%	67%	18%	44%	44%	16%
Going to beach with steady	41	40	33	12	11	21
Going to night club with steady	31	22	38	13	4	19
Group dating (parties, beach)	72	80	17	77	86	7
Going to parties with nonsteady	70	64	23	42	49	15
Going on outings (bowling, tennis) with nonsteady	58	70	21	37	52	14
Going to nightclubs with nonsteady	36	27	37	12	9	16
Going to beach with nonsteady	40	47	28	13	20	18
Group dating (movies)	61	70	22	63	77	13

Source: Pinard (1975): 106.

sex-role expectations in dating behavior. Nevertheless, the unique situation of Cebu City as the largest educational center south of Manila must be taken into consideration in evaluating these deviations, for a large part of the college population in Cebu City hails from the other provinces, and even though some may be staying with relatives while they attend college, the surveillance they receive may not always be as thorough as that exercised by parents. In other words, any changes in dating attitudes and behavior that Pinard observed may simply be superficial changes that reflect the newly acquired freedom of a special group of youngsters, rather than representing a true shift in the attitudes and behavior of the greater population. Therefore, caution is warranted in generalizing from these findings.

What is significant in Pinard's study is the confirmation that even among the most "modern" segment of the population, premarital chastity is still a highly valued norm for both sexes, and that in actual behavior a double sexual standard permits males but not females to gain sexual experience. Given the fact that the fit between normative prescriptions and actual performance in any society is never perfect, the possibility that intimacy and pregnancy may occur outside the bounds of formalized marriage must be entertained, especially when survey data presented earlier show such a short time span between reported marriage date and the first birth.

Premarital Realities

Using a gap of six or fewer months between reported marriage date and the first birth as our criterion of a premarital pregnancy, we found that the incidence of premarital pregnancies (PMP) among the respondents interviewed in our survey has increased over the years. Age cohort analysis in Table 4.12 shows that for those born between 1923 and 1928, as many as 18.9 percent of the pregnancies were premarital. The percentage increases as age decreases, so that among the youngest cohort of women, those born between 1949 and 1953, as many as 28.6 percent had had a premarital pregnancy.

When we cross-tabulated the data on premarital pregnancy with various social characteristics of the husband and wife, we found that the incidence of premarital pregnancy varied somewhat according to these characteristics. Table 4.13 shows that, in general, the higher the level or prestige of the husband's occupation or education, of the wife's education, or of the wife's father's occupation, the lower the incidence of premarital pregnancy. Presumably, families with the most resources

TABLE 4.12

PREMARITAL PREGNANCIES, BY AGE

Age Cohort	*Number*	*Marital Pregnancy*		*Premarital Pregnancy*		*No Information*	
		No.	%	*No.*	%	*No.*	%
15–19	35	25	71.4	10	28.6	0	0
20–29	798	569	71.3	223	27.9	6	0.8
30–39	1,045	777	74.4	256	24.5	12	1.1
40–45	354	280	79.1	67	18.9	7	2.0
No information	49	34	69.4	14	28.6	1	2.0
Total	2,281	1,685	73.9	570	25.0	26	1.1

TABLE 4.13

INCIDENCE OF PREMARITAL PREGNANCY, BY SOCIAL CHARACTERISTICS OF HUSBAND AND WIFE

Social Characteristics	*Number*	*No Premarital Pregnancy*		*Premarital Pregnancy*		*No Information*	
		No.	*%*	*No.*	*%*	*No.*	*%*
Total	2,281	1,685	73.9	570	25.0	26	1.1
Husband's Occupation							
Professional and managerial	311	241	77.5	66	21.2	4	1.3
White-collar	373	269	72.1	98	26.3	6	1.6
Blue-collar	1,313	960	73.1	341	26.0	2	0.9
Farmer	228	175	76.8	51	22.4	12	0.8
Other	56	40	71.4	14	25.0	2	3.6
Occupation of Wife's Father							
Professional and managerial	228	184	80.7	41	18.0	3	1.3
White-collar	313	236	75.4	76	24.3	1	0.3
Blue-collar	760	541	71.2	210	27.6	9	1.2
Farmer	925	683	73.8	229	24.8	13	1.4
Other	55	41	74.5	14	25.5	0	0
Husband's Education							
College	664	505	76.1	153	23.0	6	0.9
High school	676	498	73.7	170	25.1	8	1.2
Grade school	933	674	72.2	247	26.4	12	1.4
Wife's Education							
College	511	390	76.3	113	22.1	8	1.6
High school	549	416	75.8	130	23.7	3	0.5
Grade school	1,198	862	72.0	322	26.9	14	1.1

are able to exert more punctilious surveillance over the young and restless. An exception to this rule came among those women whose husbands were farmers. It is possible that premarital pregnancies were lower for this group because the rural environment affords fewer occasions for sexual adventure than does the urban setting with its opportunities for anonymity and privacy.

Nevertheless, when taken together, this set of findings shows that although some variation exists, there is an overall consistency in the distribution of premarital pregnancies across the spectrum of social characteristics. However they are measured, the variation between groups defined according to their social characteristics is not that great. Put differently, insofar as the norm of premarital chastity is concerned, no group is above reproach—although some groups show proportionately greater deviations than others. Conservatively speaking, between one in five and one in four Cebuano women were pregnant when they married. The slight advantage of the well-educated and highly prestigious occupational group in this regard may be attributed to their ability to monitor the behavior of their daughters better by virtue of the resources they command. Within this privileged group, daughters are scrupulously chaperoned in their social activities and are chauffeured to and from school. Alternatively, though, one could argue that the inability to recall dates of marriage or of first birth is not randomly distributed, but was more often resorted to by those who are more privileged than others. We have no way, of course, of either supporting or refuting this contention.

Comparable data for the Philippines come from an unpublished source (Concepcion, 1969), where estimates from a national sample survey of households conducted in 1968 suggested that premarital pregnancies could be as high as 63.2 percent for women in Manila aged thirty or older, and as low as 6.1 percent for the same age cohort in Central Luzon. The variability in these figures is about 10:1, which is possible, but perhaps improbable. Given the large margins of error in national sample surveys due primarily to sample size and field conditions, we are left with no reliable means of assessing the comparative significance of the figures obtained from Cebu.

Nevertheless, a quick scan of the figures on the proportion of premaritally pregnant women in other societies which are much less restrictive than the Philippines in terms of dating and courtship patterns gives us some basis for assessing the significance of the normative deviations observed. For instance, the Lewis-Faning study (1949) reported that about 22 percent of nearly a thousand English women married between 1900 and 1924 were pregnant brides. In Philadelphia, Monahan (1960:133–47) reported that in 1954, 20 percent of Whites and 45.6 percent of Blacks who married were pregnant, giving an overall proportion of about 25 percent. For Australia, using eight months instead of six months as the definition of what constitutes a premarital pregnancy, the proportion of pregnant brides reported in the 1963 General Register Office ranged from 21 to 23 percent in the early sixties. Data from the United States showed that in 1964 the premarital pregnancy rate was a little over 30 percent (Goldstein, 1967:993–1000). Therefore, the proportion of premarital pregnancies that surfaced in the Cebu data are as high as the rates found in other societies in different periods, despite the fact that dating and courtship in Cebu are very restrictive.

Yet we know that norm violations in general, and premarital pregnancies in particular, are difficult to measure, especially in a society such as the Philippines. One can thus realistically expect that the greater the social condemnation, the more extensive the efforts will be to cover up the social infraction by hastening the wedding. To the extent that this is a common solution to premarital conceptions, our cutoff point of six months may not accurately depict the true incidence of premarital pregnancies.

Pushing beyond the data base, we suspect that the true incidence of premarital pregnancy most likely represents an even more prodigious discrepancy in the behavioral conformity of Cebuano women to the ideal norm. Our suspicion is grounded on the simple sociological fact that deviance varies directly with rigid normative prescriptions, even though societies with restrictive norms also have higher proportions manifesting restrictive behavior (cf. also Christensen, 1966:65). The question arises, what underlying microprocesses contribute to the statistics on premarital pregnancies? This question cannot be answered solely on the basis of demographic analysis. In the absence of a more refined study on this topic, we have relied upon a careful scrutiny of our intensive interview data file. In general, we found that precisely because there is a strong double sexual standard and a nearly universal stress on the importance of premarital chastity, pregnancy before marriage becomes a potent weapon that both men and women can use to their advantage, even if it is not manipulated consciously with that original intention. The circumstances that precipitate premarital pregnancies vary, but a certain amount of regularity can be discerned. For instance, it is commonly resorted to by the young, as we saw earlier in this chapter, when there is strong parental opposition to their romantic relationships. Second, for the aggressive but insecure male who faces competition from other suitors—especially from a suitor who has the advantage of being unquestionably favored by the woman's parents—a premarital pregnancy may be the only way of assuring himself that his sweetheart will not be forcibly taken from him. Infraction of the chastity code means that the woman is "spoiled" or "damaged." Hence, it would be difficult for her parents to marry her off to a "better" man than the one who impregnated her. This, along with the young woman's desire to free herself from parental control, maximizes the opportunities for sexual intimacy. The following lower-class respondent is another case in point:

> *L:* I met my husband through a cousin who was vacationing in Manila with my aunt with whom I was staying. Gregorio [husband] was with him [cousin] all the time [whenever the latter came for a visit], so that as time went on we became close to each other also. *But Gregorio was not liked by my auntie, though, for they had another man in mind for me.*
>
> After one year of courtship, *we eloped because of the pressure that my*

aunt would show upon the man [husband] and besides every time Gregorio would visit me, she would spread a mat in the *sala* or intentionally banged kitchen utensils, to make Gregorio go home.

Second, getting premaritally pregnant may be the woman's only means of assuring herself that the man she loves will continue to love her. The initial compromise gestures (such as necking and petting) made in response to the man's persistent requests for physical contact may later (wittingly or unwittingly) become the woman's most powerful weapon in forcing a legitimate marriage—provided that she does not have the reputation for "sleeping around" and that she is assertive enough to fight the odds against her should such acts result in a premarital conception. Among upper-middle- and upper-class men, this is called *gi-korner* (being cornered). The following case illustrates our point very well. It involves the daughter of a poor farmer from Leyte who left home for Cebu at age sixteen in order to improve her life chances. While in Cebu City, she stayed with her older sister, who was attending the university, and supported herself by working as a salesgirl at one of the large department stores.

M: Frankly, when ______ (man who became husband] was [first] introduced to me by that lawyer friend of mine, I was attracted to him, not exactly by his good looks, though he is really handsome, but the way he carried himself and talked. Though I was only a salesgirl [at sixteen], he respected me and was not fresh like some men are.

The next day, he came again almost the closing time of the store. He invited me to dinner which I refused, because I know that it is not proper for a woman to accept an invitation from a man *right away*. I was elated by his asking me to dinner, but instead, I told him in a polite manner, I could not accept the invitation because I promised my sister to come home right after work.

From that day on, I think it was [for] almost a month, he kept on waiting for me after work and inviting me to go out, but I still refused. All the time he would accompany me home. He met my sister and brother-in-law. My sister tried to discourage me about him because she said "he is too good looking" and she was afraid that he would just take advantage of me. I was confused in my feelings, because I came to like him more as the days passed and would look forward to closing time, for us to be together.

Another month passed, and he was still persistent, and my sister kept on discouraging me. Since I knew that I loved him and wanted him, though I was not really thinking of getting married then, I accepted his love, blinded by my emotions.

We started to go out on Sundays, to movies, to picnics, and even to nightclubs, with just the two of us and all the time against the wishes of my sister. As we became closer and closer, I forgot myself one time and gave in to his lovemaking. From then on, we would go to a hotel to give vent to our passion for each other. *I know what will happen to me*, but I love him so that I never come to think of being neglected by him in case of what will happen [pregnancy], besides I trusted him so much.

Then later I knew I was pregnant. I told him one day and he assured me, never to fear for he was really going to marry me and would tell his parents. I was afraid his parents would raise objections because I am poor, and besides, his sister, ______, is the "high hat" kind and I was sure she, too, would object. I tried to hide my condition from my sister, but I started to vomit already and can't take in any food. We had a big fight over it and she sent for our mother [who was in Leyte] who came right away. Though she did not scold me, the way she cried was enough to make me repent what I have done. I assured them that ______ would marry me and that his parents will come on Sunday. But Sunday came and another passed, and all the time also ______ did not come to see me anymore.

One time I did not report for work and went to his office in ______ Hardware. He was surprised to see me and I lost all my pride and in front of everybody started to ask him what were his intentions. He calmed me down and we went to ______ Restaurant, and alone upstairs, he told me what his parents intended to do. That they were coming to see me and would give me any amount I would ask. *I told him right there and then that I can't be bought and if they were really fixed in their decision and he too would let it be, I would do everything that they would be ashamed* [I would do everything to shame them]. ______ told me that he really loved me so, but he had to follow the wishes of his parents. Because I was not able to control myself anymore, *I banged on the table and almost shouted, that if that was his decision, I'd rather kill him.* People from downstairs looked up and because he maybe was ashamed, tried to comfort me by telling me that we were really going to marry with or without his parents' approval.

The next day, he called me up in the store, to meet him after work. When we met, he told me that his parents were coming over with him to my sister's house the next night.

The next night came and my mother and ______'s parents came to an agreement that we were to get married in a very simple ceremony, without any other people but only the immediate relatives.

The next afternoon, his sister, ______, came to the store and was telling me things fit for irrationals. I just kept quiet, because there was nothing I can do at that moment, besides the manager came to my counter. Because I was so ashamed, I resigned from my work right at that moment.

Three weeks later we were married and we rented this house to be away from them. I was happy then.

These events are familiar to those who have lived in Cebu. While it is not our intention to judge either the man or the woman, we do wish to stress that there is widespread belief in the Philippines that men seek to maximize sexual pleasure and minimize permanent entanglements, especially with women from lower socioeconomic classes. Despite the shame and condemnation that a woman can suffer from the unrestrained expression of passions before marriage, premarital pregnancy does vitiate parental disapproval and guarantee family reconciliation in a country where sexual intimacy short of marriage is not acceptable (even though it is practiced), conception before marriage is not permissible (even though it happens), and marriage itself is irreversible (even though separations are possible).

One can hazard a guess that because of the normative expectations which allow men to gain sexual experience, for every woman who succeeded in "cornering" a man into marriage (to use the male chauvinist coinage) after having had sexual intercourse with him, there must be a number of other women—more obedient, less alert, and less assertive—who failed, either because their silence was purchased at a price, or because the man had deviously "covered his trail." Or worse, because they died while attempting an illegal abortion. Not uncommonly, too, the man may already be legally married to another woman, for the *querida* (mistress) system is not unusual in the Philippines (a point we shall broach again in Chapter 8).

Spacing After the First Child

We began this chapter by examining the Cebuano reproductive profile and noted that children are born to Cebuano women in rapid succession. The finding that there is a very small time gap between reported marriage date and the birth of the first child led us to digress into a lengthy discussion of the peculiarities of Cebuano courtship which, in turn, fan our suspicion that a discrepancy exists between the ideal norm of premarital chastity and actual behavior. This suspicion was confirmed by the incidence of premarital pregnancies among the women we interviewed. Now one last question remains: is there any difference in the spacing of children after the first child between women who have had a premarital pregnancy and those who have not? The question can be answered by examining Table 4.14.

Using both the mean and the median measures of averages, we find that the differences in child-spacing after the first child between women who had conceived premaritally and those who had conceived

TABLE 4.14

BIRTH INTERVALS (Months) AFTER THE FIRST CHILD, PREMARITALLY PREGNANT AND NONPREMARITALLY PREGNANT WOMEN

	Total N = 2,255		*Premaritally Pregnant*		*Nonpremaritally Pregnant*	
Between	*Median*	*Mean*	*Median*	*Mean*	*Median*	*Mean*
1st & 2nd	21	25.0	21	25.7	21	24.8
2nd & 3rd	23	26.0	23	25.8	23	26.0
3rd & 4th	24	26.3	23	25.2	24	26.7
4th & 5th	24	27.0	24	26.2	24	27.2
5th & 6th	25	27.8	24	26.4	25	28.3

postmaritally is so slight as to be almost imperceptible. Thus, the family-building processes of premaritally pregnant women bear such a striking resemblance to those of postmaritally pregnant women that one must ask a further question: what underlying cultural currents account for their similarities? Certainly, a most logical follow-up inquiry would concern contraceptive knowledge and use. It is here that the statistical techniques employed extensively by sociologists to manipulate relationships between discrete variables must give way to the ethnographic insights of anthropologists whose penchant for participant observation techniques can better encapsulate the *uniformities* (rather than analyze the *differences*) among people. In the next chapter, we shall combine these two disciplinary approaches in our effort to understand the contributory roles of contraceptive knowledge and use in the family-building processes of the Cebuanos.

5 / Contraceptive Knowledge and Use

The use or nonuse of *modern* contraception, although not the sole determinant of the reproductive patterns and fertility rates in any country, is generally used by family planning researchers to give an approximate idea of the extent to which married couples are consciously regulating the timing, or limiting the number, of births. However, the usefulness of this kind of data is circumscribed as much by the legal accessibility of modern contraception as by other institutional, sociocultural, psychological, and economic forces. Moreover, the use of contraception presupposes knowledge of at least one method, if not an assortment of methods. It further presupposes that married couples have a definite idea of how many children they want, and are motivated to achieve their desired family size by putting their knowledge of contraception into practice. In this chapter, we shall discuss our findings in these areas and pinpoint some of the difficulties in interpreting such data, collected through surveys, in countries where modern contraceptive technology has only recently been imported.

Legal Accessibility of Contraceptives

In the Philippines, the Revised Penal Code and the New Civil Code contain numerous laws bearing on family formation and planning. In the opinion of at least one legal expert (Sison, 1973), they are unmistakably pronatalistic in orientation. The Postal Law and the Customs and Tariff Code had, for a number of years, effectively curtailed the dissemination of family planning material. More specifically, the Postal Law unequivocally stated the forfeiture of the following items if mailed through the postal system:

> 1. Articles, instruments, drugs, and substances designed, intended, or adapted for preventing conception or producing abortion, or for any indecent or immoral use, or which are advertised or described in a manner calculated to lead another to use or apply them for preventing conception or producing abortion, or for any indecent or immoral purposes.

2. Written or printed matter and photographs, engravings, lithographs, and other representations, of an obscene, lewd, lascivious, filthy, indecent, or libelous character, including all such matter which advertises or describes or gives directly or indirectly, information where, how, from whom, or by what means an article, instrument, drug, or substance enumerated in the preceding subsection hereof may be obtained or made, or where or by whom any act or operation of any kind for the procuring or producing of abortion will be done or performed, or how and by what means conception may be prevented or abortion produced.

This was further supported by the Customs and Tariff Code, Republic Act No. 1937 (1957), which prohibits the importation of contraceptives, abortifacients, or any information on contraception and abortion. It was not until 1966 that the sections of these laws pertaining to contraceptives were *implicitly* repealed in an opinion rendered by the secretary of justice when he stipulated that contraceptives could be dispensed only by a licensed drugstore or pharmaceutical company *with* the prescription of a qualified medical practitioner. However, the portions of the law pertaining to abortifacients or abortion information remained in effect (Sison, 1973). In the words of one law professor (Ortega, 1973:677), "Philippine law prohibits abortion absolutely, for whatever reason, however and by whomever committed." But there are gradations of penalty for abortion. For instance, a woman who aborts a fetus to conceal her dishonor may receive only *prision correccional* in its minimum and medium periods, which is imprisonment ranging from six months and one day to four years and two months. However, physicians and midwives receive the maximum penalty for committing intentional abortion.

By 1969, the Pharmacy Law (Republic Act No. 5921) was finally passed to regulate the delivery or sale of contraceptives and abortion agents by prescription from a licensed physician. This means, of course, that unlike the United States and other countries where the dispensation of contraceptives had been legalized earlier, the Philippines has had only a decade's exposure to modern contraception. Under these circumstances, it can be surmised that at the time we conducted our study, most well-educated people had just barely begun to entertain the idea of regulating or limiting births. This is supported by our findings.

Desired Family Size

Attitudes toward desired family size are one of the pieces of information most universally sought on standard fertility surveys. Although a number of demographers with research experience in developing countries have criticized the meaningfulness of asking questions on this topic (for instance, Stycos and Back, 1964; Concepcion and Flieger, 1968; Hauser, 1967), others are convinced of their usefulness (Terhune, 1972:100; Gustavus and Nam, 1970).

It appears that confidence in the predictive value of desired family size rests on various common-sense assumptions which stem from the demographic researchers' own cultural background, supported perhaps by their perceptions of situations in other countries. However, the conceptualization of the variable itself takes for granted several suppositions. First of all, it presupposes that the sample selected for fertility research has reflected on ideal family size. Second, it imputes the salience of the issue in the cognitive structure of the population under study. Third, in interrelating the variable desired family size to another variable, fertility outcome, demographic researchers have assumed that the population studied perceived pregnancies as being in the realm of human activities that can be controlled deliberately and rationally. Fourth, it also presupposes that a majority of the married couples comprehend the biological process of conception, including a working knowledge of the rhythm and functions of the menstrual cycle, and the "scientific" (as opposed to "folk") version of the process by which the spermatozoon fertilizes the egg. Our data from Cebu cast doubt on the applicability of these assumptions.

Table 5.1 shows that the desired family size among the Cebuanos sampled is fairly uniform across social class. The range for both rich and poor, urban and rural respondents is between four and five children. More specifically, prior to the birth of the first child, the desired family size for the urban upper class was close to 5 children whereas the actual child-woman ratio was about 6.4. By contrast, the urban lower-class respondents reported only a slightly smaller desired family size (4.4 children), but actually had a much larger completed family size (7.4 children). The discrepancy between these two figures is most pronounced among the rural lower class.

It is easy to offer widely accepted explanations for these figures and discrepancies by arguing, for instance, that the urban upper class is more efficient in family planning than the poor, but such a hasty conclusion may be misleading. It obscures the unequal sample sizes of the different social classes and overlooks the fact that for many of the middle- and lower-class couples, the question of family planning was never given serious thought prior to marriage, or immediately after its consummation. This, of course, is not surprising given that since 1954, the law had prohibited dissemination of contraceptive information, and that despite the passage of the Pharmacy Law, the Presidential Decree which explicitly counteracts the prohibition against importing and disseminating contraceptives and contraception information was not in-

TABLE 5.1

MEAN NUMBER OF CHILDREN DESIRED
PRIOR TO FIRST CHILD, N = 2,094

Social Class	*Mean Number of Children Desired*	*Completed Family Size*
Urban		
Upper class	4.9	6.4
Middle class	4.1	6.8
Lower class	4.4	7.4
Rural		
Middle class	4.1	7.3
Lower class	4.1	10.2

troduced until 1972. The lack of communication on family planning was aggravated further by the circumstances that not infrequently precipitated the young to enter into a marital relationship and by their ignorance about conception, as illustrated in the following four cases:

> *L:* Before we got married, we never discussed this topic [the number of children desired]. But my parents kept on badgering me about ______ (Hu). So, we eloped. We were not really planning on getting married just then, but the circumstances were such that we had to. . . . No, it was not that I got pregnant. . . . It was just that my parents were very much against the idea of my affair with ______. So when he asked me to go with him, I did . . . we had no plans whatsoever about the future or the number of children.

> *M:* My first pregnancy was neither planned, nor was it avoided. When you get married, you expect to have babies . . . a home is not complete without a baby.

> *L:* We never seriously discussed the number of children before we got married. Sometimes, during his visits, and we have many relatives coming around with several of their children, I would point this out to him. That there was a great possibility we would have many [children] because it was *in the blood* [hereditary]. He would only smile and say: "That's up to God." As to the number of children and what birth control method to use, nothing was further from our mind.

> *L:* Neither my husband nor I knew of any contraceptive method at the time we got married. We never even heard of those things! After we got married, I indicated to my husband that I wanted to have only two children: one boy and one girl. But he simply said: "Let God be our Guide. His will will be done. He will decide for us how many children we will have."

Thus, not only did couples not seriously discuss desired family size, but modern contraceptive devices were unknown to some of our respondents. This suggests that at the time they formed their marital union, there was almost no possibility of limiting or planning the number of children other than by means of abstinence. The next case, involving a lower-lower-class housewife, captures the extent of contraceptive ignorance even after marriage and the seriousness with which both husband and wife had sought to cope with their increasing number of pregnancies by the only method they know—abstinence:

> *L:* I was pregnant every year [after marriage]. But after my third baby, we decided to stop having babies. I am afraid I might be like my own mother and uncle who each had sixteen children. I think it is in our blood to produce so many children. My husband slept in the kitchen and I stayed here with my children, but there are times when we were together. Anyway, that helped. There was an interval of two years between my third and fourth babies. We are trying it again—this time, really in earnest. We have not been together since November of last year [five months before this interview]. He sleeps in the kitchen, while I sleep in here [the only other room in the house] with the children.
>
> I told my sister about this and she asked me if I did not feel uneasy with this kind of relationship. I told her, even if I wanted to, I could not possibly make the initial move [to make love to husband]. He is dead serious. I feel very bad for him. He is not strong anymore, and he works hard, comes home late, tired and hungry. He just goes on to his place in the kitchen and sleeps it off.

For all couples, the alternative of a childless marriage was practically never entertained (barring physiological reasons causing infertility). In the Cebuano culture, children are expected to come with marriage. As one respondent said, "A home is not complete without a baby." Moreover, it is apparent that some respondents perceive rapid successions of pregnancies as something hereditary, "in their blood." Other respondents never even knew (at the time of their marriage) that the number of children a couple has could be controlled mechanically or chemically. Still others were confused as to how babies are conceived. The following statements made by one of our respondents reflects the extent of this ignorance:

> *L:* Children nowadays are really different. . . . Before, when I was young, I never dared to question things like how I came to this world. Now, my oldest daughter and the next two children have asked me already. The oldest was only eleven years old when she asked me. It seems that she learned something about it in her science class, and so with the other children, they became curious about it all, and tried to verify what their teacher said in the classroom by asking me. . . . I was surprised at first, how they learned such things. But after they told me, I was lost. I couldn't explain it fully to them either, because you see, I myself did not have any real knowledge of the mystery of life. I tried to tell them only of what I know also from my biology class in high school. But that was a long time ago.

Another respondent, also from the lower class, described the extent of her sex education when she was a young lady. Her remarks corroborate the lack of proper sex education among Cebuanos:

> *L:* I have no substantial knowledge about things like that [sex] because I never received any formal education about it. My mother did not tell me anything about it either. But I did learn something from friends, stories about how one gets pregnant. They say a woman will get pregnant if she establishes a *relasyon* [gets on steady friendly terms] with a man. There were even stories about a woman getting pregnant because she had taken a bath in a swimming pool where a man had just taken a bath, and something about a woman who got pregnant because she used a toilet used by a man. . . . With my children, I just have to depend upon what they learn in school, because I am afraid I might give the wrong ideas to them. Especially that children nowadays are so smart. You need to explain things to them fully before they would leave you.

This general ignorance about sexuality and fertilization is common among the lower class, but it is not restricted to them, as evidenced by some middle-class cases presented in Chapter 4.

Evidently, the educational attainment of some of these respondents did not always help them in understanding the human fertilization process. The "respectable" normative courtship pattern, which stresses chaperonage and favors group dating over single-pair dating, deprives prospective couples of opportunities to explore privately very intimate issues in advance, much less to discuss desired family size. In this sociocultural context the possibility of contraception could not be more peripheral to their cognitive stucture unless, of course, a man seeks to maximize sexual pleasure while avoiding, at all costs, any permanent entanglements (in which case the thought of contraception would be central to him). This renders the predictive value of desired family size somewhat dubious.

Knowledge and Use of Modern Contraception

Turning our attention now to the Cebuanos' knowledge and use of modern contraception, we find that the rhythm method was by far the most widely practiced. Among the urban respondents, appreciable class differences are evident as one moves from the upper class, where 55.5 percent knew how to use it and had used it, to the middle class, where the corresponding figure is 29.7 percent, and down to the lower class, where an even lower percentage (13.7 percent) is found. The fact that the rich have access to modern technology is evident in their wider use of the Pill (see Table 5.2). At least one out of five upper-class women

TABLE 5.2

KNOWLEDGE AND USE OF CONTRACEPTIVE METHODS, URBAN SAMPLE

Contraceptive Method	*Upper (N = 101)*			*Middle (N = 720)*			*Lower (N = 700)*		
	Heard about it only	*Knows how to use it but never used it*	*Knows how to use it and has used it*	*Heard about it only*	*Knows how to use it but never used it*	*Knows how to use it and has used it*	*Heard about it only*	*Knows how to use it but never used it*	*Knows how to use it and has used it*
Rhythm	12.9%	29.7%	55.5%	35.0%	20.6%	29.7%	43.1%	15.7%	13.7%
Withdrawal	26.7	31.7	10.9	34.2	21.1	16.8	29.0	11.1	12.6
Ligation	77.2	10.9	3.0	67.9	3.9	3.2	51.4	1.5	0.9
Vasectomy	35.6	6.9	0.0	30.4	1.9	0.0	23.3	0.5	0.0
Condom	34.7	34.7	9.9	54.6	19.2	4.0	51.3	11.4	0.7
Diaphragm	50.4	16.8	5.0	28.8	6.4	0.3	15.3	0.9	0.1
Pill	41.6	34.7	21.8	62.4	19.7	10.6	72.7	10.1	4.3
IUD	43.6	11.9	3.0	36.1	5.7	2.5	22.9	1.3	1.1
Abstinence	—	—	14.9	—	—	10.6	—	—	8.3

claimed to have used the Pill, and the percentage halves as one moves down the socioeconomic ladder (10.6 percent for the middle class and 4.3 percent for the lower class).

Likewise, for the rural sample, proportionally more respondents had used the rhythm method than had taken the Pill. However, while the percentage of rural middle-class respondents who had used the rhythm method did not differ significantly from that of the urban middle class, use of the Pill is considerably lower among the rural population in general (see Table 5.3). No doubt the dissemination of contraceptive information has not been uniform in different sectors of the country.

Instead of the Pill, proportionally more rural (22.4 percent) than urban middle-class women (16.8 percent) apparently relied upon *coitus interruptus*, a cost-free but unreliable method. In contrast, only 10.9 percent of the upper class had used withdrawal. Curiously enough, proportionally more upper-class women claimed to have used abstinence (14.9 percent) than the other classes of urban and rural women. Figures for the use of other contraceptive methods, including the condom, reveal some consistency: they tend to be small. However, a substantial proportion of upper- and middle-class respondents from both rural and urban backgrounds had generally heard of these other methods although they had not used them.[1]

Quite impressive is the high percentage of lower-class respondents

TABLE 5.3

KNOWLEDGE AND USE OF CONTRACEPTIVE METHODS, RURAL SAMPLE

Contraceptive Method	*Middle (N = 179)*			*Lower (N = 415)*		
	Heard about it only	*Knows how to use it but never used it*	*Knows how to use it and has used it*	*Heard about it only*	*Knows how to use it but never used it*	*Knows how to use it and has used it*
Rhythm	43.0%	12.9%	25.1%	40.2%	11.8%	8.7%
Withdrawal	25.1	18.4	22.4	24.1	8.2	12.8
Ligation	59.2	1.7	2.8	44.3	0.2	0.2
Vasectomy	33.0	1.1	0.0	20.7	0.2	0.0
Condom	51.4	15.6	2.8	37.8	7.5	0.5
Diaphragm	10.1	4.0	0.0	3.6	1.5	0.0
Pill	71.5	8.9	3.9	61.0	5.1	1.7
IUD	26.8	1.7	1.1	17.4	1.7	0.2
Abstinence	—	—	8.9	—	—	9.4

in both the urban and rural areas who claimed to have heard of the Pill. Considering that the ban on contraception was implicitly lifted only two years before the Cebu study was started, this suggests the swiftness with which news of the Pill has filtered down to the bottom social stratum. Yet, if information on one new technology had diffused so quickly, why was the IUD, another new technology, less well known?

Our examination of the respondents' sources of information on contraceptive use reveals that among the urban lower class, only 8.9 percent of the respondents gave physicians, nurses, and trained midwives as the sources of their information. This is to be expected, since at the time our study was conducted, medical schools in the city (there were none outside the city) did not dispense such information routinely, although one university-affiliated medical unit stationed in a slum area was already dispensing the Pill and the IUD (as revealed in our intensive interviews with some of the women). In the rural areas, the scarcity of trained health personnel makes it virtually impossible for a majority of the people to have heard of the Pill through these sources. Furthermore, since the lower class as a whole are much too preoccupied in their struggle for subsistence, it is unlikely that magazines and newspapers would be their primary sources of information: these reading materials cost money, whether they are old or newly published. Indeed, Table 5.4 shows that only 1 percent of the lower class reported

TABLE 5.4

SOURCES OF INFORMATION ON CONTRACEPTIVE USE, URBAN SAMPLE, N = 1,521

		Source of Information				
Method	*Social Class*	*Relatives*	*Friends*	*Mananabangs*	*Physicians, Nurses, and Trained Midwives*	*Magazines and Newspapers*
Rhythm	lower	4.6%	58.0%	0.4%	5.9%	2.0%
	middle	8.9	51.5	0.6	14.6	6.0
	upper	5.9	46.5	0.0	26.7	11.8
Withdrawal	lower	7.6	42.0	0.1	0.7	0.3
	middle	12.1	50.1	0.3	3.2	3.1
	upper	7.9	39.6	0.0	3.0	10.9
Ligation	lower	3.4	44.1	0.1	5.4	0.1
	middle	6.9	52.8	0.4	11.3	1.5
	upper	6.9	58.4	0.0	11.9	9.9
Vasectomy	lower	1.6	20.1	0.1	2.0	0.1
	middle	1.5	23.3	0.4	3.8	2.2
	upper	1.0	28.7	0.0	2.0	9.9
Condom	lower	6.1	54.7	0.6	0.4	0.4
	middle	12.1	58.8	0.1	1.9	2.1
	upper	6.9	48.5	3.0	9.9	6.9
Diaphragm	lower	0.7	13.1	0.4	1.3	0.1
	middle	3.5	22.5	0.4	7.2	1.8
	upper	5.9	42.6	1.0	11.9	10.9
Pill	lower	4.4	69.7	1.4	8.9	1.0
	middle	5.8	65.6	0.7	14.2	4.9
	upper	4.0	48.5	1.0	28.7	9.9
IUD	lower	1.9	17.6	0.1	5.1	0.3
	middle	4.4	24.9	1.1	10.2	3.2
	upper	3.0	26.7	0.0	12.9	11.9

magazines and newspapers as their source of information on the use of the Pill. The majority claimed that they received their information through friends and neighbors. Thus, the possibility exists that a two-step communication flow was operating whereby physicians and other trained health personnel passed the information to some key members of the lower-class community, who in turn diffused that information to a wider audience. This was the hypothesis entertained by Duff and Liu (1975). However, we now suspect that our own interviewers might also have acted as traveling gazettes of family planning information as they conducted their interviews.[2]

What is striking in Tables 5.2 and 5.3 is the very small percentage of lower-class respondents who, though they had the knowledge, ever used withdrawal or the condom. The majority of respondents had only heard of these methods. Friends and neighbors were by far the single most important source of their information.

Reasons for Never Using Contraceptives

One recurring question often raised in KAP studies is: if one has knowledge of contraceptives, why does one not apply that knowledge by using any one of the methods known? Undoubtedly, there are many complex reasons for not using any contraceptive method. In order to gain a general picture of the reasons for being a "never user," we sorted out those women who may be considered normally fecund and who possessed knowledge of contraception, but who reported never having used any method at all. Their answers, coded by primary reason, are grouped into seven categories, as shown in Table 5.5. We found that "wanting to have more children" was by far the most frequently given answer, followed by religious reasons. Aside from the positive sanctions provided by the Catholic church's official stand on "artificial" birth control as "unnatural," the negative sanction inherent in the Filipino folk belief called *gaba* in Cebuano is a very real fear. *Gaba*, or divine retribution, befalls any person who dares to go against nature's will. No doubt this concept has its origins in animistic beliefs reaching far into the pre-Hispanic days, and is reinforced by the masses' syncretic interpretation of Catholicism.

The next important reason was the fear of side effects, which is followed by fear of losing one's husband if one should decide to prevent conception. Note, however, that not one of the upper-class women expressed this fear of losing her husband, whereas for about 13 percent of the lower-class and middle-class women, both rural and urban, this fear is quite real. In the words of one lower-class respondent: "It's not

TABLE 5.5

REASONS FOR NEVER USING CONTRACEPTIVES, N = 2,094

	Want More Children	*Religious Reasons*	*Economic Reasons*	*Fear of Losing Husband*	*Fear of Side Effects*	*Misc. Reasons*	*Don't Know*
Urban							
Upper	56.5%	17.4%	0%	0%	8.7%	8.7%	0%
Middle	36.7	16.4	0	12.4	20.9	7.9	4.5
Lower	18.3	17.7	5.3	13.4	26.3	8.9	8.4
Rural							
Middle	28.4	22.7	2.3	12.5	14.8	9.1	3.4
Lower	16.8	28.2	3.4	12.7	14.4	6.8	15.1

easy to use contraception, you know. It's the husband who decides. I am afraid that I might drive him to another woman. . . . I don't want this to be the cause of his philandering."

No doubt the Catholic precept that marriage is for procreation is widely accepted in the Philippines, even though the population may consider that not part of being "Catholic" but simply a requisite of married life. As one woman said: "*Tinuyo nimo ang pagminyo, unya hinuon!*" (You intended the marriage [in order to have children], and then [you avoid conceptions. What sense does that make?]). For this reason, not only are children desired, but they are desired in large numbers.

Fear of side effects is unmistakably an important concern to a number of the middle- and lower-class respondents. Since friends rather than physicians, nurses, or midwives constituted the main source of contraceptive information in Cebu, it can be surmised that information on side effects is probably obtained from similar sources, especially in the case of the middle and lower classes. For the Pill, the most commonly feared side effects are getting sick, becoming weak, frigidity, growing pale, cancer, headaches, and insanity (presumably from the headaches). For the withdrawal method, the fear that the man will become "nervous" was often expressed, and to some respondents this has the same meaning as a "nervous breakdown." Others believe that withdrawal can cause pain in the man's loins. Women are also believed to become pale and sickly from using this method. Similar reasons are also reported for the use of abstinence. For the IUD, fear of cancer is common, because "it rubs against the uterus," although the folk concept of what constitutes cancer is extremely broad. For the rhythm method, and among those who correctly understood the reproductive cycle, menstrual pollution was a common concern. According to their folk belief, if the husband's sexual organ touches so much as a speck of the woman's menstrual blood, the contact will cause him to become physically weak and to fall ill with some disease (such as tuberculosis). One must, therefore, abstain from sex for some time after the menstrual period is over. If abstention in turn "causes" nervousness or nervous breakdown, this makes rhythm unworkable.

It is a mistake to presume that women who choose not to use contraception are being irrational. A number of these couples had discussed the various methods they knew of, and often when the choice narrowed down to any one method, they decided against it because, as they saw it, the costs of side effects from any one of these contraceptive measures did not offset the advantages they could reap from using them. As one man put it, "It will be even more difficult to care for the sickly [mother] than it will be to have more children." To take care of a sick mother not only entails the cost of medicine to cure the illness, the doctor's fee, and the hospital expenses (if the illness gets worse), but also means that the children will not be attended to and the daily routine of household chores will not be performed.

Added to this is the fact that the "cost" of children is a relative concept. For the lower-class woman an additional child is a financial "burden" only because it means that she would have to spend for a few more baby clothes and rags, a small tin can of milk a week, and as the child grows older an additional cup of corn grits daily. Childbirth in the lower-class neighborhood, if attended by untrained and unlicensed midwives, need not cost much, for the folk practitioners are willing to accept delayed payments and sometimes even token payments of 50 centavos. If the patient can afford it, delivery normally costs only 10 pesos, and this was the price of an IUD that some women in the lower-class neighborhood tried to peddle for profit (obviously an illegal practice). The Pill costs 2.75 to 2.85 pesos for one month's supply. For lower-class families whose monthly income, if there was any steady flow at all, was sometimes only 1 peso a day, that is an extremely expensive method of birth control. Besides, the poorer the family, the less the expenditure required to raise children, for the poor do not measure themselves by the standard of child care and educational services to which the better-off families aspire. They stick to what they can afford. Furthermore, one should not forget that children are intrinsically valued, and by the time they are seven or eight years old, they can become an economic asset. They can scavenge the dumps, collect and sell old newspapers, pop bottles, and tin cans, shine shoes, or beg on busy streets. They can also keep their mother company at home and run errands. Thus, when one adds up both sides of the equation—the cost and gain of delivering a baby versus the advantages and disadvantages of preventing a conception—a precarious balance exists which is sufficient to keep many of the informed couples in a state of indecision about adopting any contraceptive measures.

Contraceptive Failures

Knowledge of contraceptive methods in and of itself did not necessarily infuse couples with the foresight to use contraceptives *decisively*. More often than not, a joint decision to practice contraception was reached only after the maximum number of children they felt could be supported had been born. At that point, the execution of their plan to curb further conception was complicated by the search for an acceptable method and the painstaking task of making it work. Our data show that for the urban samples rhythm was the method first used by all social classes. It was also the very last method tried. For the upper class, the Pill represented a variant contraceptive method, but for the other classes the alternative to rhythm generally was withdrawal. Data from the rural samples showed a pattern similar to that of the urban middle and lower classes. Hence, it is evident that the small proportion of Cebuano women who have ever used any contraception have used high-risk methods. In view of this, one can reasonably expect that contraceptive failures must be common.

We asked our respondents whether they had experienced contraceptive failure while using some kind of contraceptive device. Not at all surprising to us is the fact that in all social classes, for both the rural and the urban samples, the failure rate ranged from two out of five to *one out of every two* women. More specifically, 43 percent of the urban upper-class respondents reported that they became pregnant while using a contraceptive method, compared to 49 percent of the middle class respondents. Similarly, the lower class, both rural and urban, experienced a failure rate of about 40 percent. Altogether, the rural middle class respondents had the highest percentage of failure (52 percent).

Even in those very rare cases where the married couples had agreed right after marriage or at their first birth to limit the number of children, the strong motivation did not produce the desired results. Take the following case, for instance:

> *M:* ______ [husband] initiated the step to limit the [number of] children after my difficult first childbirth [where R started labor on a Wednesday and did not deliver until Friday], and for economic reasons. We depend on both our salaries . . . no specific income from other sources [besides a U.S. Veterans Administration pension]. . . . My type of work [public school teacher] discourages frequent maternity leaves.

Subsequent interviews with this woman showed that they tried abstinence after her first child was born, but failed to carry it through long enough to make it work. As a result she was pregnant in less than two years. She and her husband then changed to the rhythm method, but she became pregnant a third time owing to "mistakes in calculations," as she put it. Although they were acquainted with two other contraceptives, the condom and a jelly, they had never used them for aesthetic reasons. After the birth of their third child, they tried using the rhythm method again, but in another two years, another pregnancy occurred. The couple had four children when we interviewed them and were still using the rhythm method, hoping that it would prevent a fifth pregnancy. The woman was only forty-one years old, and her reproductive years were certainly not over. One wonders whether the ardent proponents of the rhythm method realize that for each failure, a child is the outcome.

How many couples overshot their mark by three or more children while using a contraceptive method? This we will never know for sure, since it had not occurred to us then to ask the question in the survey phase. But one can only imagine that if the majority of the people rely heavily upon the rhythm method, as was the case in Cebu at the turn of the last decade, the "mistakes in calculation" must have been numerically enormous.

Furthermore, the incongruity of the rhythm method with the folk system of beliefs concerning menstrual pollution deserves to be emphasized. The following interview is illustrative:

> *Q:* I understand you are trying to limit your number of children. What [contraceptive method] did you use?
>
> *H* (very shy and hardly audible): Just refrain from using the wife [abstention].
>
> *Q:* I thought you were using the rhythm method.
>
> *H:* Yes, [but] it is not good for the man.
>
> *Q:* Why?
>
> *H* (blushes and answers in an almost inaudible voice): It makes the husband weak . . . you [have to] wait before the wife's blood [menstruation] comes out. . . . We did it a few times and the blood is already there by accident . . . and it is not good if the man's . . . the woman's blood—that will make him less active [impotent and physically weak]. [Probe.] I think that made me sick. My urine was unclear, I even consulted a doctor and he thought I visited prostitutes. But no, that's the truth [I did not see any prostitute]. He [the doctor] gave me a pill and told me to boil *banaba* and corn silk and drink the broth from these substances. From that time on, I stopped rhythm.

In other words, in addition to the general lack of knowledge about human anatomy and biological reproduction, there also exists a cultural taboo against having sex just prior to the onset of a menstrual cycle or immediately following, for fear that contact with the woman's menstrual flow would render the husband impotent or generally physically weak. Such beliefs are said to be deeply rooted and pervasive.

There is further competition between the use of "modern" contraceptives and the folk methods that abound in the Cebuano culture. Since some lower-class respondents do not see any difference in effectiveness between these two classes of birth control measures, they rely upon the folk methods without realizing that the risks of another pregnancy are very high. Two lower-class women describe their contraceptive histories as follows:

> *L:* I hope that I won't have any more children. . . . I had my womb inverted by a *hilot* [a folk healer]. My sister-in-law accompanied me to this *hilot*. I felt we had too many children already. When we were newly married, I sort of talk about two children as the ideal . . . one boy and one girl. But this was just wishful thinking. We did nothing [positive] about it. We hadn't heard then about birth control. After our third child, some neighbors talked to me about the rhythm method. I thought this was fine. But it was impossible with my husband. He thinks it is unnatural. *Ay sus!* He is the [sexually] aggressive type. He likes to have sexual intercourse more often. I'm beginning to believe those stories about skinny men being more sexually aggressive than the other kind. My husband would sulk in the mornings and refuse to eat if the night before I refuse his advances. What could I do? Under those circumstances, I had to get pregnant again. I did! It was then that I decided to see the *hilot*. It's a good thing that my husband did not object. Most probably because it does not affect his sexual habits anyway.

> *L:* Withdrawal worked for some time, but it does not serve the purpose. I became pregnant. It was my husband's decision to use withdrawal. I did not know until later [in our marriage], I noticed what he was doing and I asked him and he said it was to prevent me from getting pregnant. We used this *after the fourth child*. We knew no other [methods] except this and *hilot* [folk curative massage], but did not use the *hilot* until later. This was because I did not know where the *hilot* lives and was ashamed to ask because of what I heard, that only those *desgracia* [euphemism for women who are pregnant out of wedlock] resort to them. The *hilot* does not always work. A neighbor across the street *magpaga-am* [has herself ministered] by a *mananabang* [folk midwife] every time she is not menstruating but got pregnant anyway. I don't really believe that I stopped having children because of the *hilot* but *because our family does not have many children* [emphasis added]. My brothers have only four [children] each. I cannot understand why the poor have so many children while the rich have few, like two, or three only. People living along the sea have so many children. In Simala [hometown, about 57 kilometers south of Cebu City] most couples have more than ten. *Mag-itom lang ang agi* [they form a dark streak of shadows on the street]. They say that these people have so many children because of their diet of fish roe which makes people fertile. *Sus! Ang babaye dili matandogan* [Jesus! The women cannot be touched (sexually without resulting in pregnancy)].

These remarks further support our observation that some lower-class Cebuanos view pregnancy as a trait that may be carried along family lines. Or, if it is not "in their blood," it is in their diet. Such an attitude obscures the need for birth control, since pregnancies so understood fall outside the realm of human activities that can be controlled. Even diet per se is difficult for poor families to control. Since they live along the sea, fish is the least expensive and most available food.

The failure rates for contraceptive use merit additional comment. Since the most common contraceptive methods for Cebuanos are rhythm and withdrawal, improper use of such methods should constitute the most frequent reason for failure. This is borne out by the data shown in Table 5.6. About 60 percent across all social strata (plus or minus 5 percent) reported that the reason for failure was the improper application of the method.

For the rhythm method to succeed, the woman, if not the couple, must have a rough idea of the length of her menstrual cycle, and a clear idea of the rationale behind the method. For many lower-class and some middle-class respondents, however, there was widespread confusion on how to count the days:

> *Q:* In what way is the rhythm method harmful?
> *H:* Just like I told you—you count the days, and it so happened that I went to my wife on the first day of her menstruation and my penis touched this dirty blood, so I got sick. Pale and weak.
> *Q:* How do you count the days?
> *H:* From the bathday.[3] You count fifteen days, only then you can sleep with your wife.

In at least one instance, one of our perceptive interviewers found out after repeated visits and explanations of the rhythm method to a lower-class respondent that the woman had avoided sexual contacts with her husband on all days of the month except one day—her ovulation day. In other words, she had "reversed" the procedure. (An unwanted pregnancy ensued.) After much discussion with the couple, the interviewer soon learned that since they had previously known only of abstinence, and the logic behind it was interpreted as "avoidance prevents pregnancy," they figured it did not make sense for them to have sex for so many days of the month without her getting pregnant. How could having sex for just one day be so detrimental as to result in a pregnancy, and so quickly at that? If one takes the perspective of a lower-class woman whose only knowledge of birth control prior to the rhythm method was abstention, and whose cultural experience had precluded general knowledge about female anatomy and biological reproduction, such questions are very intelligent. After all, is not the linkage between

TABLE 5.6

REASONS FOR STOPPING CONTRACEPTIVE USE, N = 2,094

Social Class	*Child-Spacing*	*Health*	*Side Effects*	*Religious Reasons*	*Husband Not Cooperating*	*Other*
Urban						
Upper	55.2%	0.0%	3.4%	6.9%	3.4%	13.8%
Middle	51.5	2.0	15.8	3.0	4.0	15.8
Lower	38.7	2.1	15.5	0.7	13.4	23.9
Rural						
Middle	43.5	0.0	21.7	0.0	17.4	8.7
Lower	38.3	0.0	8.5	0.0	23.4	25.5

frequency of sexual intercourse and pregnancy the logic behind the use of abstinence?

Even in the case of the Pill, where the rule should be "easier" to apply because one need only remember to take it daily for a certain number of days, some women had difficulty understanding *when* to take it or why it should be taken regularly for a stretch of days every month—especially after being told that one can get pregnant only on ovulating days. To quote one respondent: "She [referring to her BrWi] gave me four [of her] Pills to be taken after each bathday [of the month]. It did not work. I wonder why?" Apparently the relative had magnanimously shared her resources by dividing a month's supply of the Pill with four married women, one of whom was our respondent! After finishing up the shortened supply of pills, they each found that they were bleeding. That confirmed their belief that the Pill caused cancer. Other women reportedly took the Pill for only a few days and then stopped, believing that "that should be enough to do it."

One may ask why such problems exist when the medical practitioners who work with lower-class Cebuanos must surely know how to speak the dialect. In a comment to one of Concepcion's papers (1970: 224), Flavier provided some indirect answers by calling our attention to the fact that there are no equivalent words available to translate much of the English terminology and nomenclature on family planning and fertilization processes. Although his own observations and experience are drawn from Tagalog-speaking areas, the situation in Cebu is no different, for insofar as biological concepts are concerned, both Tagalog and Cebuano have borrowed the same "hispanized" vocabulary. In his own words, Flavier asked:

> Do you know for example that there is no translation for IUD. . . . Field workers refer to the IUD as *plastik* or occasionally *alambre* . . . the connotation

> of *alambre* or wire, is one of rigidity or pain. Yet when dropouts occur we wonder why. Do you know that there is no local word for hormones? How can you explain fully and adequately the hormone basis for the suppression of ovulation as the mechanism of action of birth-control pills? Someone said hormone is *harmonika* in Tagalog (which means "harmonica," the musical organ!). Why, we are not even attuned to our own needs! Do you know also that we have no word in Pilipino for ovulation—that is, a word understandable and in common use. We should not be surprised when the women who stop taking the pill do not realize that the ovulatory suppression has been lifted. An intelligent nurse once lectured to the rural women and in defining the reproduction physiology, she spoke as follows:
>
> *Alam ninyo, ang bawat babaye ay may dalawang obario. Buwan-buwan ay linalabasan ito ng itlog. Ito ang tinatawag na obulasyon. Ang itlog ngayon ay dadaan sa palopiya at pag nakita ang sperma ay ang tawag ay pertilisasyon!*[4]
>
> She said *sperma* as a translation for "sperm," forgetting that to the listeners it meant "candle," and not the male seed.

Indeed, in both the Tagalog and Cebuano languages, words such as *obario, obulasyon, sperma,* and *pertilisasyon* are either borrowed or had to be invented to translate the reproductive concepts of ovary, ovulation, sperm, and fertilization, respectively. But they either have no meaning to the masses, who possess very little "scientific" knowledge about human reproduction, or they have different denotations and connotations in the indigenous language. *Sperma* is candle and *alambre* is wire, regardless of what they may mean to the scientifically trained health practitioner. Failure to apply a contraceptive method properly naturally runs high in such cases. By contrast, the folk contraceptive methods seem to make sense to some respondents even though they are of questionable effectiveness.

A second reason commonly given for failure in carrying out a contraceptive regimen is the husband's refusal to cooperate. The large proportions of middle- and lower-class respondents, both rural and urban, reporting that their husbands were not cooperative comports with our finding reported earlier which showed that the rhythm method and *coitus interruptus* were the major and variant contraceptive methods used in these social classes. Both procedures, after all, require considerable cooperation from the husband, whereas the upper-class wives, who have more access to trained health care practitioners and who can afford the Pill, are not restricted in their contraceptive efforts by their husbands. Their husbands might also be more receptive to the use of contraception, but this is pure speculation. We need more research to find out whether there are class differences in men's attitudes toward contraception.

Progression of Contraceptive Methods

Survey questions, by their very nature, can yield only a static picture of contraceptive knowledge and use. They do not enable us to gain insight into the individual couple's anxious search for a suitable method. However, intensive interviews, by design, are much more effective in getting at the dynamic progressions in the use of contraceptive methods.

From our intensive interviews, we found that such progressions of methods, from low-risk to high-risk or vice versa, are common among those who have attempted to limit births. The reasons behind a couple's switch from one method to another are often complex. In the following example, although the decision to use contraception was made early enough—immediately after the first pregnancy—successive contraceptive failures yielded three more children. The lengthy remarks made by the wife illustrate the kind of problems a lower-class Cebuano family faces in trying to limit their family size:

> *L:* After the arrival of our first baby, I began to realize for the first time how tight our financial condition was. I was afraid of having more children, because the salary of my husband was barely enough for our subsistence. And he was the only person working between the two of us, and his salary was very low. So we abstained from sex. But it did not work out. My husband did not want to be controlled. I was pregnant again.

After the second pregnancy, the respondent was even more determined not to have any more children. She learned from her neighbors about withdrawal. She told her husband about it, and they tried it. But as she said:

> We tried withdrawal, but it did not last long. My husband did not enjoy the act. He was frustrated and nervous every time he went to bed with me. So I got pregnant the third time. [Probe.] My husband consoled me by saying that God is merciful. He will provide; we will manage somehow.
>
> During this pregnancy, I heard that there was a Mother's Class being conducted in Pasil [where R used to live], so I inquired and decided to attend the class, *faithfully*. There, I learned about the rhythm method. I came home and told my husband about it, and after the third child was born, we tried it. But somehow we calculated it wrong. And not long afterwards, I was pregnant again.
>
> I was on my fourth pregnancy when a group of medical interns from Southwestern [University, College of Medicine] conducted a campaign on family planning and the IUD. I told my husband about it. But he said: "*What if you get sick from the IUD? Who will pay the medical expenses? Where would we get the money to see the doctor?*" But I insisted on trying it, so my husband finally agreed, on one condition. He said: "I don't want to have any complaint from you, be it physical or otherwise." I decided I would suffer the consequences and use the IUD. [Probe.] Four months after our [fourth]

child was born, I went to see Dra. Alfonso for IUD. The *doctora* charged me a minimal fee, and allowed me to pay her on an installment basis. That was the only way I could afford to use the IUD. I haven't been pregnant for two years now. I feel very good. I have gained weight and acquired confidence. I can sleep soundly now without the fear of getting pregnant.

[Probe.] My husband's relatives are opposed to my using IUD. *They are afraid that it might be harmful for me, so that it would turn out to be even more expensive [than getting pregnant] as I would have to be brought to a doctor again* [emphasis added]. But we stuck to our decision despite their objections. [Probe.] My own mother has no objection to my using IUD. She believed that it has done me some good, because I have gained a little weight, and look very healthy and contented. My mother also thinks that I should not have any more children because of our financial situation.

[Probe.] Yes [R heard about the Pill], but only after I started using IUD. But even if I had known then, I still would not be able to use it *because it is too expensive for me* [emphasis added].

Again, we observe that the fear of side effects is often a very common reason for couples who have decided upon contraception to rescind their plan. This is even more likely to happen if it is complicated further by financial difficulties, as evinced in the following family. Both the husband and wife happened to be interviewed together:

Q: Did you plan your family before marriage?

W: No, we didn't know about that before.

Q: Have you thought of limiting your children after you got married?

H: Yes, *after the fourth child* [emphasis added]. I thought of abstaining from my wife, because it is hard to have so many children.

Q: Did you discuss your plan with your wife?

H (looks at wife): No, because I was afraid she will not understand and she will be jealous again. I just kept it to myself. Because she will suspect me again. [The husband did have a history of philandering.]

Q: What happened to your plans?

H: Gave it up. It would not work. My wife will get jealous if I don't touch her.

Q (to wife): Have you thought of stopping childbearing?

W: Yes. After I got sick [VD] and had a miscarriage because of what I got from him [Hu]. I was afraid my children would be lame or without ears or cross-eyed.

Q: Did you tell your husband about this?

W: Yes, we agreed to use the IUD, but then we were afraid we would get cancer. We used the condom instead. I was the one who had to buy it from the *botica* [drugstore] because he was ashamed to buy it himself. It costs 25 centavos each.

Q (to husband): How many times did you use the condom?

H: Many times.

Q (to both): Why did you stop using it?

W: *Ay! Kalas!* [Gosh, it's expensive!] Imagine, we have to spend 25 centavos every day?

Q (to husband): Do you have any other reason why you stopped using the condom?

H: Well, because there is less pleasure with it also.

Q: From whom or where did you know about these methods of birth control?

H: From my friends. We talked about that and they know it because they use it.

Q: Did your employer ever talk to you about birth control devices? Or teach you to control?

H: Yes, when I have to ask for an advanced salary—at the time when we got sick [from VD].

Q: What did he say?

H: I think he was just joking. . . . He said: "So that you won't have to spend for more babies, why don't you use your neighbor's wife or pay a few pesos for a prostitute?"

Q: What did you tell him?

H: I was ashamed to continue the conversation. I just laughed. He was only joking.

Q: Did you ever use withdrawal?

H (after a pause): Ah, yes. I know about that. No, I did not use it. It is not good.

W: *That will cause nervous breakdown* [emphasis added]. Like our neighbor —he is a distant relative of ours—he got sick—*trembling of hands and body because of that.* Now that they stop practicing it, they have many children.

Q: How did you know?

W: *Ay!* The wife told me about it. [Switching focus.] Tita [a neighbor] told me that she told her husband to go to a prostitute *nalang* [tag word suggesting decision based on lesser of two evils] because the doctor said she could not have another child anymore. She knows that her husband goes to other women, but it's better that way, because if she gets pregnant, that will be the end of her.

Q (to husband): What other method do you know?

H: I heard this from my friends—you put one-half of a Cortal tablet [brand name of a locally manufactured aspirin] into the vagina before intercourse to kill the *kuan* [those things, whatever is inside the vagina].

Q: Why didn't you use the jelly which your friend gave you?

H: I was afraid to use it. I have not tried it before.

On another interview occasion, the wife revealed her fear of the IUD and the extent of her folk contraceptive knowledge:

Q: Why do you think you would get cancer from IUD?

W: I heard that from our neighbors. A friend of mine died of cancer of the uterus because she used the IUD.

Q: What other methods of birth control did you know?

W: The *habak* which I told you last time and the "gold coin" [condom]. There is also another kind of *habak*, called *habak sa lana*. The roots of the *panaktak* tree are soaked in coconut oil and the oil is rubbed over the stomach of the pregnant woman.

Q: How did you know this?

W: From the *mananambal* [folk healer].

Q: What else do you know?

W: ______ [Hu's] cousin told us about the Cortal. It is powdered and placed into the vagina before intercourse. This is different from the Pill. Sister Louisa also told us about ergot. We can buy that from the drugstore.

Q: Do you know about rhythm?

W: Yes. A cousin of mine from ______ taught me. She is a teacher. But I did not practice it.

Q: What other methods do you know?

W: No more. Ah, yes, withdrawal. We used it.

Likewise, fear of the IUD and a parallel progression in the utilization of contraceptive devices is evident in the following example:

M: There was no such thing as birth control methods then, or maybe there was, but we never heard of anything about those then. We just thought it would be nice to have two boys and two girls. But after our second child, we were already practicing withdrawal. Johnny [Hu] had a better-paying job then. We were not really decided on having just two, but we used withdrawal to space the children. Now, this withdrawal thing, which Johnny learned from a friend of his, was bothering him. He never seemed to get full satisfaction from the intercourse, so we stopped using it. And that's why we had this third child. We went to a doctor at St. Vincent Clinic who advised us to use the IUD. *The wires scared me.* I thought it too dangerous. There was the alternative—the Pill. The one I was asked to take was Lyndiol. I took the tablets for six months, each bottle costs 5.80 pesos, but we did not mind. It was the side effects that made us break the habit [of taking the Lyndiol]. *I got so heated up from the inside; my stomach got hot and it seemed that this heat emanated from the vagina* [emphasis added]. My head got so hot. I was temperamental and when Johnny complained, we said this was too much. Every time we made love, the heat from my vagina would irritate his penis. At first I thought he was joking, but when we examined his penis after an intercourse, we found out that it really got irritated—like it was bruised. So we had to use some cream to cure it. You can imagine all the trouble and all the pain [we had]. The doctor next prescribed a cheaper pill, Anovlar. Unless anything happens, we intend to continue using this.

Even though side effects from the Pill were not publicized in the late sixties, quite a few Cebuano women who used it reported that they had suffered side effects. In the light of more recent research, there may have been a basis for our respondents' complaints.

L: I learned about the Pill from a friend, a nightclub hostess who was married. We became friends in 1962–1963 when I used to sell ladies' handbags and she was my *suki* [regular customer]. When we became friends, we used to chat . . . about what to do in order not to have any more children. She was already using the Pill and she gave me a pack. After I finished it I went with her to the doctor who prescribed it for her and the doctor told me to continue taking the C-Quens since it seems to agree with me. After five or six months I developed an allergy to the Pill . . . thick black spots appeared on both my cheeks so I stopped and told my neighbor to stop also. The doctor didn't say that the spots were allergic reactions . . . just my own deductions. The doctor had me change from C-Quens to Oracon, then to Orthonovum, then to Lyndiol.

[In subsequent interviews, we were to learn that the woman finally gave up the use of all modern contraceptive methods and resorted to the folk method of "inverting the uterus."]

Obstacles to Procuring Contraceptives

The two preceding respondents are lucky to be able to afford the Pill. For most lower-class Cebuanos, it represents the most expensive method. Our interviewer reported that one respondent treasured a pamphlet describing the Pill (called Minovlar) in the bottom of her wooden trunk:

Q: Have you decided now on what method you will use for limiting your children?

L: I was at the Centro [a "free" clinic] last Friday and I was given this [R proudly opened her trunk and showed the pamphlet describing Minovlar]. I am keeping this in case we can afford . . . anyway, that is a long time yet. . . . I will deliver perhaps at the end of this month, and then there will be a year before my menstruation comes. There's enough time.

Q: Have you decided to use this [the Pill]?

L: If we can afford, we will buy. They say it costs 2.75 pesos per month and that means much to us. Imagine 2.75 pesos every month! We have to pay attention to food first—feed our five children before we can pay for this.

Q: Don't you think it will come out more economical in the long run than postponing [the purchase of the Pill]?

L: Yes, I know. *But do you expect us to miss our meals to buy it?*

Q: What does your husband say about it?

L: He just told me to keep this pamphlet so that we could use it when my time is near.

The Pill, besides being expensive and beyond the reach of lower-class respondents, is also one of the most inaccessible methods (along with the IUD) because it is largely controlled by medical prescription (even though some women were apparently black-marketing them in lower-class neighborhoods). This requires a personal visit to a licensed physician's "modern" office, rather than the familiar nipa hut of a folk healer in the neighborhood. Such an experience is both uncomfortable and expensive for lower-class women. Moreover, ignorance about the professional and impersonal code of ethics adhered to by modern physicians sustains misunderstanding of the conditions under which the Pill may be prescribed. This is most clearly demonstrated in the following:

> *Q:* Have you tried other means [of contraception]?
>
> *L:* I would like to try the Pill. But I am ashamed to tell the doctor. *They said the doctor will not give unless you are his friend. I am ashamed to consult the doctor.*
>
> *Q:* Did you try the local methods which you told me about—like the *habak* and the *pamaktak*?
>
> *L:* *Ay,* no *oy! Susmariosep!* I might die because of that.

A reluctance to see physicians and a certain amount of hesitation in making inquiries from the sources of contraceptive information are not uncommon among lower-class respondents. One woman articulated her fear of what the neighbors might think if she made inquiries about contraception. Her remarks reflect further her sense of modesty:

> *Q:* Have you ever tried asking anybody like your neighbor or sister-in-law how to stop bearing children?
>
> *L:* No, *oy!* Anyway, I don't think she will tell. I know she is using something because she has stopped having children . . . [but] she wouldn't tell. I also would not tell [anyone] if they ask me.
>
> *Q:* Why won't you or the others tell [anyone about it]?
>
> *L:* *Ay!* Because this neighborhood—they will start to talk about you and *biay-biay* [poke fun at you with malice]. Besides it is *mahilas* [scandalous, indecent to talk about birth control devices].
>
> *Q:* How will your neighbors poke fun?
>
> *L:* Hmm! They will say, "So and so, you know, she is using this . . ." and then they will look at you when you pass by.
>
> *Q:* Why don't you want [to use] the IUD—you pay only once whereas the Pill you have to buy every month.
>
> *L:* Our neighbor who had this IUD got sick, but if I had money at that time when those women came to sell the IUD to me, I would be using it now. The IUD, it is shameful, *no?* You have to spread your legs [for insertion]. I think the Pill is okay.
>
> *Q:* How did your husband know that IUD causes cancer?
>
> *L:* Because I told him—maybe if I use the IUD I will need to have special substance [nourishment] so that I will not get sick.

The difficulty in procuring contraceptive supplies (along with an inadequate knowledge of the rhythm method) is reiterated in the following interview with a different lower-class family. In this case, the husband, who was around the house, is the respondent:

> *Q:* Were you worried when your wife was not pregnant for two years after your marriage? Did you do something about it?
>
> *H:* No. I know such delays happen. I just thought, maybe I was not able to connect well, or did not hit the right spot, or maybe our blood did not mix well at that time. I just waited for God's will.
>
> *Q:* I remember from our first interview that your ideal number of children is two. When did you agree on this?
>
> *H:* After our first baby. [But] I am not really sure if we can make it only two. We are still young. [Both Hu and Wi are twenty-seven years old, and they now have two children.]
>
> *Q:* How do you plan to go about it? Do you know of any method?
>
> *H:* Just figure out the days by counting seventeen days before the bathday.
>
> *Q:* Where and from whom did you learn this?
>
> *H:* I knew that when I was still a bachelor from a friend who has studied biology; I think he is a doctor now. I did not forget what he told me.
>
> *Q:* When did you start the rhythm method?
>
> *H:* After the second child. I thought of this when the baby was eight months old. . . . Oh! You must excuse my wife, she has to go to Nang Goring's [HuMoSi] to ask for vegetable and banana for the baby.
>
> *Q:* Do you know of another way?
>
> *H:* Mrs. Torres [neighbor] was using the Pill—then, they change to the *pukot* [literally, "net"; here referring to the condom]. I saw it because it fell from their outhouse. The husband also jokes about it with the neighbors. Of course, it is only a joke, but parts of his jokes are true. . . . Ma'am, how much does it [the condom] cost? Tsk, tsk, tsk, it's expensive. [Interviewer replied.]
>
> *Q:* Why do you want to control?
>
> *H:* It is very hard when you have no money. Also, so that my wife can work if she wants to. You see, the number of children will depend on what kind of work one has. If he has a good job, he can have many.
>
> *Q:* Do you think you will use the condom?
>
> *H:* Ah, no. We have no money yet. Until now, I do not have a regular job. I am only a casual worker at the pier.
>
> *Q:* If your wife becomes pregnant again, would you accept the child?
>
> *H:* Yes, of course. *I expect we would make a mistake—impossible to be perfect in this thing.* If my wife does not accept it, it's up to her. If she wants to abort it, I can only tell her it's not good for her health. If she insists . . . she is no longer a child. Let her decide for herself.

This interview illustrates a number of important points. First of all, although the husband was fortunate enough to obtain some information on contraception, it is not certain how clearly the instructions were given to him, or how effective his method of counting the fertile period is. Second, it is evident that there is a discrepancy between the husband's knowledge of how babies are produced and the "scientific" version of how conception takes place. To him, apparently, a child is conceived if a man could "connect well" with his wife or "hit the right spot," or if the couple's blood "mixes well." Third, for the lower class, economic difficulties are still the greatest obstacle to the use of birth control devices, even after the motivational and cognitive factors are overcome. Their poverty leaves them with no choice but to employ the most low-cost contraceptive method, which not only involves a great deal of risk, but generates considerable frustration. The following interview with the wife shows that in order to lessen their anxiety about additional pregnancies, the couple sometimes resort to abstinence:

Q: Do you plan to have more babies?

W: *Ay,* no more. They are troublesome. I get tired easily with them.

Q: Did you talk about this with your husband?

W: Yes, he wants only two because he cannot feed more than two mouths.

Q: How do you intend to go about this? Do you know some methods?

W: *Ay, no oy!* We would just stop sleeping together and I will not let him touch me. Maybe my husband knows [some methods of contraception].

Q: How do you manage to sleep separately when you have only this one room?

W: *Ay!* He sleeps there with our older boy and I sleep here with our younger child [pointing to opposite ends of their one-room nipa hut].

The extent to which poverty, modesty, and lack of adequate contraceptive information can frustrate a couple's attempts at contraception is reiterated by the woman below, who originally wanted to have only two children, but ended up with five:

Q: Did you do something about limiting your number of children after your second child?

L: At my third pregnancy, I wanted to abort it. Then I decided to consult with the doctor at the Centro [a "free clinic"] how to go about it, but he advised me against it. He said it was sinful and bad for my health.

Q: What was your husband's reaction when he learned of your third pregnancy?

L: He was resigned. He said: "*I hope it is a boy.*"

Q: Why does your husband want a boy?

L: Because a boy can help him in his work more than the girls.

Q: Was he disappointed when you gave birth to a girl?

L: He just said: "It's all right. You are safe. I only wished it were a boy."

Q: Do you know other means of birth control aside from abortion?

L: No, except what I heard from [a] social worker—by counting days [rhythm], but it did not work.

Q: From the first interview I learned that your husband knew about the condom. Did he ever use it?

L: No. I don't know what that is. [Interviewer explained what a condom is.] Oh, yes, that one! I know one of our neighbors who is using it. I think it probably works because their youngest is already six years old and the wife is not yet pregnant, *but I am ashamed to ask my neighbor about it.* Where can you buy that? [Interviewer gave details of where to purchase the condom.]

Q: Have you tried other means of birth control?

L: Like I told you, we just sleep separately. My husband used to joke about it with his brother when they drink in the kitchen. He would say "We'll just abstain from our wives and *mag-abang* [rent] other women." Of course, I laughed with them because I know he would not do that.

Q: Tell me, why does your husband go to the mountain [his hometown in Carcar, 40.3 kilometers south of Cebu City] periodically?

L: He goes there during harvest time, to help harvest [the crops] and get a sack of maize in return.

Q: Is that the only reason? Why did he stay there for five months as you told me before?

L: Because he was afraid we might have sexual intercourse and he is afraid he might have a relapse [of tuberculosis].

Q: What made him come home after five months?

L: His former employer sent word that he could have his old job again. We started sleeping together again and we had Arturo [fourth pregnancy], and then when Arturo was one year and nine months old, I was pregnant again.

Q: I think your husband knows about withdrawal. Did he use it with you?

L: I don't remember.

Q: Would you object if he uses it?

L: It is all right with me. I would not mind. It's really the husband who enjoys it most.

Q: Are you still thinking of using the Pill?

L: There is very little hope [of using the Pill] really. Yesterday, my husband came home empty-handed [with no earnings]. I will have to see that doctor at the Charity Center of your school for the rhythm. Maybe this time it will work, with the doctor's help.

Q: Who took care of you while you were at the hospital [delivering the baby]?

L: My husband. He did not work for two days to be with me.

Q: Did you have enough food that week?

L: Well, we managed. It was barely enough but it was the Holy Week anyway —exact timing for fasting.

Q: How did you manage with the expenses?

L: *Na!* It was really hard. I wanted to call you up from the hospital to borrow money but the nurse did not allow us to use the phone. We wanted to borrow just for capital so that my husband could start buying and selling bottles again.

Q: To whom did you go then?

L: My husband went to Rosing [HuSi] to borrow capital. She lent us five pesos and gave us a *ganta* of corn meal.

Q: Do you pay interest for that money [you borrowed]?

L: No, *oy!* We just pay back the five pesos.

Q: How do you think you will manage to pay back the five pesos you borrowed from your sister-in-law?

L: We will have to pay by installment—maybe a peso now and then, until it is paid off.

Q: Are you afraid or feel guilty to borrow money from her or your other relatives?

L: No, *ma-ikog lang* [just feel a bit embarrassed], but they do not refuse if they have [it].

Q: Do they also borrow [money] from you?

L: *Ay!* No! We have nothing to lend. If we have, we would gladly lend, but they are better off than us.

Q: Do you feed the baby on schedule?

L: No, only when it wakes up and cries.

Q: Do you give any supplementary diet [to the baby]?

L: No, I want to give him *Tiki-Tiki* [a locally manufactured Vitamin B supplement) but it costs sixty centavos![5] It is too expensive. Thank God, I have plenty of [breast] milk.

From this interview, it is clear that although the family, living well below subsistence level, was motivated toward contraception, they were largely ignorant about the ways to realize their goal. It was not until after more than the desired number of pregnancies had occurred that they actively sought methods of contraception. Their first thought was abortion, but the wife was soon convinced by a clinic practitioner about its religious consequences and alleged harmful effects on her body. They tried the rhythm method, but it did not work. As a result, the couple resorted to the most fundamental and drastic birth control method they know of—abstinence. Its success was short-lived. The wife soon became pregnant. The Pill is ruled out by their extreme poverty.

A major factor contributing to the couple's unsuccessful trials at birth control is their reluctance to ask neighbors who are not relatives for information. The woman has repeatedly reiterated a desire to become less dependent upon others in their struggle for a living, and yet they are also aware that with average monthly earnings of thirty pesos they have not been able to make ends meet. They are sustained by borrowing on their future earnings from relatives who are also their neighbors. Although they have always been able to receive monetary aid from their relatives, the husband (on other occasions) reported feeling very ashamed about having to ask for help, and of being always on the receiving end of social exchange. As poor as they are, this family has a need to maintain their sense of dignity and self-respect. While the wife says she only feels a bit embarrassed, the husband is especially sensitive about seeking assistance from others, particularly from nonrelatives, since such gestures reflect badly on him and his ability as a breadwinner. Hence, unless the wife herself is physically ill, he prefers that she do the asking. Over the year in which we observed and interviewed this family, only once did the husband approach their relative-neighbors for assistance. This was when his wife returned from the "charity" hospital after a delivery and there was not a single grain of rice in the house, much less any other kind of food. Since the wife was physically weak, the husband in desperation sought his sister's assistance and was able to borrow five pesos—as narrated above.

Second, there is also the cultural valuation regarding women seeking contraceptive information. In a subculture (and possibly in the larger society as well) where women are not supposed to enjoy sex, but serve mainly to satisfy men's needs and to produce babies, it would not reflect well on the woman if she were to approach a neighbor who is not her relative for the purpose of seeking contraceptive information. This would imply that she enjoys the marital act and is doing it for more than procreation, in a regular fashion, so as to warrant a search for contraceptive measures. The risk of being shamed as "that kind of a woman" is too great, especially since the neighbors are not all one's kindred, and hence under no moral obligation to render assistance.

Third, long accustomed to poverty and deprivation, the lower-class Cebuanos have come to see goods in this world as existing only in limited quantities. Therefore, these possessions must be carefully apportioned. Contraceptive knowledge, insofar as some lower-class Cebuanos are concerned, appears to fall within the realm of limited goods. Hence there is the expectation that individuals who possess such a scarce resource may not want to share it with others. Not being able to cultivate friendship ties beyond the most geographically proximate and elemental kindred network, this lower-class family felt that they could not rightfully expect to obtain scarce contraceptive information from neighbors who are not their relatives. Even if one of them is a relative, it is still "shameful" to inquire whether condoms really work and where one may purchase them. The risk of being denied access to that scarce knowledge is perceived to be too great.

Desire for an Additional Child of a Specific Sex

At times, the decision to employ contraception may be countered by other motives. In spite of physical discomfort or complaints about the cost of additional pregnancies, the desire to have another child of a specific sex is still uppermost in the minds of some respondents, and may undermine their previously strong motivation to prevent pregnancies completely. The woman below is quite satisfied with the IUD. She has had various complications during every pregnancy. Added to that, she and her husband realize that their financial situation does not allow them to entertain seriously the idea of another child; yet after she had found an acceptable and effective contraceptive method her husband started to have second thoughts about preventing all pregnancies:

> *L:* My husband wants another boy as there is only one in the family. He is begging me to have another baby. I told him: "Good if we can be sure of the sex of the child. *Then I would be willing to have one more child*" [emphasis added]. Sometimes, I tell him we will have another child when our lot improves. I am afraid that if I have another child and the baby does not turn out to be a boy, my husband would keep hoping that the next one would be a boy, and we will keep on having babies.

Three other women eloquently articulated the conflict they and their husbands experience between the need to limit births so as to provide an adequate education for their children, and the desire to have another child of a certain sex to make *at least a pair* of boys or girls. In the lower-middle-class example below, the woman, aged thirty-three, stated that she simply cannot afford more than the five children she now has. Yet after one contraceptive failure, they have decided to abandon the idea. They hope that the wife will not get pregnant, but if she does they hope it will turn out to be a girl:

> *Q:* Does it bother you that you have to do so much work around the house? [R was ironing a big pile of clothes when I arrived, and insisted that I stay on so that we can talk as she irons.]
>
> *M:* No. I don't mind this work at all. It's all for the family.
>
> *Q:* Do you sometimes regret that you have so many children? [R has five children.]
>
> *M:* No. No regrets at all. In fact, *I would even have wanted some more.* Seven is the ideal number of children. I would like to have seven kids, but we simply cannot afford that. [Although husband is a graduate in marine engineering, his salary was only seventy pesos a week. R was working up until a few months previous to this interview.] I would have wanted another daughter, but I guess five [children] is just enough. Every time I get pregnant, my mind goes ahead to the time when I will deliver and that means money. Then, the caring of the child, that also means money. Then, the feeding. . . . The cost of living today is very high. At breakfast when the children ask for eggs, there are so many mouths to feed. It becomes such a problem to be able to give them what they want. And then before you even know it, they are already of school age. This is the biggest headache of all. Education costs a lot of money, but somehow you'll just have to educate them or they don't stand a chance in this world. Without education, you are nothing. *They'll blame*

their parents for not having given them the opportunity to be able to fend for themselves [emphasis added].

Q: Did you ever think of using any contraceptive?

M: After the fourth child, we decided to space pregnancies. But there, we got all messed up. *Instead of having longer gaps between pregnancies, I immediately got pregnant.* This fourth child was especially weak, and we were afraid I would not be able to take enough care of him if I should have another one right after that [fourth child]. Too bad it happened that way. After my third pregnancy, I got the scare of my life. My stomach was extraordinarily big, I thought I would have to be operated on. As a matter of fact, they used forceps to deliver the baby. Imagine, if I had the caesarean section, that would have meant a lot of money.

Q: How did you get messed up in using a contraceptive after your fourth pregnancy?

M: It just happened that our fourth child was born sickly. On advice of a cousin of mine who is a doctor, we decided to try a birth control method. The doctor suggested IUD. I objected. Because I know a friend of mine who used this particular type of method and she got pregnant anyway. So we tried the jelly. I don't know whether we simply forgot the doctor's instruction or the doctor did not give out the instructions clearly that this had to be allowed to settle first. In other words, you are supposed to apply this [jelly] fifteen minutes before intercourse. We didn't. Naturally, I got pregnant again. And this was even worse than when we didn't use anything. *Before when we use no [contraceptive] device at all, the spacing between children was two years. This time, it was only one year.* So, the fifth child was born. After this, I again talked to my husband to use the jelly. This time, he objected, saying "*no matter what one does, it is the Lord who disposes. There is a line set for us by Fate that we must follow. And nothing can keep that from happening so that whatever one does, he must reckon with the Divine.*" And that is how it is with us now. We only wish and pray, but we also know that if God so desires, His will and not ours will be done. He [Hu] always says that that time when we used the jelly, I got pregnant even earlier than usual, because that's *gaba* [divine retribution or curse].

Q: What if you get pregnant again?

M: My husband said he wanted to have a baby girl. We only have one daughter.

Q: What would happen if the next child or children turn out to be boys?

M: After my seventh child, I'm going to see to it that I don't have any more. I don't care what my husband will think. I will try my best to convince him. This time [*after* the seventh child], I will be taking pills. They are the most effective [contraceptive].

Q: How did you know about the Pill?

M: I took a Mother's class, and that's where I got a good idea of the effectiveness of the Pill. All the other methods are either too dirty or too unreliable. The IUD is so messy, and so is the jelly. It does not feel good inside. And the condom is unreliable. It is what caused a quarrel between my friend and her husband. They were using the condom, but they did not know that it had a hole. So the wife got pregnant, and the husband got angry, thinking that his wife was bad; he accused her of being unfaithful to him. Can you imagine that?

Q: What about the *hilot*? What do you think of them?

M: That's the best way to endanger a mother's health. I don't know how the *hilot* does it but the stories that I've heard about women suffering from serious stomach ailments because of the *hilot* have scared me away. I will never go to a *hilot*.

In another case, the respondent shows some indecision about contraception, and also reveals a common attitude that any woman who does not have a baby every two years or less is not fertile, even though she already has had seven children!

L: After Ida [third pregnancy], I thought it would be a good idea not to have too many children. . . . I just thought of it myself. I did not try *pag-alam* [a folk contraceptive measure]. They say one will get tuberculosis that way. [Probe.] It was not really inverting the uterus, it is just tilting it a little bit but I don't like it . . . I might get sick. But I had decided to do something [about controlling the number of children].

Q: How did you do it?

L: My husband did the controlling. We used withdrawal. I was very happy I did not get pregnant anymore. But that was the only time we tried "control." After Ben [fourth pregnancy], we no longer did anything. That is why I had Mario soon after Ben. Then after that, I was pregnant again, the fifth time. However, after the fifth pregnancy, I did not get [easily] pregnant anymore. We did not try to prevent pregnancy. And from Julio [sixth] to José [seventh pregnancy], I did not get pregnant easily either. There was a period of three years between Julio and José. Perhaps, I am just not *sundanon* [very fertile]. All my sisters are. They have so many children.

After my seventh pregnancy, my husband said he wanted me to become pregnant so we might have a girl because we have only one girl now [emphasis added]. I did not become pregnant. Now, last October, my menstruation did not show up. But November, it did. Now again, looks like I am late. Perhaps I am already getting old. That's why my menses *nagkabuang* [are going haywire]. And I was also thinking, José is now about three years old. Another nine months would make four years—[the spacing is] just like it has been with the two previous pregnancies.

When I delivered José, I went to the hospital because I was afraid something might go wrong because I was already *idaran* [getting older]. Looks like I might be pregnant again this time! And just this month, a fortune teller read my palm and said that if I deliver a baby when I am aged forty, I will die. I am worried. My husband says for me not to believe that kind of talk but I am really scared.

Another lower-class woman manifested her indecisiveness by first stating that she would feel miserable if she were to get pregnant again, yet she hopes that if this happens, the next child will be a boy. The couple's feelings are captured very well in the following discussion:

Q: What do you think about additional children?

L: To tell you the truth, *I would feel miserable if I were to get pregnant again.* It isn't like it was in the beginning. Then, it was all heavenly and thrilling. Imagine, having a child of your own. Your own flesh and blood born in love and understanding. When you think about the economics of it, you will surely think several times before wanting any more children. They are your responsibility. I was a little disappointed when my first child turned out to be a girl. *Now, if I must get pregnant again, I would want this to be a son* [R has four children: one boy and three girls.]

Q: Why a son?

L: I've heard it said that if the oldest is a boy it means good luck. [This belief is most likely due to the Chinese influence in the Philippines.] So that with this in mind, I wanted so much to have a boy when I had my first child. That being impossible [since the first child turned out to be a girl], *I would like to have a boy next time.* In my anxiety to have a son—I think this was all psychological—one day I looked at the sexual organ of my daughter, I thought I saw a penis.

Q: How did you feel on your third pregnancy?

L: I felt miserable. There and then I told my husband that we would use a birth control method. I was thinking of the expenses. Maternity alone costs twenty-seven pesos. Add to that the fact that I do not have enough milk for breastfeeding, so that it [milk] will have to be bought. And that means more expenses. When the children get sick, that's another expense. The doctor, the medicine . . . everything means money! And where am I supposed to get all that money? And the more children you have, the more risks you take and the more chances of their getting sick and the more effort you will have to put into it. When one gets sick, you will have to care for him and you cannot do anything else. Besides, how about dresses? And food and other incidental expenses and later on, their education? This is the most ticklish problem of all. Your children will blame you later if they do not get the proper education that they need to get on in this challenging world.

[*Husband interjecting*] This matter about the children and what would be the ideal number depends on the parents. If the parents do not care at all what happens to their children later, then they can have all the children they can make. After all, *by the time these children reach the age of eight, they can already fend for themselves:* selling newspapers, ice candy or shining shoes . . . or even begging on the streets. But if the parents think very seriously of their responsibility to feed these children, bring them up in a decent environment, and give them the necessary education, then, that calls for controlling the number of children. In my case, I have already learned my lesson. Look at me. I don't have any education to speak of. So the kinds of jobs I can get are those which call for people who cannot think very well, or those that do not call for technical knowledge. These jobs are heavy manual labor. And I wouldn't want my children to grow up that way. I would like to give them a fighting chance in this world. That's why we have decided to stop having any more children.

L: After my fourth child, I knew we had to do something about it. And we did. I went to a *hilot* to have my uterus inverted. It has been three years now and we haven't had another pregnancy. Moreover, we are also using withdrawal now [because] my friends told me that after three years, the inverted uterus will get back into its proper place. So that there is a risk of another pregnancy. I have been looking for the same *hilot* . . . don't know where she lives now.

Q: Why not take the Pill?

L: Pills are expensive. I have heard several stories about the pills. *If one takes them for a long period of time, there is every chance she gets frigid or goes insane* [emphasis added]. I am not sure if these stories are true. But *I do not want to take chances.* When I am already thirty-five years of age, that's when I intend to start taking pills. That way, I won't have to take pills for too long. When my menopause period comes I won't have to worry anymore about birth control.

If it were up to ______ (Hu) and me to decide, we would not want any more chilrdren. Originally, we thought two would be the ideal number. But that was when we were still too young to know the full impact of birth control. And birth control at that time was not as widespread as it is today. Even when we already had our third child, ______ (Hu) was still not so serious about birth control. It is only when our fourth child was born that we decided very seriously this was it. Our youngest is already old enough. I haven't had another pregnancy as yet. And that's good. We hope and pray that our wishes will be granted. *In the last analysis, you still have to reckon with the Almighty God. While we do not want another child, we also pray that none of those we have will be taken away from us.*

In those instances where the couple decided before marriage to limit the number of children, their foresight was not always rewarded with the desired result. The Rozaleses are a good example. Anita Rozales, thirty-two, has been married for twelve years to Juan Rozales, also thirty-two. The wife has had eight pregnancies, of which six children are living. Unlike other lower-class families, they had discussed their family size before they got married. They agreed on two children because Juan at that time had no permanent position. He was drifting from one casual job to another. As Anita said: "We wanted only two children, but God had other plans for us. He gave us three children!" After the third child, the husband decided that they should practice contraception. Each of Anita's pregnancies had been difficult, and according to Juan, this affected him in his job because he was always worried that something might happen to his wife while he was at work, especially since she has *kabuhi* (folk illness loosely translated as gas pain) and was always weak when she was pregnant. After the fourth child, Anita's sister Rosario and Juan's maternal aunt simply told them to practice contraception. This aunt suggested a hysterectomy because one of Juan's nieces who was a nurse had had that operation. But the couple had also heard of a woman who had the same operation and afterwards became very stout and moody. As a result they ruled out a hysterectomy. The aunt also suggested using an IUD. Juan was agreeable to that, but Anita was afraid to use the IUD. The couple finally used the condom for two successive years. It was an effective method, but when they had to transfer to a distant town in Bohol because of the husband's job, they found that they could not procure prophylactics, since there was no drugstore in the area. It was under these conditions that their fifth child (a son) was born but died soon afterward from a congenital defect. Not long after that she was pregnant again. After her sixth child, the Rozaleses decided to try another contraceptive method—rhythm. But somehow they made a mistake and she was pregnant for the seventh time. The infant died of the same congenital defect, imperforate anus, two years later. Not wanting to have another child, the couple practiced abstinence, or as the husband put it "*nag*-self-control *kami.*" But Anita became pregnant again. This time they thought seriously about aborting the fetus. The husband went to see his company's physician and the doctor gave him a prescription which would allegedly abort the fetus. When he went home, however, he thought things over more carefully:

> On the one hand, I knew it would be financially difficult to bring up a large family if the pregnancy is allowed to follow its course; we had no money to bring another child into this world. But on the other hand, I asked myself, what if this one turns out to be a girl [all the children were boys]? It would be the greatest mistake of my life!

With these thoughts, Juan threw away the doctor's prescription, and as our interview with this family progressed, we learned on our second to the last visit that Anita had given birth to a girl. They were the happiest couple in the neighborhood. As the husband put it: "She will be the guardian angel of my boys when they grow up. She will correct them if they make any mistakes."

On one of our last visits to this family, Anita was taking a Mother's Class together with her neighbors. The course teaches them how to use different contraceptive methods, and a sample of the Pill called Minovlar was distributed to them free. Would Anita use the Pill from now on? Here is her answer:

> We were taught how to use the Pill. But I won't use it. I heard it causes tuberculosis. My neighbor, Oping, tried using the Pill. But after less than a month, she had to discontinue using it because she felt weak and could not breathe. Another neighbor of mine, Erundina, also wanted to take the Pill, but after what happened to Oping, Erundina's husband would not let her take it.

Thus, on the basis of what Anita has heard about the side effects of the Pill, it is apparent that she would likely try other methods. On our last interview, Anita disclosed their contraceptive decision: they would try the rhythm method again. In this lower-class neighborhood, what the next-door housewife says seems to carry more weight than the instructions of a middle-class contraceptive "teacher" who does not live in the area.

Desire for More Children

There are also several cases where one spouse or both may earnestly decide before marriage upon a certain number of children, but the desired size is not always small, and the reasons for limiting pregnancies may be farfetched. In the two verbatim interview records below, the husband has definite ideas about family planning and realizes the high risk involved in having girls in view of the existing sex-role structure and the perceived sexual division of labor. This, however, did not necessarily result in a smaller family. The first family (lower-class) has had twelve pregnancies, of which eleven children are living, mostly boys. For this, the wife at one time proudly proclaimed that among her relatives, "I am the champion!" The second family (middle-class) overshot their mark by two pregnancies:

> *L:* When my husband was courting me, he said that he wanted to have a dozen children immediately. Before our first child was born he said he wanted it to be a boy. I wanted a girl. I did not think about how many I wanted. He preferred them to be boys. With my folks [in Luzon] boys are preferred—any number. They said that boys can help sooner than girls; boys are bigger help; girls will just be taken away by men. People here in Cebu prefer girls. They say that girls are of more help to the mother and can be talked into not marrying yet [delaying marriage]. Most mothers here complain that boys are hard to manage, always out of the house, and even [when they are] without a job, [they] bring a girl to their mothers, saying they want to get married. Who's going to support them? The parents, of course! When they say they want to get married, they'll get married and you have to do what's necessary.

> *M:* When I got married, I never heard of anything such as the Pill, or other things that can control births. Dodong [Hu], who had been married previously, had definite ideas [about the number of children]. He wanted only two more children. Not only that, he even wanted to dictate the kind [gender] of children he wanted to have: both boys. Because, he says, he fears the birth of a daughter. He thinks it is too risky, especially when she is grown up and starts dating. He would not want a daughter going astray. And all that stuff about virginity and the fact that it is always the woman's reputation that gets ruined in premarital sexual relations, or in the case of unwed mothers. It's a good thing that the daughter we have is still very dear to him. I guess that's the way with all fathers. They all talk a lot about this and that, but when it's your own flesh and blood, you'll have to take care of her just as well as the others. Boys are freer in our society. [Pause.]

> His age also had a lot to do with his wish to have only two more children. [Hu is forty-four, twelve years older than Wi.] He wants very much to see them educated and finished with their courses and live as men on their way to success. And he did not want to leave young children behind when he dies. Me, I was ignorant in these matters, and I wanted all the children I could possibly have. Later on, I knew better. With the arrival of my third child, this was the time when we really had problems about making ends meet, I went to see a doctor. After my fourth child, I was desperately in need of advice on the use of contraceptives and I was advised to take Oracon for six pesos a set. But it worked. I didn't get pregnant. It was only when it got to be so expensive, I remember that time when it costs eight pesos a set. I thought this was too much. When I complained to my husband, he suggested that I go back to the doctor. But I thought I had a better idea and not an expensive one—the rhythm method. He was completely in agreement. Only, he said, he had to travel a lot, and he still does, and it would be just dandy if he should come home at a fertile period. He might not want to be refused. My neighbors were not of any help either. They told me to go to a *hilot*. I know of one woman who got tuberculosis because of this. So I said a firm "No!" The doctor prescribed Feminal, which costs some three pesos, and that's what I use up to now.

In two other cases, the stated reason for limiting the number of children was to complete the letters of a certain name, or of a theme song the couple enjoyed during their courtship years. For the Cinco family (middle-class), the topic of children was brought up before their marriage, but the husband did not say a definite number. Instead, all he said was that he would accept as many as God wants him to have. The wife never really gave the matter any serious thought. After their marriage and before the birth of their first child, they agreed to have "only five children"—a number that would complete the husband's family name (*C I N C O*) and "enough to educate, feed, and clothe them." When we interviewed them, the couple had four children (Carmen, Ignacio, Nenita, and Carlos). There is no indication that they will change their plan and stop with the fourth child. The next child's name will begin with *O* to complete the family name. That, they hope, will be their last child.

For another family (lower-class), there are more letters to be completed: *E V E R L O V E*. It is their theme song and the husband, especially, wanted to complete it. He further wanted to have five boys and three girls, "the boys to form a complete team for basketball [Hu's favorite sport], and the three girls to help out their mother." Although the wife was only twenty-nine at the time of the interview, they already had had six children in nine years of marriage. They need two more to complete the letters of their favorite song.

As idiosyncratic as their reasons for wanting to have a certain number of children may be, these couples nevertheless illustrate the parameters of motivation for birth control among a selected group of

Cebuano families. To refuse to accept their stated reasons as "serious," "rational," or "intelligent" grounds for family planning is to impose our own ethnocentric interpretations on their personal values. The existence of two such cases, each from a different social class, simply highlights how culture-bound our perceptions of the costs of childbearing are. Research on the perceived costs of children have overemphasized the economic component and failed to grasp the paramount importance of noneconomic factors. In these two cases, the couples realized the economic burden of added pregnancies, and it was precisely for this reason that they wanted to restrict the number of children to those specific figures, not more! Both wives are taking contraceptives to space children, but not to terminate conception. This statement by Mrs. Cinco provides a clearer understanding of her perspective on the matter:

> *M:* I only want five children, if possible. My husband also said we will complete the letters of the family name. After this one [the fourth infant], the next one would be the last, I hope. I intend to use the rhythm method which I learned from a Mother's Class in the neighborhood. . . . *I don't want more than five children. It's not easy to be pregnant. Besides I am afraid we might not be able to give the children the best education we can afford if they are many.* My family does not have any say regarding the number of children we plan to have. It's my husband's say. It's his responsibility. Besides, *he is doing everything to give us the best he can afford.* I won't use other methods aside from the rhythm. *I am afraid those* [other methods] *will be harmful to my body. I am afraid to commit a sin besides* [emphasis added].

The lower-class family that wanted to complete the words "Ever Love" said:

> *Q:* What do you think about having additional children?
>
> *L:* *Sus!* I don't know.
>
> *Q:* What do you mean by that?
>
> *L:* I just don't know what to do. We really *don't intend to have more than we plan for* [eight]. As you know, I am even using the Pill now *to have some spacing before I have the next child* [emphasis added].
>
> *Q:* What is really your reason for having such a number only?
>
> *L:* You can say that eight is "only?" That is even more than enough. Frankly, I really wanted to have four only, but *because he* [pointing to husband] *wants that many, well, as a good wife and because we had agreed already, I can't do anything.* [Husband interjecting] You know, I really want to have five boys and three girls. The boys to form a complete team for basketball and three girls to help out their mother.
>
> *Q:* Supposing you have more than your planned number or in case you change your mind, what would you do?
>
> *L:* It's impossible because I have the pills. [Husband interjecting] Yes, and I won't allow her also to have more [than eight].

> *Q:* Do you find therefore that this number is enough for you to be able to give them all the things they need? [I asked this to find out what the husband would answer, *as he does not have a fixed income.*]
>
> *L* (reluctantly): Ah . . . Ah . . . *ambot lang na niya.* [Literally:I don't know with him.] [Husband, head was bowed when he answered, as if in shame] *Tingali* [Maybe].
>
> *Q:* Don't you find them a financial burden?
>
> *L:* Yes, of course we do. *But they give us joy also* and my children are all very good in their school work, so I have faith that *someday they could help one another even if they could not help us* [emphasis added].
>
> *Q:* Which of the two, the Pill or the children, do you think cost you more?
>
> *L:* Of course, the children, for since they are babies they need a lot of care, much more so when they are bigger or older.
>
> *Q:* Do you rely or do you have confidence that by using the Pill you would not get pregnant?
>
> *L:* Yes, very much. I take it every evening before going to bed. [Husband interjecting] I remind her also every night, or if I come home late, I never fail to ask her if she has taken it.

A number of insights are immediately apparent from these cases. First of all, the wives worry about the economic burden of an unlimited number of children. It is for this reason that they are taking contraceptive measures—not to prevent pregnancy completely, but simply to space the forthcoming conceptions until they have the planned number of children. Second, for both wives—but for the lower-class wife especially—*the fulfillment of desired family size is part of the role of a dutiful wife*, who must go along with the husband's wishes in order not to alienate him or jeopardize the marital relationship.

Third, the number of children planned has a symbolic meaning of its own: they are a reminder to the married couple of their conjugal commitment and affective involvement, however much it might have waned from time to time. To stop conceptions before the desired number of children is attained would leave the letters that they cherished in limbo; it would be tantamount to symbolically admitting a reduced conjugal commitment—an admission that might just go beyond the symbolic level, especially when the wife in each family has repeatedly reported that her husband has not been so romantically inclined as he once was. In the case of the Cinco family, the husband had—for six to eight months—neglected his conjugal and parental role obligations as he became more involved with his *barkada*, men whom he met at work and some of whom became his children's godparents. In the Ever-Loves' case, the husband had also become more involved with his peer group as he needed them to "cover up" his cockfighting activities from his wife. As a result of his inability to find a steady job other than through cock-breeding and fighting, he has also unwittingly forfeited his role as the breadwinner of his family. This has created a sense of unease between husband and wife, as inferred from his answer to the interviewer's query about their financial ability to support such a large number of children. The wife is fully aware that her sixty pesos' monthly earnings derived from washing other people's laundry is the family's only source of steady income. From the record of previous interviews with her, it is also clear that she knows her monthly income is not enough to support their planned number of children. Yet she neither sought to dissuade her husband nor attempted to "shame" him by answering the interviewer's question with a flat admission of their economic inability to rear so many children. Instead, she simply shifted the burden of answering that question to her husband by saying "*ambot lang na niya*," which gives a hint of her displeasure at having to go along with her husband's plans, but at the same time acknowledges that *he* is the head of the household and the official breadwinner. As in the Cincos' case, the wife credits the husband with the responsibility of family planning and economic support. The husband's posture and answer convey that his economic dependence on his wife is certainly nothing to be proud of. His monosyllabic reply suggests his uncertainty in fulfilling his economic role in the family, but it also carries a certain degree of wishful thinking —the hope that perhaps, *maybe*, things will turn good for a change. The ambivalence the couple experiences regarding their large number of children is reflected in the wife's remark that although children are admittedly a financial burden, they are also a source of joy to the parents and their hope for a better future.

In studying the reproductive patterns of the Cebuanos, the importance of children cannot be overemphasized. As one woman said: "There is a big difference between the expense of a child and the cost of a pill. *A child belongs to you, is yours. You do not count the expenses. You do not think of the expenses of a child.*" This family is in fact destitute.

Other respondents vehemently opposed the thought of giving their children up for adoption just to free themselves of their tight financial situation:

> *Q:* Would you be willing to give your children for adoption to be free of [financial] burden?
>
> *H&W* (emphatic and together): NEVER!
>
> *H:* That will happen only when we are dead. It is our obligation to bring them up—it's part of marriage. *You're happy because you have children.* It is also difficult to bring them up. I must give them a good example. That's just like an inheritance that I give them.
>
> *W:* I will miss my children if I give them away.

Thus, quite often the woman who complained in one moment about the economic burden of child care would in the next moment express a desire for another one—a small "baby" who can keep them company at home while the older ones are in school. In our interviews with Cebuano women, the "joy" of children is constantly being emphasized. Consider, for instance, the following case:

> *Q:* What do you think of having additional children to the ones you have now?
>
> *L:* I don't think we can afford it anymore, we are even financially hard up with this seven, how much more if more will be added. I just can't imagine how we would get along. With two in high school, oh! My God, maybe I won't sleep anymore, just so that I could earn more to help in supporting them.
>
> *Q:* But, is it not that some of your brothers-in-law are helping you?
>
> *L:* Yes, but it is a shame if you would just depend on them. Besides, it is not much, they have their own family to think of, too.
>
> *Q:* Do you consider children as a burden then?
>
> *L:* Financially, yes. With the high cost of living and education nowadays, even if you could earn five hundred pesos a month, it is hard to get by. Just look at those rich people, they even have more debts because they have to see to it that their children *dili mapere* [will not fall behind others] in things they need and the kind of school they attend.
>
> *Q:* You mean emotionally you love having them?
>
> *L:* Yes, that is why *I am spacing them in such a way that one or two is left with me while the others are in school* [emphasis added].
>
> *Q:* So, are you thinking of having additional children then?
>
> *L* [pause]: Yes. *We feel that eight children would be just the right number for us, in accordance with my husband's salary* [husband actually earns less than four hundred pesos a month]. We have been spacing our children since after the second pregnancy by withdrawal *so that when the older ones are in school, I will have the smallest one as a companion in the house. Also, the older children could help with the younger ones' education this way.* My husband gets some benefits from the Philippine Constabulary, for the more children you have, the more you are provided with these benefits like clothing, allowances, canned goods.
>
> *Q:* What would you do if someday all of them are going to school and you can't have more children, because as you said you can't afford them anymore?
>
> *L:* Oh, for sure by that time I would have many customers already [R does sewing at home] and I would then devote my time to sewing [for profit].
>
> *Q:* What would you do to prevent any more conception?
>
> *L:* I think I would use the rhythm method for it won't cost you anything.
>
> *Q:* But there is a risk of getting pregnant, if you make a mistake in counting or when you can't control your husband.
>
> *L:* I guess the best thing to do would be to mark the calendar and see to it that my husband would also keep track of the days to avoid the risk. Anyway, he is not so aggressive also.

Children are a source of joy, and a hedge against want. They are loved for what they are, and for what they can become—the parents' main (if not their *only*) hope for a better future. These values are even more clearly articulated in the following case, involving another family:

> *Q:* What do you think if God gives you more children even if you are using the IUD for contraceptive purposes?
>
> *L:* Well, if it is really God's will that I have more children even with the IUD, there is nothing I think I can do about it.
>
> *Q:* Would you consider them a blessing then?
>
> *L:* I guess I could, for it is only God who knows what is good for us and what is not. It might be He has some reasons for doing it. *Who knows that the children would not only give us glory and prestige in the future but also some financial security?*
>
> *Q:* Do you think of them as an economic burden?
>
> *L:* If we will have more than we have now, it would really be very hard to give them the things they will need and a better education. Unless they themselves would consider working their way to college. I don't think we could afford to give them that higher education, with just the salary that my husband is receiving. *Sus!* I just don't know what I would do then.
>
> *Q:* After your first child, did you ever think that children are liabilities or an asset? I mean to say, if they would be a help in the future for your family or a burden?
>
> *L: I never think of them, of course, in that way.* It was only when I had my sixth child that I decided that I should do something, because we are a little tight financially. *In some ways, they can be called a help, because if all of them, God willing, will be able to finish a course and then have a good job, they surely would not turn their back against us and maybe we will be a little comfortable then.*
>
> *Q:* Do you feel that having more children would cost you more than using the IUD?
>
> *L:* Of course, I do! I only spent twenty-five pesos to have this IUD. To have babies, my God! You will not only spend while you are conceiving, like me for example, I always become very sick when I am pregnant, and I spent a lot for medical care. Then when you deliver, you pay the hospital fees. While they are growing up, you must give them good food and vitamins. When they get sick, you spend so much for the doctor and the medicine. When they start going to school, even if you send them to a public school, there are many *amut* [contributions or collections of money from students for charitable causes]; you have to buy presentable dresses [for the children], you have to provide them with school supplies. I think you very well know what the rest are. If I enumerate them all, we won't finish until tomorrow.
>
> *Q:* In short, then, do you consider them as an economic burden?
>
> *L:* Yes, *but to have children is also fun*, especially when you are tired and they would start singing or dancing, *especially the younger ones. They are a joy to see.*

The reader might argue that surely these cannot be typical cases, and that the proportion of couples who knew how to use and were practicing contraception but who stopped in order to have another child could not be large. To answer this question, we direct the reader's attention to Table 5.6. For the urban upper class, the single largest reason for stopping contraceptive use was that the measure was undertaken for "spacing only." Only about 7 percent said that the reason for discontinuation was "religious." Within this class, only a little over 3 percent did not wish to continue the practice of birth control for fear of side effects or because they could not obtain cooperation from their husbands.

For the urban middle class, one out of every two also listed child-spacing as the main reason for stopping the use of a birth control method, while about 15 percent stated that continuation of contraceptive use might have side effects or cause illness. Among urban lower-class respondents, the number who used contraceptives for spacing is a little over one out of every three. However, about 13 percent reported that continuation met with resistance from their husbands—a 10 percent difference between the lower class and the other two classes in the urban group.

Among rural dwellers, those who reported that husbands refused to cooperate are about 17 percent for the middle class (compared to the urban middle class of 4 percent) and 23.4 percent for the lower class (compared to 13.4 percent for the urban lower class). Other reasons, including the belief in *gaba*, differ by social class: from about 25 percent for the lower class to about 9 percent for the rural middle class.

Contraceptive Effectiveness in Child-Spacing

Another way of understanding the contraception predicament of Cebuano couples is to study the child-spacing patterns of the users and nonusers of modern contraceptives. Table 5.7 presents these data by age cohort and parity up until the seventh child. In addition, the number of pregnancy wastages for each parity and age cohort was sorted out. Based on a total of 2,094 cases, from both the rural and urban areas of Cebu, Table 5.7 shows that the average length of time between marriage and the birth of the first child was 13.3 months. For those who had used contraceptives, the mean was 15 months. However, the total number of users prior to the first birth is only 38 persons, which is rather small.

With the second parity, for the total count of 1,916 cases, the average length of child-spacing is 23.6 months, or almost two years. For the 174 contraceptive users, the birth of the second child is delayed by only 5.4 months compared to the nonusers. Those who reported an exclusive reliance on prolonged breastfeeding for contraceptive purposes had a gap of 27.6 months between the first and second child.

Even for subsequent parities, the child-spacing patterns of users do not significantly differ from those of nonusers. At the very best, the use of contraceptives merely delays the birth of a child by 5.2 months. In fact, during the seventh parity the contraceptive users succeeded in spacing their child by merely 2.1 months longer than the nonusers. In some age groups, such as the fifteen to twenty-four cohort during the fourth, fifth, and sixth parities, the nonusers exhibited a longer interval between births than the contraceptive users. Little wonder that many Cebuanos remain unconvinced about the effectiveness of modern contraceptive methods.

The figures on pregnancy wastage present another interesting observation. In every parity and for every age cohort, the occurrence of a pregnancy wastage (due to miscarriage, stillbirth, or spontaneous abortion) was swiftly followed by another pregnancy which resulted in live birth. In such cases, the birth intervals are quite short, ranging from 8.6 to 18 months only.

Finally, in examining the data on lactation, one cannot help but note that compared to contraceptive users, those who deliberately stretched their breastfeeding period in the belief that it would "prevent rapid births" might have a point. Judging from the differences in months between lactating mothers and contraceptive users in Table 5.7, lactation seems just as effective for child-spacing as the use of modern contraceptive devices. Table 5.8 compares the child-spacing patterns of lactating and nonlactating mothers. The table suggests that, at least empirically, the folk belief that prolonged lactation has a contraceptive effect appears to be supported.

Table 5.8 shows that women who lactated nine months or less do not seem to differ from nonlactating mothers in terms of child-spacing. A surprising finding is that those who lactated six months or less had, on the average, a shorter time span between births than those who did not lactate. However, those who lactated for more than nine months, and especially those who lactated for more than fifteen months, appear to have markedly long intervals between parities. Additional research in reproductive medicine is necessary to establish whether the Cebuano folk belief has any scientific basis.

Conclusion

Our lengthy presentation of demographic data and textual interview materials reveals the striking similarities between the "never users" and the "ever users" of contraceptives. Both groups appear to

TABLE 5.7

CHILD-SPACING PATTERNS

	All Age Groups		*15–24*		*25–34*		*35–45*	
Parity and Type of User	*(N)*	*Mean Months*	*(N)*	*Mean Months*	*(N)*	*Mean Months*	*(N)*	*Mean Months*
Marriage and 1st child								
Total	*2,094*	13.3	*310*	12.7	*1,003*	13.1	*781*	13.7
Contraceptive users	*38*	15.0	*11*	18.6	*15*	15.5	*12*	11.2
Nonusers	*1,899*	13.6	*283*	12.7	*908*	13.4	*708*	14.0
Used lactation	N/A	—	—	—	—	—	—	—
Pregnancy wastage	*155*	—	*16*	—	*78*	—	*61*	—
1st and 2nd child								
Total	*1,916*	23.6	*236*	21.3	*925*	23.2	*755*	24.7
Contraceptive users	*174*	28.7	*28*	23.5	*98*	29.9	*48*	29.4
Nonusers	*1,603*	23.3	*193*	21.4	*766*	22.7	*644*	24.5
Used lactation	*35*	27.6	*5*	20.4	*19*	24.7	*11*	36.0
Pregnancy wastage	*104*	18.2	*10*	14.9	*42*	16.8	*52*	20.0
2nd and 3rd child								
Total	*1,602*	24.2	*118*	22.2	*764*	23.7	*720*	25.2
Contraceptive users	*226*	29.0	*16*	23.9	*119*	28.8	*91*	30.2
Nonusers	*1,248*	23.8	*94*	22.1	*580*	22.8	*574*	25.1
Used lactation	*37*	29.3	*1*	40.0	*26*	30.2	*10*	25.7
Pregnancy wastage	*91*	16.4	*7*	16.7	*39*	16.3	*45*	16.4

3rd and 4th child								
Total	1,281	24.5	43	19.0	582	23.4	656	25.8
Contraceptive users	242	27.0	10	16.6	122	24.7	110	30.6
Nonusers	933	24.4	28	21.6	407	23.5	498	25.4
Used lactation	33	26.0	0	—	22	26.3	11	25.5
Pregnancy wastage	73	15.6	5	8.6	31	15.3	37	16.8
4th and 5th child								
Total	974	25.0	14	29.5	388	23.6	572	25.7
Contraceptive users	193	28.2	4	24.0	77	24.6	112	30.9
Nonusers	685	24.7	10	31.7	270	23.6	405	25.3
Used lactation	29	26.5	0	—	19	28.4	10	23.0
Pregnancy wastage	67	17.3	0	—	22	16.4	45	17.8
5th and 6th child								
Total	727	25.5	9	27.4	234	24.0	484	26.2
Contraceptive users	170	28.5	2	18.5	54	23.7	114	31.0
Nonusers	489	25.3	6	32.8	159	24.3	324	25.6
Used lactation	18	24.4	0	—	11	25.9	7	22.1
Pregnancy wastage	50	17.5	1	13.0	10	18.9	39	17.3
6th and 7th child								
Total	508	24.3	4	17.8	121	23.0	383	24.8
Contraceptive users	117	26.6	0	—	31	23.3	86	27.8
Nonusers	345	24.5	3	18.3	81	23.9	261	24.8
Used lactation	9	27.9	0	—	2	33.5	7	26.3
Pregnancy wastage	37	14.7	1	16.0	7	8.6	29	16.2

TABLE 5.8

CHILD-SPACING PATTERNS OF LACTATING AND NONLACTATING MOTHERS

Parity	Mothers Not Lactating	Lactating Mothers				
		3 months or less	4–6 months	7–9 months	10–12 months	Over 15 months
1st–2nd	23.4	21.0	19.9	22.3	25.0	32.4
2nd–3rd	24.2	21.4	21.6	22.6	25.9	32.5
3rd–4th	24.6	22.9	20.1	24.8	27.1	31.9
4th–5th	24.8	23.8	24.6	24.4	26.3	34.0
5th–6th	25.5	24.1	23.7	25.0	27.6	34.8

base their decision on a common premise—the desire for more children. No doubt, the predominant attitude in Cebu is pronatalistic and supportive of large families. The intrinsic psychological and social rewards of children are not offset by the economic burden of child care, even among the very poor.

Furthermore, underlying the difficulties that some of our respondents had in preventing conceptions is a thick layer of cultural beliefs, concepts, and fears which not even the most effective contraceptive device invented so far can dispel or counteract. The fact that more recent studies on family planning in the Philippines (Laing, 1973; Ballweg and MacCorquodale, 1974) continue to report that the incidence of accidental pregnancies even among Pill users is as high as among IUD users suggests that ovulation may not be well understood by many. This makes the rhythm method even more risky, since it depends critically on the correct identification of the woman's fertile period.

With the ban on contraceptives now lifted, the problem is no longer so much the lack of information on contraception (although this still exists) as it is the clash between folk beliefs and modern technologies and unfamiliar concepts. Scientifically trained health practitioners generally give very little credence to folk beliefs on sexuality and reproduction, although continued ignorance of this conflict can seriously hamper provider-client communication. While there are women who do not have faith in folk healers or in folk contraceptive measures, there are those who do, and there are even those who would switch from the most reliable modern method to folk measures of unknown effectiveness. The proliferation of these measures suggests that a supply of folk practitioners must exist in the environs of Cebu to disseminate their knowledge and usage. This is explored in the next chapter.

6 / Folk Methods of Birth Control

An analysis of Cebuano reproduction is not complete without some understanding of the extent to which pregnancies, contraception, and abortion are still partly handled by traditional healers who possess a bewilderingly rich body of knowledge on reproductive physiology and folk methods of birth control. Because this facet of human behavior is so intimately associated with being female and married, it is largely outside the purview of male anthropologists and unmarried female researchers. Hence, empirical data are especially hard to come by. The sparsity is reinforced by the fact that most KAP studies apparently do not emphasize the competition of ideas or methods offered by systems of folk belief. In our own survey questionnaire, for instance, we paid no attention to folk methods specifically but cast them in a residual "other" category. Fortunately, through the use of in-depth interviews in Phases II and III of our study, we were able to fill in some of the gaps in our knowledge. Moreover, a few researchers have been able to collect data on this subject among the Cebuanos in Negros (Hart, 1965) and in Cebu (Demetria, 1969; Damo, 1969; Rubel et al., 1971; 1975). The study conducted by Demetria was made in consultation with the Cebu Family Health Project, and the ones by Damo and Rubel et al. were integral components of our research project. Their materials are, therefore, contemporaneous with the survey data we collected, whereas Hart's study was based on an earlier report. Despite this time difference, there is a great deal of similarity in these data sets.

In this chapter, we shall briefly describe the folk concept of reproduction and the cultural repertoire of birth control methods, after a quick inventory of traditional or folk healers in the Cebuano medical system.

Folk Practitioners

The consensus among researchers is that there are three broad types of Cebuano folk healers: the *manghihilot* (masseur), the *mananam-*

bal (general practitioner), and the *mananabang* (midwife).[1] These terms should not be confused with the *hilot* practitioner in Tagalog-speaking areas, which includes the traditional unscientific midwife as well as the massager-healer (cf. Jimenez, 1955:29).

One may become a folk healer through apprenticeship under a lineal or ascending collateral relative, alleged patronage with a certain supernatural power or spiritual figure, or formal training (in the case of midwifery). Alternatively, the abilities may be fortuitiously ascribed ("born with it") if not imposed by desperate clients as a result of great urgency combined with a shortage of nearby competent paramedical attendants. Information on the geographic or demographic distributions of these folk practitioners and on the type of patients who are inclined to seek their service is almost nonexistent, since there is no exhaustive central listing for any one of the different types of folk practitioners. Lieban (1967), however, provides a preliminary profile of the educational level of those who seek the services of physicians[2] versus those who visit *mananambals*.[3] He found that 65 percent of the 327 patients of the *mananambals* he observed had attended (but not necessarily completed) fourth grade or less, 17 percent had between a fifth- and a seventh-grade education, another 13 percent went to high school, and only 5 percent ever attended college. This is in contrast with the educational level of those who seek physicians' services, which tended to be evenly spread out in the four categories.

In an investigation into the background of the *mananabangs*, Demetria (1969) reported that of the eighteen barrio midwives she was able to contact, half had no formal education at all, and of the twenty *mananabangs* she studied who were working in Cebu City, close to half ($n = 8$) also had no education. Of those who had attended school, most had had four years or less of primary education. Only one of the twenty urban *mananabangs* she interviewed had ever attended college.

There are a number of reasons why folk medicine has persisted in Cebu and elsewhere in the Philippines. These include: (1) extreme poverty, (2) insufficient modern health service units, (3) inadequate transportation and communication facilities, (4) lack of rapport between modern "scientifically trained" health workers and the masses, (5) personalized services and the familistic-*gemeinschaft* manner of folk healers, (6) the ability of folk healers to work within the cultural universe of deep-rooted superstitions and ethnomedical etiologies, (7) the overdifferentiation of modern "scientific" health care systems that compartmentalize services into medical, psychiatric, and social categories, (8) the corresponding lack of differentiation in the folk healer roles which enables them to treat the "whole" person—spiritual, psychiatric, medical, social, and even interpersonal or intrafamilial problems, (9) the lack of mass health education programs, and (10) government inertia in inducing change.

The oft-repeated line that "the doctor cures but we cannot afford to buy his '*receta*' [prescribed medication] since all the money we have is only enough to cover his consultation fee" is widely acknowledged. Another grim reality is the small number of Filipino physicians willing to serve the rural population. Of those who do, most practice in the *poblacion*—the smallest political division which is the seat of government administration. This means that barrio dwellers, many of whom live outside the *poblacion*, must be willing to spend as much as five to twenty pesos for transportation and meals on their way to seek modern medical advice. According to the Annual Statistical Report for Cebu in 1966, the whole province, with a population of 1,148,125 at that time, had only fifty-three rural health units, thirty-six health centers, and two government hospitals. Ruiz (1968:137) noted that in her personal communication with Dr. Solon, head of the Rural Internship in Pakna-an, Mandawe, she learned that in one year, and in that area alone, the local midwife delivered as many as 423 babies, whereas the rural health personnel assisted in 21 deliveries, the hospital had 32, and private physicians attended only 3 cases.

Other researchers, ourselves included, believe that even if geographical insularity and socioeconomic disadvantages are overcome or neutralized, these folk healers will not necessarily be consulted less frequently, for their roles are rooted in the folk medical belief system and in the people's ability to avoid cognitive dissonance when a cure is not effected through folk healing. While Ruiz (1968) stressed the importance of rapport between the patient and the medical attendant, Lieban expressed some doubts about the importance of this factor (1967:93), basing his position on the observations he made that two of the most successful *mananambals* in Cebu City were in fact overbearing and harsh with their lower-class patients, even going so far as to accuse them of "moral lapses." The precise reasons behind their popularity we leave to future students of social anthropology to argue. What is pertinent is that a complex system of folk beliefs and practices still thrives in Cebu. This system is sustained by three folk medical roles: the *manghihilot*, the *mananambal*, and the *mananabang*.

The *manghihilot* specializes in treating sprains, fractures, and bone dislocations primarily by massaging them into place (Lieban, 1967:81; Ruiz, 1968:21). However, because of the differences in the attribution of illness between Cebuanos and North Americans, the *manghihilot* attends to more than just "bone" problems. He or she may also attend to female reproductive problems and provide prenatal care, especially if the patient's complaint is attributable to "dislocation" of the uterus, or of the unborn child. Likewise, the *manghihilot* also treats respiratory symptoms, since in their folk etiology coughing and chest pains can be caused by "the child falling on its chest, pushing in or curving the soft bones of the rib cage, which adversely affects the lungs" (Lieban, 1967:97); hence the need to massage the bones back to their place or into their normal shape.

The *mananambal* is considered a general practitioner. Within this category there are finer distinctions, depending on the predominant style of treating an ailment or ailments. Ruiz (1968) classified five types of *mananambal*: (1) the *herbolario* (herb doctor), whose treatment utilizes herbal medicine; (2) the *orasyonan*, who relies on the miraculous power of a special incantation, usually verses in (adulterated) Latin, in the treatment of illnesses, particularly those attributed to sorcery (Lieban, 1967:31); (3) the *diwatahan*, who invokes a cure by propitiating the spirits (*diwata*) through offerings and rituals (for example, a child who becomes ill after playing under a big tree may require the services of a *diwatahan*, since the Cebuanos believe that spirits live in trees and they may be angered by the child's playing there); (4) the *spiritista*, a medium who treats illness by making conjurations to spirit doctors, saints, heroes, or dead ancestors; and (5) the *mananambal*, who treats illnesses attributed to sorcery, as aptly described by Lieban (1967).

The third kind of folk healer, the *mananabang*, specializes in midwifery, which is essentially a female "profession," although there are a few men in this field. Because of their vital role in reproduction, we shall accord this group of folk practitioners a lengthier discussion than the other two.

The Mananabang as Reproductive Practitioner

The word *mananabang* means "one who helps." In the Cebuano culture, it is specifically applied to those who help during births. *Mananabangs* may be licensed or unlicensed. Researchers are not at all consistent in their use of the term. Some apply the concept to unlicensed folk midwives only; others use it to encompass both the licensed and the unlicensed practitioners. Insofar as the poor Cebuanos are concerned, both types are called *mananabangs*. Hence, in the absence of a less confusing alternative, we shall follow the folk usage.

To become a licensed midwife, the *mananabang* must complete an eighteen-month training course administered by the government, pass the examination given by the Board of Examiners for Midwives, and obtain a certificate of registration issued by the Board of Examiners, which requires a nominal fee. In spite of the free midwifery training program established by the government, a number of *mananabangs* still fail to take advantage of this opportunity. Older, practicing *mananabangs* feel "ashamed" (*ulaw*) to be with the younger ones, whom they believe to be smarter than they. Also, even though the course is free, many cannot afford to purchase the "modern" equipment (such as scissors, curved or straight forceps, gloves, medicine kit, syringes, and sponges) to replace their improvised bamboo instruments, even if they were to do it by installment. Finally, those *mananabangs* who can afford to buy the equipment often find themselves without money to pay for the permit after they have passed the course. They become what is generally called "trained but unlicensed" midwives.

How important the *mananabangs* are in Cebuano reproduction can only be inferred from published statistics, however imperfect these may be. The following figures obtained from the City Health Office show the total number of births in Cebu City and the types of attendants, for the years 1961 to 1967 (see Table 6.1).

On the basis of these figures, at least one researcher (Damo, 1969) has concluded that the role of the *mananabang* in reproduction is not important. It is easy to understand why such a hasty conclusion can be drawn, since the table shows that at the very most, the *mananabang* handled only 18 percent of the deliveries during the reported period. Physicians delivered nearly three-quarters of the reported births in some years. Nevertheless, the fact that these figures, collected from Cebu City, represent only a partial picture prompted us to investigate whether the same proportion of birth attendants would prevail for the province of Cebu, or for the Philippines as a whole.

TABLE 6.1

REPORTED BIRTHS AND TYPE OF ATTENDANT,
CEBU CITY

Year	Number of Reported Births	Type of Attendant (Percentage)			
		Doctors	Nurses	Licensed Midwives	(Unlicensed) Mananabangs
1961	12,954 (100.0%)	63.0%	10.0%	9.0%	18.0%
1962	13,209 (100.0)	64.1	10.0	8.6	17.4
1963	13,138 (100.0)	64.7	11.2	10.1	14.1
1964	15,537 (100.0)	56.0	16.0	11.4	16.6
1965	15,435 (100.0)	59.0	16.4	12.4	12.1
1966	17,036 (100.0)	72.4	9.3	8.7	9.7
1967	18,747 (100.0)	73.7	6.9	7.6	11.9

Source: City Health Office of Cebu City, courtesy of Damo (1969:5).
Note: The percentages may not add up to 100 because of rounding.

Table 6.2 shows the type of practitioners who delivered the lastborn child for our survey respondents. Hence, it may be taken to reflect "recent" trends, since all the women we sampled were still in their childbearing years. For all age groups, physicians play a leading role, followed by the unlicensed *hilot* or *mananabang*. Age breakdowns show that the overall distribution is not drastically affected by the women's ages. However, if one were to follow the folk concept of *mananabang* at the time we did our study—which does not distinguish between licensed and unlicensed midwives—then, in every age group, about half of the lastborn children of our respondents were delivered by nonmedical folk practitioners. The older the women are, the more likely it is that their lastborns were delivered by these traditional birth attendants.

TABLE 6.2

ATTENDANT AT BIRTH FOR LASTBORN CHILD

Lastborn Delivered by	*Total Cases (N)*	*Social Class*				
		Urban			*Rural*	
		Upper	*Middle*	*Lower*	*Middle*	*Lower*
All age groups	2,358	76	506	1,133	73	570
Physician	1,012	68	365	514	21	44
Nurse	63	0	19	28	8	8
Licensed midwife	500	0	75	289	22	114
Hilot or *mananabang*	674	1	27	247	21	378
Others	109	7	20	55	1	26
15–24	302	4	45	166	9	78
Physician	134	4	33	88	0	9
Nurse	14	0	3	5	1	5
Licensed midwife	69	0	6	40	4	19
Hilot or *mananabang*	83	0	2	32	4	45
Others	2	0	1	1	0	0
25–34	1,172	25	246	571	35	295
Physician	552	25	204	288	13	22
Nurse	23	0	3	15	3	2
Licensed midwife	247	0	30	137	11	69
Hilot or *mananabang*	325	0	7	118	8	192
Others	25	0	2	13	0	10
35–45	884	47	215	396	29	197
Physician	326	39	128	138	8	13
Nurse	26	0	13	8	4	1
Licensed midwife	184	0	39	112	7	26
Hilot or *mananabang*	266	1	18	97	9	141
Others	82	7	17	41	1	16

Table 6.2 also shows the rural-urban difference in child delivery. While the urban lower class are able to avail themselves of physicians' care, the rural dwellers must rely rather heavily upon the *hilot* or *mananabang*, especially the lower class. Disturbed by the thought that we had undersampled the rural segment of the Cebuano population because of formidable field conditions, we conducted a search through several major libraries in the United States, hoping to find data that could give us another look into the role of the *mananabang*. Our efforts yielded some useful information, which is presented in Tables 6.3 and 6.4.

For the province of Cebu, Table 6.3 shows that unlicensed midwives attended more reported births than any other type of attendant for every year between 1967 and 1973. Fewer reported deliveries were handled by licensed midwives than were assisted by physicians. To understand the magnitude of the *mananabang*'s role in Cebuano reproduction, one needs to group the licensed midwives in the tables with the unlicensed ones, since the legal distinction between the two does not exist in the original folk terminology the Cebuanos use. In so doing, one finds that except for 1971, when the *mananabangs* attended 43 percent of the total reported deliveries in Cebu, they had consistently handled more than half of all reported births.

Data for the country as a whole suggest an even more significant role played by folk birth attendants in Filipino reproduction (see Table 6.4). By and large, they assisted in the deliveries of close to one-third of the reported births ever submitted by the local civil registrars to the Manila head office. By comparison, physicians handled at most only one-quarter of such deliveries.[4] Since unlicensed midwifery is in fact an outlawed or illegitimate activity frowned upon by trained professionals and legislative bodies in the Philippines, the possibility of underreporting is great. The available figures have barely scratched the tip of the iceberg. The true situation is impossible to determine.

At any rate, this brief digression highlights the prominence of folk birth attendants. Although more systematic studies on *mananabangs* await future students of social anthropology, we shall attempt to piece together a summary of the characteristics of folk midwifery in Cebu City, on the basis of unpublished works made available to us by their authors.

By means of snowball sampling, Damo (1969) obtained the names of ninety-five *mananabangs* (licensed and unlicensed) who worked within the streets and urban barrios of Cebu City. Only nine of them were males. Most came from lower- or middle-class backgrounds. Follow-up interviews into the background of forty-four of these folk practitioners (licensure not specified by Damo) indicated that twenty-four were married, nineteen were widowed, and one was separated. Not one was sin-

TABLE 6.3

NUMBER OF BIRTHS, BY ATTENDANCE AT BIRTH, CEBU PROVINCE

Year	*Total Births*		*Attendance at Birth (percentage)*					
	No.	*%*	*Physician*	*Nurse*	*Midwife*	*Unlicensed*	*Others*	*Not Stated*
1967	47,527	100.0%	23.5%	5.2%	21.1%	37.8%	8.3%	4.1%
1968	52,219	100.0	27.9	4.7	16.3	39.1	9.4	2.6
1969	54,205	100.0	30.6	3.5	16.1	38.7	8.0	3.0
1970	54,444	100.0	29.1	4.0	16.6	41.0	5.9	3.3
1971	55,723	100.0	32.1	18.2	3.5	39.9	3.8	2.5
1972	53,101	100.0	30.9	2.2	20.1	42.9	2.3	1.5
1973	58,895	100.0	29.3	3.4	18.7	35.7	7.8	5.2

Source: Department of Commerce and Industry, Demography and Vital Statistics Division. Calculated from figures in *Journal of Philippine Statistics*, 1969–1975.

TABLE 6.4

NUMBER OF BIRTHS, BY ATTENDANCE AT BIRTH, PHILIPPINES

	Total		*Attendance at birth (percentage)*				
Year	*No.*	%	*Physician*	*Nurse*	*Midwife*	*Unlicensed*	*Others*
1965	727,653	100.0%	24.4%	6.0%	24.0%	34.9%	10.6%
1966	753,558	100.0	22.8	5.7	26.4	35.5	9.6
1967	779,673	100.0	22.4	5.2	29.1	35.1	8.3
1968	837,493	100.0	24.9	4.9	26.8	35.4	8.0
1969	887,268	100.0	25.0	4.7	26.3	36.3	7.8
1970	915,941	100.0	25.2	4.5	26.6	35.6	8.2
1971	1,248,695	100.0	19.5	29.6	18.8	26.0	6.0
1972	919,638	100.0	26.4	3.5	25.3	37.3	7.5
1973	997,766	100.0	24.0	3.3	25.6	38.5	8.6

Source: Department of Commerce and Industry, Demography and Vital Statistics Division. Calculated from figures in *Journal of Philippine Statistics*, 1967–1975.

gle. Twenty-two of them each had six to ten children of their own; sixteen had between one and five children each. Five had more than ten children each. Only one *mananabang* had no offspring.

Data on the age distribution of *mananabangs* are not available in Damo's write-up, but Demetria's interview (1969) with eighteen rural and twenty urban *mananabangs* in Cebu revealed that their ages ranged from thirty-two to eighty-four years. Over half of the total sample started their practice between the ages of twenty and forty. One city *mananabang* started doing midwifery work before she was even fifteen years old. Five did not start their practice until they were between fifty and sixty years old.

The majority of the *mananabangs* (52.1 percent of Damo's urban midwives and 55 percent of Demetria's rural birth attendants) credited their close relatives as the major source of their knowledge, followed by friends and neighbors (29.5 percent of Damo's respondents). A few claimed to have learned their trade through *tuga sa langit* (knowledge given by God through dreams), with more rural practitioners (four out of eighteen) making this claim than urban ones (one out of forty-four). In addition, four of Damo's forty-four *mananabangs* maintained that they always had this special talent (that is, the skills were ascribed, not achieved).

More than half of the forty-four urban *mananabangs* (or 61.3 percent) stated that their first patient was not related to them through kinship ties, while only a few reported that their first patient was a relative. Prolonged residence in the community where they practiced seems to be an important characteristic of *mananabangs*. Thirty of them (68 percent) had lived in the community for more than fifteen years. Not one of them had lived there for less than a year. The rest were almost equally divided into residencies of five or ten years.

The amounts they charged their clients varied, depending, among other factors, on whether it was a first-parity delivery or subsequent birth. First-child deliveries are generally more expensive than subsequent births, and the city rate is usually higher than the barrio rate. The majority of the rural *mananabangs* charge ten pesos for first-birth delivery, while their city counterparts charge fifteen pesos. For subsequent deliveries, the fee is generally about five pesos less in both the rural and urban samples. If the client's pregnancy resulted in a miscarriage, or if the client is too poor to pay, the *mananabangs* customarily do not demand any payment. In some cases, they may receive as little as fifty centavos, which is the price normally charged for folk prenatal or postnatal care. These price ranges are incredibly low compared to what one would pay in modern hospitals.

A thorough inquiry about the kinds of services these *mananabangs* offer provides us with some insights into the popularity of folk practitioners. Damo (1969) lists the types of pre- and postnatal care that were normally, occasionally, or never performed by the *mananabangs*. Ninety percent or more of them normally performed the following types of care: (1) give massage to the pregnant woman; (2) check the uterus or do something to make sure it is in the right place; (3) check the umbilical cord; (4) take care of the mother after delivery; and (5) give postnatal bath and *lihi*[5] for both mother and child. Another three-quarters or more of these *mananabangs* normally prepare for the arrival of the child, as well as prepare or supervise the preparation of special food for the mother and infant. Furthermore, about half of the *mananabangs* also engage in other types of services, such as preparing food which is good for the expectant mother (tonics), helping her take care of her other children or with housework if needed, and actually washing diapers, cooking, and doing the household chores. This contrasts sharply with the kind of pre- and postnatal care that scientifically trained physicians are willing to perform for their patients.

Damo's data also show that the midwives have a pro-natalistic orientation. The majority claimed that they never gave advice on how to avoid or delay pregnancy (66 percent), nor did they ever give advice on how to get rid of a pregnancy when the woman did not want to carry it to full term (91 percent). Available evidence also show that they do not just attend to births. Sixty-one percent of the *mananabangs* give advice on marital and sexual matters, 95 percent give instructions on how to conceive, and 70 percent counsel women on how to be good wives or how to control their husbands. Thus, as folk reproductive practitioners, the *mananabang* as a social type represents the woman's, rather than the husband's, interest. Such functions are vital in a society characterized by a pronounced double standard where women are continually faced with the threat of losing their primary wage earners to other women, and where men are perceived to be innately incapable of controlling their sexual urges when thrown in the company of women who innocently or intentionally flaunt their femininity. Hence, in their indigenous medical setting, the *mananabang* performs three essential roles: psychiatric, medical, and social. This makes it all the more important to understand their ideas about reproduction, and to appraise the potential advantages to be gained from mobilizing their legitimated functions in the folk community for family planning purposes.

To date, our sources of knowledge on the *mananabang*'s view of reproductive physiology, conception, gestation, and delivery are very limited. Rather than reproduce what has already been published, we shall briefly outline the folk conception of reproduction that Rubel et al. (1975) and others unraveled.

Folk Knowledge of Conception

According to five *mananabangs* (licensure not specified) that Rubel et al. (1975) interviewed in Cebu City, conception requires at least two acts of intercourse performed at the request of the husband. *The wife should not seek such activity*. It should not take place when she is menstruating since both the man and the woman will contract illness if they do: he from contamination with the woman's hot blood, and she from inducing the blood to flow up to her head as a result of penetration. In the process of intercourse, the man spills his *similya sa lalaki* (man's seed) or *tus* (juice) into the woman's inside. Four of the five *mananabangs* maintained that the woman also has her *similya sa babaye* (female seed) which is thinner than the man's. The couple's seeds must mix well for conception to take place. Performing the sex act three times every night for five consecutive nights increases the probability of conception, according to one *mananabang*. Nevertheless, conception may still fail to take place for assorted reasons: (1) God does not bless the sex act or the seed, (2) the man's *kabuhi* (pulsation found near the navel) is out of place, (3) the male and female seeds are incompatible, (4) seed is lost by either the man or the woman as a result of sickness or fainting spells (for the man) and lack of blood (for the woman), (5) the *matris* (uterus) is bent or low, and (6) the woman's lack of desire closes her "womb tip."

Needless to say, the kinds of treatment that each *mananabang* recommends for clients who cannot conceive varies with their attributions of etiology. A common folk method of helping conception is called "*pag-alam*," which literally means "to take care of." It consists primarily of applying manual massage to the woman's abdominal region, which will presumably push the uterus down. For this reason, it is also called *i-us-os ang matris*, which means "to lower the uterus." Conducted forcefully, this method is believed to be capable of preventing conception by blocking fertilization, since the male's substance would be easily drained out of the female reproductive system. But applied lightly and slowly, the same method can put a misplaced uterus into its proper place. To be effective, it is performed three or five days after menstruation, for three consecutive days. Either *hapas*[6] or *hampol*[7] is used as the lubricant for massage (Demetria, 1969:54).

That there may be other reasons for conception difficulty besides those mentioned by Rubel et al. is apparent in the observations noted in other unpublished works. For instance, instead of the *pag-alam*, a different treatment was recommended by an unlicensed but trained female *mananabang* to women who want to conceive but were unable to: "What you lack is love-making. You should be able to arouse your husband well enough. To prevent the semen from flowing out immediately after the intercourse, support your buttocks with a small pillow. Play with the penis and he will work stronger." This *mananabang* further claimed that she once dragged a childless couple into her room and locked them there, telling them "to work" while she stayed outside to listen (Damo, 1969).

Another *mananabang* (unlicensed and untrained) advised women who cannot conceive: "Keep patience and pray hard. No matter how long a procession is, it always winds up in the church where it started. Stay where you are and show him that you are a good wife. Be faithful even if your husband becomes unfaithful" (Damo, 1969).

Other *mananabangs* believed that sterility is caused by the hardness of the loins. This problem, they said, can be treated with a poultice made from finely shredded *dapdap* leaves (*Erythrina indica*).

After conception has taken place, it is believed that the fetus goes through two phases of change. First, it takes on the resemblance of a blood clot; this is the "beginning-of-a-child." Then, it grows bigger and bigger, sufficient to be referred to as a child. Through the nine-month gestation period, the fetus moves from the first room (*unang kwartu*) of the *matris* during the first month to the next room within the *matris* during the second month. By the third month, the fetus is a child, with differentiated human forms. Some *mananabangs* who believe that a woman's *matris* consists of three rooms (instead of two) state that during the third month, the fetus moves to the third room, there to stay and grow until ready to be born.

Normal delivery may be impeded by "falling-off" (miscarriage), induced abortion, or early birth. The *mananabangs* believe that falling-off and early birth happen only during odd-numbered months. Falling-off is attributed to disease, unfulfilled cravings, defective male seed, falling down, or being struck.

After the child is delivered, the father of the child must silently bury the *inunlan* (placenta), *lumawig* (connecting filament), and cord, preferably at night. This is to keep the child from knowing of the burial (cf. Rubel et al., 1975, for additional details).

The Mananabangs' Knowledge of Modern Contraceptives

Given the *mananabangs*' unique role as folk reproductive counselors, they are the poor masses' natural sources of contraceptive knowledge. What do they know about the different methods of birth control? The question seems so simple that one wonders why research in this area has been unusually sparse. Yet at the turn of the decade, such questions could only be asked clandestinely, for the general attitude of most people was (and still is) pronatalistic. Unlicensed *mananabangs* who must protect themselves against being prosecuted for illegitimately practicing midwifery could not afford to increase their risk further by admitting that they know of any way to *prevent* conception or to arrest the growth of an unborn child. To do so would mean that the gap between knowledge and use could be bridged easily. Consequently, all we can do here is piece together information scattered in a few unpublished works and one published paper.

Damo (1969:52) asked 41 of her urban *mananabangs* for their knowledge of birth control, and obtained the answers in Table 6.5. The table shows that very few *mananabangs* were familiar with the "Western-scientific" methods of contraception. Only three appeared to claim knowledge of either the Pill or "tablet." Strictly speaking, the latter is a different contraceptive device whose application and effectiveness differ from those of the Pill. Hence, the actual number of midwives who knew about the Pill is most likely fewer than three. A careful rereading of Damo's paper confirmed this suspicion. Only one woman *mananabang* was described as having prescribed Lyndiol and Femenal, local brand names of the Pill (1969:55). Most claimed to know of "other" birth control procedures, and only seven maintained that they knew about the rhythm method. Exactly what they knew about the rhythm method, and how well they really knew that method, can be gleaned from the verbatim illustrations provided by the following *mananabangs*, one of whom is male and the other female. The male midwife advised that if a couple wants to prevent conception, intercourse should be limited to the first two weeks after menstruation because that is the sterile period. He explained: "The woman would not get pregnant because the semen of the man would not be able to fertilize the eggs. At this time, the ovary is closed. There should be no contact anytime before the menstrual flow because the egg is on its way out and might be met by the sperm." The female midwife had different advice which would probably produce the same results as the previous counsel if followed to the letter: "Intercourse should be confined to the period immediately before the menstrual period. Should intercourse be done then the man should withdraw before ejaculation to prevent his "dirt" from entering the woman. *A woman is sterile during the second week after menstruation* [emphasis added] and immediately after the first postpartum bath."[8]

We lack precise empirical data as to what "*after* menstruation" means. Casual observations indicate that to some people, the phrase means after the cessation of the menstrual flow; to others it means the onset of the menstrual cycle. In both cases, however, the proverb that "a little knowledge is dangerous" could not be more appropriate.

The fact that a majority of the *mananabangs* who worked in the city

TABLE 6.5

MANANABANGS' KNOWLEDGE OF BIRTH CONTROL

Method	*Number of Mananabangs Claiming Knowledge*
IUD	3
Pill or "tablet"	3
Foam	0
Withdrawal	2
Abstinence	3
Rhythm	7
Abortion	3
Others	17
None	3

Source: Courtesy of Damo (1969).

professed knowledge of "other" birth control methods deserves further consideration. A review of the literature suggests that, indeed, a cultural repertoire of folk contraceptive procedures and abortifacients does exist, even though the masses are predominantly Catholic and many folk practitioners stressed that it is sinful to use them.

Cultural Repertoire of Folk Contraceptive Methods

There is a much greater assortment of folk contraceptive methods than the limited array of modern scientific devices. They range from manual, herbal, and chemical applications to inanimate objects. Some substances are for external use only, others are to be consumed, and still others may be used both ways.[9] Among the external procedures are:

1. *Pag-alam* or *i-us-os ang matris*—forceful and painful massage applied for thirty minutes in the woman's abdominal area, for three consecutive days. Some *mananabangs* maintain that it should be done right after menstruation; others recommend two or five days later; and still others claim that it can be performed on any day.

2. *Lisu-on ang matris*—literally, "to turn the *matris*." It entails unidirectional massage (either to the left or to the right) for the purpose of "tipping" or misplacing the uterus. Three such sessions are needed to be effective, but they do not have to be on consecutive days. As in *pag-alam*, coconut oil is used as the lubricant in the massage. Both this and the preceding procedure are commonly recommended by *mananabangs*. Their widespread use is surpassed only by that of the *bato-balani*.

3. *Bato-balani*—believed to be magnetized stone. It is placed in a small cloth pouch which is worn around the belt as a *habak* (charm) for as long as the woman does not wish to conceive. It is believed to be so powerful that unmarried women should not even possess it, for it can cause permanent sterility.[10] The *mananabangs* believe that it works by weakening the sperm or preventing the sperm from being active, and also by "eating up the egg-producing cells of the woman." This is the most widely used contraceptive device in Cebu, equally popular in both rural and urban areas.

4. Tablets—referred to by *mananabangs* as "the brand usually only used by prostitutes" which they said can be purchased over the counter in drugstores (Demetria, 1969). By inserting one tablet into the vagina before intercourse, a woman can prevent conception because of the toxic effect of the pill. Through our own intensive interviews, we found that the tablet most often used is Cortal, a locally produced aspirin product. Hart (1965) mentioned that, besides aspirins, quinine is sometimes used in its pulverized form.

5. *Asin*—the common (coarse) "table" salt used in cooking. If a pinch of salt is placed on the woman's navel, the man's semen will presumably "pass out" of the woman's reproductive system, like urine.

6. *Panaktak*—a plant (*Rhinacanthes nasuta*) that folk practitioners claim is found only in the forest of Antique, Iloilo. Its bark or leaves are pounded, heated, and then placed in a cloth pouch tied around the waist like a belt. It makes the semen "drop out" of the vaginal canal.

Rubel et al. (1975) mentioned two other techniques for preventing conception without resorting to sexual abstinence. One technique is for the woman to urinate frequently after sexual intercourse, thereby expelling the man's seed before it mixes with her own. The second method is for the man to remove his organ from the woman's *pwirta* ("door") before he expels his seed or for the woman to kick him away at the appropriate time.

Similarly, for internal consumption, the miscellany includes herbal and chemical substances as well as inanimate objects, soaked in water. These are:

1. *Bato-balani*—a special stone which is soaked in water that is then drunk *before* intercourse. It appears that the decoction may be imbibed by both men and women (Hart, 1965).

2. *Asugi*—described by one *mananabang* as "a small solid object found in electric bulbs and radios," but a sample obtained from a *mananambal* by Demetria shows it to be mercury. The word *asugi* means mercury in Cebuano. It is prepared by soaking a few drops in water, and drinking the water but not the *asugi* itself. This will presumably "magnetize" the semen.

3. *Essencia Maravillosa*, or *Crown Essence*. According to Deme-

tria, this is a common liquid medicine sold in drugstores which is usually taken for stomachache caused by constipation and indigestion, and is also used as a laxative during epidemics. This is taken three times a day at mealtime, for three consecutive days, starting three days before a woman's menstruation. Its effect is to make the semen "pass out" of the vaginal canal.

4. *Panaktak*—the seeds of the *panaktak* plant (*Rhinacanthes nasuta*) are steeped in water and the decoction is drunk by the woman before intercourse.

All the thirty-eight rural and urban *mananabangs* whom Demetria interviewed professed to know some folk contraceptive methods, but most maintained that they themselves do not use them[11] because it is against the will of God to delay or avoid pregnancies; because they are financially able to support the number of children they have; and because they are concerned about side effects, physical or psychological, which always accompany these techniques.

If they did give contraceptive treatment, the majority of the *mananabangs* charged fifty centavos only; others charged as little as ten centavos. The *habak* (charm) costs more (about four pesos) because it must be procured from a *mananambal* who in turn charges a mark-up to the *mananabang* (Demetria, 1969:88).

When queried as to the actual effectiveness of these folk methods of birth control, the *mananabangs* were quick to ask, if they were not effective, why have they lasted for so long, from generation to generation?

Folk Abortifacients

The assortment of contraceptive methods just described is surpassed only by the diverse abortifacients that researchers (Demetria, 1969; Damo, 1969) have uncovered—as many as thirty-seven. They range from internal intrusion to external pressure; from the use of herbs and chemicals to the use of inanimate objects. Briefly summarized, these methods are:

1. *External applications with herbal concoctions.* The bark of the *kalamungay* tree (*Moringa oleifera*) is scraped, pounded, wrapped in a banana leaf, heated over a slow fire, and placed in a cloth pouch which is then tied around the waist (directly over the abdomen) or attached to the sole of one foot. Its strong odor supposedly poisons the fetus, causing it to be discharged together with the menstrual blood.

2. *External pressure.* There are four different ways of using this method, all of which involve the application of very strong pressure directly on the woman's abdomen so as to crush the fetus.

a) The first technique is called simply *kumot* (meaning "to squeeze"). In some areas, the person who performs this procedure (called the *mangungumot*) is referred to as *berdugo sa mga anghel* (executioner of angels). It requires repeated forceful massage on the woman's abdomen, using coconut oil as the lubricant. A strong and sudden squeeze is made in the final stage of the massage to force internal bleeding.

b) A variation consists of using a poultice (*hampol*) made from the bark of the *kalamungay* tree (*Moringa oleifera*) and applying it on the woman's abdomen *after* the forceful and sudden squeeze.

c) A third way is to give the woman an ergot tablet after the squeeze, instead of using the *hampol* or poultice.

d) The last technique requires the use of a thirty-six inch bamboo pole, which is placed on the woman's abdomen while she lies down in supine position. Weight is applied to the pole by having four or five persons sit on it.

3. *Internal intrusions.* Foreign objects or substances are inserted into the woman's body to induce abortion. Four such objects or substances have been identified:

a) Catheter. Any of the commonly used tubular medical devices is inserted into the vaginal canal to scrape the uterus and detach the fetal membranes from the wall.

b) Wire. Any ordinary wire cut into the desired length is sometimes used, if a catheter is not available.

c) Fingers. One *mananabang* claimed that by letting the fingernail of her ring finger grow, she is able to reach into the uterus and "break the bag of waters . . . [then] pierce or scrape the walls of the uterus with her fingernail" (Demetria, 1969:66).

d) Enema. *Essencia Maravillosa*, a laxative, is heated and infused into the rectum, after the woman has fasted. The hotter the enema, the more effective the abortive action is believed to be. It is recommended as soon as the woman misses her period.

4. *Chemicals.* Chemicals are better known to urban *mananabangs* than to rural midwives. The following drugs or substances, when taken in large doses, are believed to be abortifacients: Cortal (brand name of a locally produced aspirin), quinine, ergot tablet, *Essencia Maravillosa*, paregoric, and alcoholic drinks. In addition, *asugi* (or mercury) mixed with water and drunk every morning for two weeks is also believed to have abortive effects. Finally, *apog* (lime mineral), mixed with water and boiled, is believed to be effective but only during the first month of pregnancy.

5. *Use of inanimate objects.* The presumably magnetic stone, *bato-balani,* is either soaked in water for at least a day or ground before it is mixed with water. The solution is believed to be powerful enough to induce abortion.

6. *Herbal preparations for internal consumption.* The roots, barks, seeds, or leaves of a number of plants, when prepared according to instructions, are felt to be capable of effecting abortions. Among these are:

a) The roots of *kalamungay* (*Moringa oleifera*), *kumintang* (*Lochnera rosea*), *humay* (*Oryza sativa Linn.*), *gabon* (*Blumea balsamifera*), *dita* (scientific name not known), *panaktak* (*Rhinacanthes nasuta*), *malbas* (*Abutilom indicum*), and *bangkal* (*Nauclea orientalis L.*) —each of which is considered to be an abortifacient.

b) The bark of *panaktak*, *margos* (scientific name not known), *kalachuche* (*Plumiera acuminata*), and *panghushos* (scientific name not known).

c) The seeds of *kabalingga* (*Brassica integrifolia*).

d) The leaves of *gabon* (*Blumea balsamifera*).

e) The roots and bark of *kalachuche* (*Plumiera acuminata*) mixed together.

f) The roots of *atay-atay morado* (*Gratophyllum pictum*) mixed with *apog* (lime), or *gabon* leaves mixed with lime.

g) *Camias*, a mixture of herbs peddled on the streets. It is mixed with water and boiled. The preparation may be drunk as it is, or fortified with liquor, the common brands of which are Siok-Thong or Kulafu.

h) The leaves of *gabon* may be combined with *ampalaya* (*Momordica charantia Linn.*) and *bangkal* (*Nauclea Orientalis L.*), or the roots of *gabon* and *tubli* (*Derris elliptica Roxb.*), and the leaves of *ahito* (*Tagetes erecta Linn.*), *mustasa* (*Brassica integrifolia*), and *kumintang* (*Lochnera rosea*) may be combined into one preparation.

7. *External pressures combined with herbal consumption.* The use of either the *lisu-on ang matris* or *i-us-os ang matris* massage techniques combined with drinking decoctions made from either the roots of *kumintang* (*Lochnera rosea*) or *gabon* (*Blumea balsamifera*), some *mananabangs* believed, could abort even a four-month-old fetus.

The fees charged for abortion are much higher than those for contraception. Herbal preparations ranged from ten to twenty pesos. But generally the client is encouraged to secure the ingredients herself after the *mananabang* has given her the instructions for preparation.

For all manual methods (such as squeezing or massage), the lowest fee in both rural and urban Cebu was thirty pesos, going as high as sixty pesos in some cases (Demetria, 1969:89).

By far the most commonly known method of abortion is the use of *kalamungay* roots and *kumintang*, followed by the squeezing technique. There is almost no difference between the rural and the urban practitioners in this regard (Demetria, 1969). Rubel et al. (1975:140) described a rather gruesome squeezing procedure for abortion in late pregnancy which apparently involves reaching into the woman's reproductive system and breaking or cutting to pieces the fetus. "The arms, legs, etc. are then forcibly pulled out." Accordingly, *mananabangs* who perform abortions are called *makapakuha* ("the removers"). Damo (1969:56) has noted that they do not make any distinction between legal, therapeutic and illegal abortions. Furthermore, she found that:

> When the word was broached before the informants, a feeling of contempt and fear of the word was pictured on their faces. They say that they would rather not have anything to do with abortion, but further probing showed that if necessity arises, they knew of other persons who would perform the job. . . . Some even knew of ways of aborting a child but still would refuse to do it. . . . However, others believe that teaching a method (to a client) is a paler shade of evil.

Demetria (1969) learned that most of the women who seek abortions are the "mistresses of some rich men in the city" or students from the schools clustered in the city. Generally, a verbal agreement is struck between the *mananabang* and her client who seeks an abortion. Most women reportedly abide by their promise never to reveal the *mananabang*'s identity so that she will not be apprehended. The most widely employed strategy is to have the woman take an ergot tablet as soon as she starts to bleed, and ask her to go home. From then on, the patient is on her own. If she still has her senses, she can go to the local hospital for emergency treatment, labeling her sufferings as due to an accident.

Because any procedure which is capable of aborting the fetus is also capable of harming the mother, death from profuse bleeding or infection is a common outcome of abortion attempts, and the *mananabangs* are not unaware of this risk.

When we examined our survey data on fetal deaths, we found that strangely enough, there is very little social class variation in the percent of fetal deaths reported by the Cebuano respondents we interviewed. Among the rural respondents, 21 percent of the middle class as compared to 19 percent of the lower class reported having had one fetal death. Among the urban respondents, 22 percent of the lower class, 20 percent of the middle class and 21 percent of the upper class women admitted having had one fetal death. Moreover, an additional six to seven percent from each social class in the urban sample, and four to six percent from the middle and lower classes, respectively, in the rural sample had had two fetal deaths.

Considering the wide gulf between the rich and the poor, and the vast differences between the urban and the rural sectors of Philippine society, this finding came as a surprise to us. Most research in the United States shows that fetal death rates tend to be higher among the poor and the underprivileged because of material deprivation, inadequate health care, and other disadvantageous environmental factors.

Furthermore, it is noteworthy that the percentage of women who gave no information on fetal deaths is highest for the urban upper class (7 percent) and the rural middle class (5 percent), than for the other classes (2 percent each). These differences may or may not be significant. But since our data on fetal deaths is arrived at by summing up the number of women who reported having had a spontaneous or "accidental" abortion, along with those who candidly admitted to having "done something" which might have caused the expulsion of the fetus, it is understandable why certain classes of respondents may be less reluctant than others to answer our questions on this topic. Sampling variability aside, we know for certain that because of the restrictive sexual mores in the Philippines, our inquiries into such a sensitive subject have uncovered only the tip of the iceberg. We are reminded of an interview case involving a politician's wife who had unusually long gaps between the births of her children. Persistent probings by the interviewer revealed that the couple was neither physiologically impaired nor using any contraceptives. However, the wife reported having used "hot water enema" whenever she missed her period. That, she explained, was used "only" to regulate her period.

Implications for Family Planning

In the very brief time during which family planning programs have been established in the Philippines, much attention has gone into the demography of contraceptive knowledge and use, so that nearly all research in this area is still aimed at obtaining the percentages of acceptors every year. The findings have been consistent: while the number of acceptors looks encouraging, the dropout rates are also substantial. Our own findings in Cebu have been indirectly confirmed in Laing's more recent National Acceptor Survey (1973:150) where he reported that nearly half of all bona fide acceptors in the Philippines can be expected to terminate the use of their first contraceptive method within a year, and that about one-third stop using any kind of contraceptives at all. He further estimated that more than 20 percent of acceptors are likely to become pregnant within a year after acceptance, and 30 percent of these pregnancies occur while the first method is still in use. It is obvious that an overemphasis on family planning *methods* alone will not be adequate in dealing with the population growth of the country.

More specifically, our intensive interview data highlight the importance of children to male-female roles, and underscore the existence of competing folk paradigms of sexuality, reproduction, health, and illness which frequently subvert the effective utilization of modern contraceptive methods. Our review of published and unpublished literature shows that in disseminating contraception information, scientifically trained physicians and nurses face additional competition from folk practitioners who function best in a *gemeinschaft* environment by serving not only as healers and midwives, but also as psychiatric counselors. Even though only a small percentage of respondents from each class appeared to have given the untrained *mananabang* as the source of contraceptive information, the fact that in rural Cebu (which we have undersampled)—and in the rural Philippines—folk healers may be the only source of medical care makes them potentially powerful resources in the community. Rather than driving them underground and keeping the fatalities of folk contraception and abortion attempts unknown, efforts should be made to educate these folk practitioners in a non-threatening way. Reducing the family size of the poor will make a significant difference in the overall aggregate growth of the country, and it is the poor who are forced to use the services of folk practitioners in their search for ways to cope with their rapid succession of births.

Given the present state of economic underdevelopment and sociopolitical struggle, perhaps no other health practitioner has quite the same opportunity for disseminating knowledge of family planning as the *mananabangs*. They are established members of the folk community who are sympathetic to the problems of women in a sex-segregated society with a strong double standard, and they know from experience the frustrations of poverty. By tradition they have been the ones to whom the lower and the lower-middle classes turn in times of illness and family crisis. Now that there is growing mass awareness of a population explosion in the country, new responsibilities can be added to the *mananabang*'s traditional roles, in order to strengthen the effectiveness of family planning programs.

Our observations from this chapter lead us to redirect our focus away from the individual woman and her contraceptive methods to marital and extramarital relationships, as well as family and kinship networks, in order to understand how the individual woman and her family have coped (and will continue to cope) with successive pregnancies and family-building processes.

7 / Marital Relationships

Of all the variables that have been brought to bear on fertility studies in general, marital and extramarital relationships are by far the most enigmatic. On the one hand, the technical competence of demographers and sociologists has illustrated how particular age cohorts, religious groups, or social classes contribute to high fertility. Applied to highly industrialized societies which manifest uneven contraceptive motivations and systematic variations in the fertility rates of different subgroups, such sociodemographic analyses have produced enlightening results. On the other hand, in preindustrial societies where modern contraceptive technology has had only a brief history, and the poor and the not-so-poor alike so far appear to share more similarities than differences in fertility outcome, the continued application of sociodemographic techniques is not only myopic but unproductive. What is needed is not an explanatory model for religious, cohort, or class differences in fertility outcome, but insights into the meaning of reproduction for men and women who, as husbands and wives or as illicit lovers, produce babies. Unfortunately, the curious omission of conjugal relationships in major fertility studies has not been sufficiently balanced by Rainwater's fine description (1960) of working-class sexual behavior and attitudes in the midwestern United States, primarily because in the years following the publication of his work, writings about empirical findings in this area have generally been more substantial than the findings themselves. In this and the following chapters, we shall discuss what we know and do not know about marital and extramarital relationships in the central Philippines, and ponder their significance in family planning decisions and fertility outcome.

Conjugal Relations Through the Revealed-Difference Method

In an effort to analyze the quality of conjugal interactions among families characterized by varying degrees of motivation and effectiveness in contraception, one of the staff on our Cebu Project experimented with a total of forty-five families who were specifically screened for this purpose from the urban respondents included in the survey phase of the study (Hutchison, 1970). The original intention was to select from among a group of highly motivated contraceptors two types of families: those which manifested low effectiveness despite their high motivation, and those which showed great effectiveness. This, however, turned out to be infeasible because the number of highly effective couples, particularly among the urban poor, was too small to allow for anticipated sample attrition and to control for other relevant variables (such as social class, age, years married, and knowledge of contraceptive methods). Consequently, an alternative design was employed to compare (1) *middle class* couples who exhibited high motivation but varying effectiveness (MhEh vis-à-vis MhEl), and (2) *lower-class* couples with varying motivations but consistently low effectiveness in fertility outcome (MhEl vis-à-vis M1El). From these four groups, it was possible to examine *interclass* differences by comparing the lower-class MhEl group with the corresponding middle-class group.[1] Conjugal interaction patterns were measured by means of the revealed-difference method (cf. Strodtbeck, 1951) and content analysis by a panel of Cebuano judges trained specifically for this purpose.

Briefly, the procedures involved: (1) presenting to a couple a series of short stories, each posing a problematic situation and offering two possible resolutions; (2) asking each couple to indicate independently their preferred solution; (3) on items where they disagreed, asking the couple to discuss the issue and reach an agreement, and (4) having these discussions tape-recorded and content-analyzed by Cebuano research assistants trained in Bale's Interaction Process Analysis (1950).

The sophistication and complexity of the research design did not produce the kind of conclusive findings we had hoped for. Many of the expected relationships that Hutchison hypothesized turned out to be statistically not significant. Nevertheless, the results are highly suggestive for future investigation, especially in the light of some of the findings that did surface. Among these are: (1) effective husbands rated significantly higher than noneffective husbands on the quality of encouragement they give to their wives; (2) positive affect in the interpersonal relationship between spouses did not significantly discriminate between the highly motivated and the low-motivated families, nor did it differentiate the highly effective group from the low-effective one; and (3) lower-class husbands were rated significantly more powerful and more domineering than middle-class husbands.

Since the research design was not meant to validate a causal sequence between interpersonal spouse relationship and fertility behavior, we cannot conclude from these findings that couples are effective or ineffective at controlling their family size *because* the husbands are more encouraging or more powerful and domineering. As Hutchison

(1975:157) sums up: "We may only say with some degree of confidence that certain interaction patterns are associated with particular groups and spouses, based on the three distinguishing criteria of social class, family size limitation effectiveness, and motivation to attempt contraception."

Pondering the implications of these results further, Liu and Hutchison (1974) noted that a major stumbling block in spousal interaction research is our acceptance of the widely held assumption that the process of problem-solving between family members is no different from that occurring among nonfamily members cast in an impersonal conference setting. In the now well-known Phases Hypothesis in small group research, Bales and Strodtbeck (1951) argue that problem-solving processes begin with orientations and information exchange, followed by socioemotional acts which end in mutual support, status-raising, and tension-releasing acts. Thus, in the course of deliberation, the whole spectrum of affective and hostile feelings, along with low-key and cool arguments, is evident. In applying this paradigm to family problem-solving processes through the revealed-difference method, scholars have neglected to take into account the extent to which familiarity and habituation among family members may in fact "short-circuit" the series of acts Bales and Strodtbeck delineated. They have also equated communications about instrumental and impersonal problems with communications about sex and contraceptives. Yet, it is obvious that even within the context of U.S. society, the opportunities for a child to learn to communicate verbally about sex are rare compared to those which deal with day-to-day issues such as family purchases, leisure time activities, or school work. For some members of the lower class, the opportunity to deliberate and make choices about a variety of issues in their day-to-day experiences may even be absent. This may account for the common observation that inability to articulate a point, lack of persuasiveness, and an inordinate proportion of socioemotional acts in relation to instrumental acts are common with lower-class respondents (cf. Strodtbeck, 1964, for instance).

After reviewing Hutchison's data on spousal interaction, Liu and Hutchison (1974) concluded that one of the salient features of communication ineffectiveness in family planning is the inability of the individual to shift perspectives, to argue on a more abstract level, and to relate a concrete problem to the generalities of a moral dilemma. There is, in addition, a minimum degree of empathy and understanding in asking pertinent questions regarding the issue, and in somehow balancing socioemotional acts with instrumental acts in the process of deliberation. Two illustrations from the Cebuano tape-recorded protocols collected by Hutchison (1970) are presented to demonstrate this point:

Case 1. *Discussion of Who Should Use Contraceptive*

H: The wife should use birth control methods as it's easier for her. She can buy pills and take them. It is difficult for the husband. I don't think there are pills in the drug store that's for the men.

W: The husband should be strong-willed enough to control because the wife . . . there are times when the husband really insists . . . it should be the husband's role to control.

H: If the husband can't control. This is difficult.

W: For me, I think it should be the husband so there's no disagreement about controlling because . . .

H (interrupts): It would be easier for the wife. She'll just consult the doctor and take the medicine.

W: That is, if the husband agrees to control.

H: Yes, I agree.

W: Then there is no problem. So long as you agree . . . husband should be the one to control so there would be no problem.

Case 2. *Whether or Not to Contracept*

H: I would still go on having children. I don't want to use any form of birth control because that's a sin.

W: But you can also practice birth control without using any form of birth control like the pills as long as the parents come to an agreement. They themselves should control because if they add one more to the five children and if the wife is weak . . . in the nine months when the baby is growing inside her, she won't be able to nourish the baby until she gets sick . . . she will die because she can't take it.

H: If it's not using birth control methods, that would be all right. But if you use, I don't agree because that's a big sin before God.

W: That's why. The couple should come to an agreement. They agree to stop producing children as the wife is weak and can't go through another pregnancy.

H: That depends on the agreement. The husband would be crazy to allow for another child if the wife is so weak.

W: But if the husband goes on . . . he doesn't take notice of the wife's weakness.

H: There is no husband who would do that if he sees that his wife is not fit to have another child.

W: Five is enough for their family. If you add one more, the wife, especially if they're poor, can't bear it because she is so weak. It would be all right if they were rich and they can get all the doctors . . . but they are poor. The wife will die as she can't stand the labor in giving birth. What do you think of that?

H: It depends on the conditions of the husband and the wife.

Even though these are only specimens rather than representative samples randomly drawn from the Cebuano population, the material is convincing. There is, for instance, a clear indication of the couple's inability to assess a problem sharply, to engage in rational deliberations, to take the perspective of the other person during a discussion, and to make alternative suggestions about how they might cooperate and understand the problem.

However, the problem of communication about contraception does not end here. For family planning to be effective, there must be clearly stated goals and perceived choices. Our data from Cebu show that many couples perceive family size to be in the realm of "heredity" or "God's will" and hence beyond human control. To the majority of preindustrial lower-class families, therefore, the psychological ecology is as restricted as their geographic mobility and life chances.

From the viewpoint of social change, the functional relationship between effective communication and better family planning has been erroneously identified as unidirectional. Yet, it may be heavily influenced by prevailing sex-role expectations which on the one hand predicate husband-wife relationships on the principle of egalitarianism but on the other hand support a strong double standard of sexuality. Aside from this, changes in household composition, the woman's life cycle, the husband's occupational mobility, and the couple's family size and patterns of spacing, among other things, are also likely to lead to a redefinition and readjustment of conjugal role relations and to an alteration of family planning decisions. Thus, the attempt to measure conjugal interactions through the revealed-difference method has raised more questions than it has answered. What, for instance, are the similarities and differences in the style of conjugal interactions in joint decision-making between traditional societies and industrial urban groups? How do couples resolve differences and handle hostilities in different societies? What are the ideally conceived and the actual conjugal interaction patterns under various economic conditions? How do couples align with other members of the family in the process of interpersonal bargaining in general? How do couples make calculated decisions, singly or jointly, about family size and child-spacing? We do not pretend to have a set of packaged answers to these questions, but a preliminary understanding of Cebuano marital and family planning behavior can be gleaned from our intensive interview data.

The Expression of Conjugal Affection

The expression of conjugal affection is one aspect of marital relationships that is most difficult to measure quantitatively since it lies in the interstices of personality and culture, the idiosyncratic and the normative. In the Philippines, this difficulty is compounded by the obvious contradictions of beliefs and practices which allow women to achieve equally with men in certain occupational roles (cf. Hunt, 1965) but at the same time deprive them of the sexual latitude granted to men. Yet, to give up entirely all efforts to understand how conjugal affection is expressed by individuals sharing a sociocultural milieu because it is difficult to measure, is to abandon the precious insight that can be gained from even the most rudimentary attempts at collecting such data. Without doubt, we owe much of what we now know of Cebuano conjugal affect to the persistent probes of our field interviewers, one of whom succeeded in eliciting the detailed remark below from a lower-class respondent:

> *L:* It is not kissing and hugging that prove a couple are "loving" to each other. It is how much you *uyon* [agree] with each other. Many couples are very "loving" outside, *nag-agbayay, nagaparaeg ang babaye* [they put their arms on each other's shoulders, the woman is demonstrative in displaying her affection], but when they reach their house, *sus! Karambola!* You can hear plates being thrown at each other, *sinumbagay* [boxing], shouting because they are selfish and they don't understand each other.
>
> A very "loving" couple is *watchful* of what the other wants and needs, and what the other does not want. Each one should avoid doing what the other does not like. What one wants, the other should try his or her best to get or accomplish for the other.
>
> If there are problems, the couple should understand each other very well, and come to an agreement. Each should give in to the other sometimes. If I say I want a thing bought or done or decided, but I see he does not quite like it, I give in to him; if he first makes the suggestion and sees that I have second thoughts about it, he gives in to my reason. We do not *sumpaki* [argue furiously]. We never had a big quarrel. Whenever there is a difference between the two of us, I talk to him about it, and he sees the disadvantages or weaknesses and we agree. Likewise, if there are things I like but he does not like, he talks to me about it, and I agree with him. *Nobody is above the other. I don't think anybody should be above the other.*
>
> However, if one party is doing a really bad thing, like a husband's drinking or any other vices [such as gambling or women], and nobody can stop him, the spouse should let it go at that and avoid useless quarreling for the sake of the children and for some peace at home. It is firstly the wife who should talk seriously to the husband about changing his ways. If she is not successful, she can ask her husband's parents' help. If they are far away, she can write to them. Then their parents can come and *ayos* [settle things].

Although this woman is uneducated and has no occupational skill, she is able to describe succinctly the traditional Cebuano conception of an ideal husband-wife relationship (shared more strongly, we suspect, among those who came from the rural areas than among the westernized younger generation in large metropolitan cities). Several conjugal role expectations embedded in her lengthy remarks deserve additional emphasis here:

1. There is the belief, common to the older (middle-age) generation, that public display of conjugal affection, especially kissing, is not an absolute requisite of marital relationships and is at best a superficial gesture which does not necessarily represent the couple's backstage behavior or inner feelings.

2. There is also the Cebuano conception that the key factor in a happy marital relationship is the degree to which a couple agrees with each other. If there are problems, they should try to understand each other's viewpoints, and they should try to be flexible. (But as we shall see in point 8, the wife is expected to do most of the adjusting.)

3. There is also the clearly stated idea that a couple who are truly in love with each other should be sensitive to or "watchful of" each other's wants and desires.

4. The ideal quality of the husband-wife relationship is based on an egalitarian principle whereby "nobody is above the other" rather than founded on a sexist premise as it is in the Chinese patrilineal family.

5. *Sumpaki* (to argue furiously) is a far less advisable approach to marital problems than talking. Communication—verbal rather than sexual—is highly emphasized and greatly valued, at least by the female respondents.

6. In the face of serious spousal conflict where the habits or preferences ("vices," as this woman puts it) of one partner have become detrimental to the functioning of the conjugal unit, the matter should first be settled by the couple themselves.

7. Where intervention into marital discord is deemed necessary, the preferred candidates for the role of mediator are the parents or guardians of the spouse whose behavior is perceived to be the source of the conflict.

8. Finally, if all efforts to settle the matter are in vain, and the guilty party persists in his actions or behavior, the spouse (presumably the wife) should simply condone or endure the situation. Quarreling under such circumstances is considered to be fruitless. A high priority is placed on the children and on "peace at home" over the hurt feelings of the spouse (presumably the wife).

The importance of conjugal role performance over public display of affection is apparently felt by a number of our respondents, for when they were asked how feelings of love and devotion are communicated in their marital relationship, their remarks reveal considerable flexibility on the part of the husband in household task performance. Consider for a moment the following comments:

> *L:* I know my husband loves me by the various mainfestations of affection he displays. When the children were small, he used to get up in the middle of the night to change their wet diapers, because he wanted to spare me this

trouble. And he laundered the baby's soiled clothes. Before he leaves the house for work, he sees to it that there is enough wood and water in the house to last till he comes home and is back with us again. Sometimes on his way he passes by the market and buys some rice and other household needs.

L: My man has managed to be very helpful around the house. He fetches water, feeds the pigs, chops wood, and does other things that require carrying weight and exertion of effort. For my part, I cook the meals for my husband and children, clean the house, wash the dishes, the dirty clothes, and other things that require time and feminine ability such as sewing, repairing worn-out clothes, going to the market. . . . Whenever I can, I buy the food which my husband likes very much at the *carenderia* [store]. I usually just buy enough for him and for the children because of economic reasons. I myself do not eat this food because I want them to eat it. And I would behave in such a way that my husband would not notice or realize that I did not eat it, because I know he would mind if ever he finds out I am sacrificing for him this way.

L: When he comes home from work, and he sees that we don't have any water in the house, he would walk [one block] to fetch some water for me. My neighbor, Kiskis, would say "*Gikan na sa trabajo, karga pa'g tubig*" ["He just got back from work, and now he is out fetching water"]. But my husband would reply: "It is like this only because there is nobody here to *sugo*" [send around to do this errand]. Sometimes when he comes home and I am trying to chop some firewood, he would take it from me because I was not getting anywhere with my chopping. The *bolo* [cleaver or knife] always *untol* [glances off] the wood I want to cut. Some of my friends say to me: "If my husband were like your husband, I would be very happy."

L: My husband is a very good father and husband. He gives me all his salary and is always home for lunch even if he should be on duty [at the police station]. If he is at home he helps with the children in their homework, and there are times also when he helps me with the dishes, especially when I have a lot of dishes to do. *But we are not fond of showing our affection outside the bedroom for fear of influencing the children* [emphasis added]. We are still very loving and affectionate toward each other, and growing more so every day.

L: I know my husband loves me because he does not maltreat me. Whatever I ask from him, he always grants. If I have my moods and pout, he is anxious to know what is wrong and asks me what the matter is. He entrusts all his salary and only asks me money for his needs. I show my love for him by eating with him after his work even if I am already full when he arrives. I cook his favorite food. If he does not feel well, I massage his back. I call him by his nickname, and softly too. *I always abide by his wishes.*

L: I don't want to say it [affect toward husband], because he might become arrogant or he might abuse my feelings. But I show it [affection] by *attending to his needs*, prepare his food, bring it to him whenever he is not able to come home for lunch, fetch water for his bath because he is too tired to do that. I also do errands for him, like buying some cigarettes for him.

Note that the husband's willingness to turn in all his income and to assist the wife in her household chores is consistently identified as a positive sign of spousal affection, whereas the woman expresses her love by attending to the man's "needs" which, defined broadly, do not exclude the sexual aspect of married life. Being unskilled, the woman cannot possibly intrude into the man's work world as a way of expressing her affection. Her able performance of maternal and wifely duties thus becomes the logical expression of her positive feelings to her husband. From the few husbands who were at home during some of the interviews, we were able to obtain the male perspective and confirm our interpretation. The following statements are typical among the husbands:

> *H:* ______ [Wi] is a very understanding woman, a good wife and a good mother. I cannot recall an instant in which she denied me anything that I like or needed. . . . I am not sexually aggressive because I tire easily.

> *H:* I feel the same toward her now as I felt toward her when we were newly married . . . I trust her, I give her all my earnings and always ask leave when I go out. When I come home I inquire about her work. Before leaving for work, I assure her that I will take care of everything.

Among the middle class, too, egalitarianism in household task performance and the wife's faithful attendance to her husband's "needs" is a common way of expressing conjugal affection:

> *M:* He does not distinguish between which chores are his, and which are mine. When he sees me tired from laundering and ironing, he doesn't think twice about helping me. . . . He even bathes the children, helps with the cooking, tidies up the house and makes little repairs here and there. . . . My husband always accompanies me whenever I go out to buy something, even if it is only a pail or a pair of slippers or any small item.

> *M:* He helps me clean the house, tend to the children. Sometimes I think the children are closer to him. The children don't go out of the house when he is around. He looks for them first thing he gets home. I often tease him that he doesn't even look for me. He looks for the children instead.

> *M: Pinangga kaayo ako* [He loves me dearly]. . . . We both believe that we should be equal; all major decisions should be made together and even in minor household matters, we should help one another as much as possible. We share many tasks together. He often does the cooking, even though we have a maid. We relax together mostly. . . . He helps me when I need help with the children, he plays with them as well as disciplines them. He fixes things around the house. I don't know what I would do without him; he is always around when I need him. He is simply wonderful. In fact, I often tell him he is better than I am. I often wonder how I would manage without him.

> *M:* I show my affection for him by showering him with attention whenever he gets home, and *see to his needs myself*. . . . He is not demonstrative; he never grew up with love [being an illegitimate child] because he was alone most of the time with no family to care for him.

> *M:* We show our love and affection by respecting each other . . . know what each other would like, and would not like . . . adjust to each other . . . do not

take the other for granted. . . . Thoughtfulness is important. [He] calls me up when he can't come home at the time he is expected to, and [tells me] where he is. . . . I buy him his personal things, [and] *attend to his other needs.*

Even though couples from the lower and the middle classes rarely mention public display of conjugal affection, it would be incorrect to say that overt gestures are totally absent from Cebuano husband-wife interactions, for some couples do hold hands when they go shopping or take a walk in the city streets. Others put their arms around their spouses. Yet, even for such relatively mild gestures of affection, the couples are not free from onlookers' gazes. Women more than men are especially sensitive to the reaction of others around them:

Q: Does your husband show affection toward you in the presence of your children?

L: Yes, he makes *paraeg* [overt gestures of wanting affection] and _____ [oldest girl, aged nine] would laugh and say: "*Agbay-agbay na sad si Papa da. Ah, Papa da!*" [Gee, Papa is putting his arms around Mama's shoulders again!] Sometimes the children (who sleep with me) will send him out of the room if he comes to me early in the morning [husband sleeps in the kitchen for contraceptive purposes] and the children are wide awake.

M: He [Hu] shows more affection and demonstrates this [by] hugging me in other people's presence. For my part, I act passively to his outward affection.

L: Sometimes my husband shows his *paraeg* in front of the children. The children would laugh and make fun of us. It's because we are both old already [wife is forty, husband is forty-three] and maybe the children find that out of place when my husband is demonstrative in his affection.

M: He is very sensitive; if I fail to hold on to him or take his hand when we cross the street, he gets mad. And I am not joking either. He always accuses me of taking things for granted or that I am ashamed to show the public that he is my husband. Of course that is not true. But he insists on those little things. Sometimes I refuse to do it on purpose because *I am so ashamed to act romantic in public* [emphasis added], but he would not hear of it. As a matter of fact, it was only lately that he acceded to my request not to address each other the way we used to. We used to call each other by a pet name, "Chim." This is a Chinese [Hokkien dialect] word for "kiss." After some years of marriage, I felt so embarrassed being addressed that way and calling him "Chim," so one day I told him to stop it, and I gave him my reasons. But it took some time before he finally acquiesced. Now, it is only in his letters [that he sent me] whenever he is out of town on a job that he signs his name "Chim." Oh, you should see my husband!

The obvious disparity in the socioeconomic background of the respondents notwithstanding, there is a strong hesitation, especially on the part of the woman, to disclose her affection publicly and directly, either for fear of rendering herself vulnerable since the husband may "become arrogant and abuse" her feelings, or for fear of shame and ridicule from onlookers, their children included, who are not used to such outward gestures of love. References are constantly made to the husband's parental role and his willingness to perform traditionally women's work around the house as the primary criteria for determining the intensity of conjugal affectivity.

Thus, while the American notion of conjugal love is defined in terms of the marital dyad (Hsu, 1969) to the exclusion of other family relationships, and at the same time supported by the subordination of other familial dyads to the marital bond, the Cebuano husband-wife relation—as expressed consciously by the men and women we interviewed—does not signify the same degree of exclusivity. In fact, for most of the Cebuanos interviewed, *the husband-wife relationship is not sufficiently differentiated from the parent-child role constellations.* The former bond allows for and does extend lineally to include generational linkages. To do something for the children is to show affection for the spouse who helped conceive them. This is more pronounced for the lower class than for the middle class, since the economic stability of the middle class enables them to rely upon the institution of housemaids (Brandewie, 1973) to isolate parental obligations from conjugal roles, at least to a certain extent. For the lower class, poverty and the inaccessibility of gainful employment opportunities is interwoven with the *inclusivity* of conjugal relations.

The Meaning of Pregnancy to Wives

In the Cebuano culture, the conjugal system faces constant competition from the male *barkada* (informal peer group) system, especially in the early years of married life when the husband can afford the time and resources to stay away from home, simply because he does not have "too many" children to care for. Such an attitude is taken by many women as an affirmation of the belief that children solder the conjugal bond. Although the husband may be delinquent in fulfilling his spousal role, the coming of a child, especially the firstborn, is often sufficient to bring him into line. At the very least, it is reason enough for the wife to demand that the husband for once "accept" his responsibility as a married man and father (or father-to-be). Some husbands have been known to stop their heavy drinking as they prepare to become fathers, or as they begin to realize the grave burden of caring for large numbers of children; others have at least temporarily (though not always successfully) put a stop to their gambling or other vices. Comments such as the following are not unusual:

> *L:* The birth of our first child brought us together, much closer than before. Before his birth, my husband would stay away [from home] the whole day. He took his time in returning home from work, stopped at his friends' houses and played basketball. But when the baby came, he put a stop to this. . . . He literally ran home from work; brought me my favorite food. It is really different when we have children. *They bind us closer together.*

> *M:* My husband was very happy when our first baby came. Our relationship has been smoother than ever.

Pregnancy, then, has a special meaning in the Cebuano context. It entitles women to certain privileges and gives them a legitimate claim on their husbands' time and resources. A pregnant woman is considered a delicate creature whose physical and emotional state must not be upset lest it adversely affect the unborn child and result in a pregnancy wastage. Being pregnant, therefore, is far from being inconvenient or undesirable, as illustrated in comments such as these:

> *M:* I am *pinangga* [well-loved] and cared for by my husband and parents whenever I am pregnant. *Everybody adjusts to me, tries to please me.* My husband brings me to our doctor [which he doesn't do normally]. His reaction [is] very happy. My parents, when it rained, would send someone after me with an umbrella. My husband would never say anything to contradict me then. Now when I say: "Dad [term of address for husband], let's go to the movies" and he tells me he is tired, I say to him that *I wish I were in the family way; I am well loved only when I am in the family way.* Even now, I tell him this.

> *L:* [Husband] used to help around the house, *especially when I just delivered a baby.* He washed the diapers and served me food. He is a very attentive man when one of the family gets sick, especially when it is one of our children who gets sick. [Husband has been gambling again lately.]

Regardless of social class, parents or parents-in-law who live nearby "fuss over" the pregnant woman. Folk measures of precaution are generally undertaken to protect her:

> *L:* I was then two months pregnant. I was told by Mama [HuMo] not to go out if it is already six o'clock, so that I would not get gas pain. Mother fussed over me so much . . . she taught me how to rub my belly with oil treated in ginger roots to prevent gas pain and keep the evil spirits away in case I do step out of the house by chance. They say that a pregnant woman is always sought after by *mga u-ngo* [the witches] because the blood of the fetus and young children is fresher.

Husbands are more tender and gentle when the wife is pregnant. They avoid doing things that might irritate their wives. They take over more of the household chores, especially the heavy ones, and are the first to relent in conjugal squabbles. The following comments of some lower-class husbands are representative of the general attitude of most men we interviewed:

> *H:* I feel the same toward her now as I felt toward her when we were newly married—*even more attentive and concerned when she is pregnant* [emphasis added]. I always warn her not to work too hard, to take care of herself so that she won't catch cold or get sick. I also take over the household chores to give her some rest. I babysit for the other children, cook, and fetch the water from the public pump.

> *H:* I have always been the one to prepare breakfast so that my wife can rest longer *especially when she is pregnant.*

In some cases, not altogether rare, the birth of a child may infuse the marital relationship with a certain degree of affection where none existed previously. Recall that one of our respondents was in this predicament:

> *L:* I hated him and I had no affection for him at all. I used to sleep between the floor and the mat so that he would not find me. I could hear him asking his mother where I was. I started to pity him only after ______ [first child] was born. The child looked very much like his father so that when I look at my baby, I see my husband and that's when I started to pity him.

What is interesting about this family is that (according to our interview records) the husband's mother was most concerned that the wife was not pregnant "soon enough," and had used her skills as a *manghihilot* to massage the wife's abdomen in the hope of bringing about pregnancy right after their marriage. The first child was born exactly a year after their marriage, to the relief of everyone concerned. Its birth marked a turning point in the wife's attitude toward her husband. She gained access to his full paycheck, which was formerly submitted to her mother-in-law living nearby. She came to expect conjugal fidelity and parental responsibility from her husband as well. Here is how the respondent describes her mother-in-law's diligence in "putting the wife's uterus back in its place" after every delivery so as to make her body receptive to additional pregnancies:

> My mother-in-law is the *manghihilot* of the community. I do not really get pregnant if she does not massage me. You see, my uterus sags below its normal position, because I am the athletic type. It is impossible for me to get pregnant without the *hilot.* After every childbirth, my uterus sags back to its former place, so my mother-in-law has to massage me after every delivery to put it back in its right place. My mother-in-law wants me to have children, because this is the first time that she has grandchildren. But I want this pregnancy to be my last. I have a feeling this is going to be a painful delivery. I have been thinking of using the IUD, but I am afraid I might get cancer. Anyway, I don't get pregnant if my mother-in-law does not massage me. I will just not let her touch me anymore.

With a reproductive rate of six pregnancies (five live births) in eleven years of marriage, our interview record reveals that the mother-in-law still feels, and the wife herself is convinced, that she is not fertile.

That the presence of children solders a weak conjugal relationship is clear to many lower-class women we interviewed. One respondent offered the following words of wisdom:

> *L:* If there are no children, there may be no happiness in married life. Even the rich when they quarrel and they don't have children, separation almost always takes place.

Thus, children are vital links in the Cebuano conjugal unit. Given the unequal economic roles of the sexes, the birth of a child can assure the woman a "claim" on an economically productive man, however underemployed he may be. The more children she has with that man, the greater is her "claim" over him, and the less likely is their spousal relationship to be terminated quickly in the face of marital discord. Where the conjugal unit has not as yet established a separate domicile, the presence of a large number of children is a good reason to establish a neolocal household.

Conversely, the less certain a woman feels about her marital relationship, the less eager she may be to keep her pregnancy. Children, born or unborn, can also be used as a "weapon" to hurt the husband or his significant kin. It comes as no surprise, then, that a pregnancy wastage (or a near loss), particularly if it is the couple's first pregnancy, does lead to conjugal fights. One woman recounted her first quarrel with her husband as follows:

> *L:* We were already quarreling even when I was five months pregnant with our first child. I participated in a neighborhood dance and I started to bleed. He hit me because he thought I would lose the baby.

The significance of her husband's reaction stems from the fact that he was more interested in making their relationship "permanent" during the initial period of their marriage than she was. Hence, he was keenly interested in having a child to seal the union.

In another case, a premarital pregnancy resulted in a shotgun marriage, which the husband resented. Although the circumstances are unique, use of pregnancy or pregnancy wastage as a "weapon" to hurt certain key figures in the family or to protect oneself is not:

> *M:* I was so hurt by the way he [Hu] acted in just the few months that we were living together. [Husband was out almost every night with his *barkada*, and he made it known to her that he was having one *querida* after another.] I wanted to make my *panimawos* [revenge] on them [husband and his relatives], one which could hurt all of them very much.

The respondent decided to seek an abortion even though she was in the fifth month of her pregnancy. She paid a hundred pesos to a physician in the city. True enough, her husband and his family were very hurt.

They were also furious. The husband, with the explicit approval of his family, hired a private detective (paid for by his father) to investigate the matter because he did not believe the wife's alibi that she fell off the stairs while wearing a pair of wooden slippers. The respondent describes their reactions as follows:

> *M:* I was pressured by everybody. The first who came was ______ [HuSi], she was so angry and she accused me that I did not really want to have the child for fear that I would be found out that it was the child of another man. She thinks I had a low reputation and had so many boyfriends before [husband], that I also pressed him into marrying me because I was pregnant, and that I married her brother because I was after their wealth. All these I took without saying anything to contradict her for I knew I would not have a chance to give my side [of the story].
>
> The next one to come was my father-in-law; with him was the detective. He [father-in-law] did not say anything all the time that he was there, but the way he looked at me was enough to make me *kurog* [tremble in fear]. It was the detective who did all the interrogations, which I answered negatively.
>
> Then came my mother-in-law, who tried to convince me that nothing will happen to me if I will just tell the truth. But I was able to convince her that it was accidental, and since she is a very sentimental woman and sympathetic, too, she believes me.
>
> My relatives, on the other hand, were on my side and did not scold me for what happened. *My mother thought it was a waste [ka-usig] for I could have made the baby a bridge between me and my father-in-law.*
>
> I think she was right. That was the only thing that made me regret what I did. I wouldn't have suffered so much if I had used my right judgment. But I was not in my proper state of mind at that time, but was only blinded by jealousy toward my husband and spiteful toward my father-in-law. I wanted to make my *panimawos* [revenge], one that would really hurt them.
>
> *Q:* What would have happened if they had found out then?
>
> *M:* If he [Hu] knew before just right after it happened, I guess you would not be interviewing me now, for I could have been jailed for it, for murder, especially at that time my father-in-law was just waiting for a slight mistake that I would make and I would be like what they used to say at the end of a story: "*Nahulug sa lim-ao, dayong katunaw*" [like something which has fallen into a lake and disappears].
>
> *Q:* What do you think would happen if they find out now?
>
> *M:* If they find out now, I know I would be ostracized by everybody, even my own relatives. And I don't want to be away from my children, and above all, I don't want to hurt my husband, now that he has regained his confidence and trust in me. Maybe I'll just take my life if ever I find out that they know. [Probe.] I think God will forgive me [for committing suicide] for the sake of everybody's reputation, *nga dili sila ma-uwawan* [that they will not be shamed].

The respondent's story does not end here. The harsh interrogation that she suffered under her husband and her in-laws, and the marked distrust that they displayed, left her with a deep sense of anxiety and a great deal of uncertainty. Her husband avoided her sexually. And whenever he had relations with her, he did it brutally. After the pregnancy wastage:

> We had intercourse only very seldom, and that was usually when he was very drunk. The result of it would just be a failure on his part, for he couldn't finish, because he would sometimes fall asleep on top of me. I felt like throwing him off, but I calmed myself down for fear that I would only be maltreated if I did so. [Probe.] Of course, I felt insulted and dejected. I could not reprimand him also, or say anything about what had happened the night before because I feared that I would only be more insulted.

In view of this, she decided to take the Pill for the next four years after her first pregnancy, in order "to wait and see" if her relationship with her husband and her in-laws would improve. It was only when she felt that her husband had changed his ways that she decided to stop using the Pill. Everyone was jubilant over her subsequent pregnancy. Unfortunately, three days after the child was born, it died from suffocation. Her husband and in-laws were extremely angry. They suspected that the respondent played a role in the child's suffocation. Careful investigation soon revealed that it was due to the negligence of the attending nurse at the hospital. Through the father's influence, the nurse was immediately fired from her job.

A year later, she had her third pregnancy because, she said:

> *I had to stop using the Pill to make up for what happened and to prove to my husband and my father-in-law especially,* that I was not at fault, and *that I was still capable of begetting more children.* This was followed by another boy a year after but it seems that they were still not convinced of my innocence. I began taking the Pill again, because I had given up hope of "getting back" my husband. Then, I got pregnant two years later [after the fourth pregnancy]. It was only after the birth of this baby girl [fifth pregnancy] that my husband gave back his confidence and trust, and my father-in-law and ______ [HuSi] started to be friendly with me. Three years later, another boy came, and then I started on the Pill again. This time for good, because I still feel so insecure although they are all friendly [to me] now.

There is little doubt that this woman's reproductive history is intimately related with kinship pressure and tensions, even though coresidence with relatives is absent. The first pregnancy was aborted to avenge her anger and resentment at being so contemptuously treated by her in-laws and so patently rejected by her husband. The second pregnancy was deliberately delayed on account of the sexual brutality displayed by her husband. She had her second conception only after she felt a certain degree of hope in her marital relationship. Unfortunately, the nurse's negligence brought her much sadness, and revived her husband's and in-laws' distrust. However, having recognized the wisdom of her mother's advice that a baby might "bridge" the gulf between her and her father-in-law, she quickly became pregnant for the third time. Her uncertainty as to her husband's and in-laws' attitudes toward her prompted her to continue with the Pill once more, but only for a little over a year. One pregnancy followed, and another. The last one, being an only girl, caught the fancy of her parents-in-law. They always sent for her on weekends and holidays to keep them company. Needless to say, the respondent was very pleased. Nevertheless, she confided that since her last delivery, she had again started taking the Pill, because she still feels very insecure in her marital relationship and with her in-laws. She said: "I am poor and I seem not to fit anywhere in their family. I still believe that a time will come when my husband would leave me for another woman much better looking and richer than I am."

In spite of her feeling of insecurity, her children—particularly the only girl—have succeeded in "bridging" her relationship with the in-laws. Their social visits have become much more pleasant. The husband's parents are also paying for her children's education and some incidental expenses.

These case histories, though anecdotal, illustrate the meaning and function of pregnancy to the woman and affirm the general belief that children solder the conjugal bond as well as bridge relationships with in-laws. The next step is to analyze the meaning of pregnancy to the man.

The Meaning of Pregnancy to "Responsible" Husbands

In a society where sex roles are distinctly defined, it would be unusual for pregnancy to carry the same meaning for both sexes. Pregnancy entitled the woman to a "claim" on the man who fathered her child precisely because her economic role, if she works, is socially defined as secondary to all the other roles which have been assigned to her. Marriage, therefore, is a convenient mode of improving one's status and acquiring economic security. The presence of children prevents the marital relationship from disintegrating too soon. To the man, pregnancy symbolizes his willingness to "accept the male responsibility," which inevitably calls for the fulfillment of his prime adult role: that of breadwinner. To the extent that each child is an economic cost, the number of children that a man is able to support becomes a rather sensitive indicator of his financial capability—hence, of his competence in performing his economic role—not to mention the numerous social advantages of a large family that may accrue to him. Just as the number of *queridas* (mistresses) a man has attests to his virility, and the number of *querida* households he can underwrite reflects his financial status, so also does the number of children affirm his economic competence.

Given this world view, some husbands—particularly those who perceive themselves as "socially very responsible men"—are not likely to be receptive to artificial birth control. There is evidence that such men interpret the use of contraceptive devices as an open admission of their inability to perform the one vital role that every dignified adult male should carry out. When such a world view is coupled with a rich traditional folk wisdom regarding the natural order of the cosmos—and hence, the harmfulness of artificial human intervention in the inherent order of the body—one would expect that such husbands would not only resist artificial birth control, but would find it unnatural as well, if not morally reprehensible.

Consider the case of Cesar, a forty-nine-year-old lower-class husband. The series of events in his life and the kind of choices he has made convince us that he sees himself as a very affectionate, thoughtful, and responsible provider. Briefly, this is how he describes the series of events in his life: "I left Cebu for Manila as a trainee for the [U.S.] Army [in the Philippines]. After the training, still some two years before the [second world] war, I was a Philippine Scout and lived in Fort McKinley. After the war, I stayed in Manila with my wife and children until I resigned from the Army." The reason for Cesar's "resignation" was that after the war, Philippine Scouts were given the option of joining forces with the Americans and moving to Guam with an assurance of continued employment there, or remaining in Manila and receiving an allowance of U.S. $120, plus a four-year technical training course, but without assurance of reenlistment for active duty. According to his understanding, the first choice required that members of the Philippine Scouts' families stay behind in the Philippines. They were to send for the immediate family only after they had adjusted and found suitable settlement in Guam. He rejected this option because he did not want to leave his wife and two children, especially since his wife's parents had opposed their marriage—not because of any blemish in his character, but because he is from another province, Cebu. His wife is from Batangas. Furthermore, Cesar felt that the possibility of receiving an education paid for by the U.S. government was a golden opportunity. Even if he went to Guam, he felt that aside from the pain of separation from his family and relatives, he could never be completely assured of lifetime employment, since he had had a very limited education. If he stayed behind, he would receive an education that "no person can steal" from him, and besides, there was the possibility of reenlistment. He was confident that, being a hard worker, he would eventually be reenlisted.

With these thoughts in mind, Cesar received four years of training in radio mechanics, a specialization he chose because that seemed like a very promising technological product to him. After his training and prolonged waiting for his application for reenlistment, he found out that by not moving to Guam he had lost his chance to reenlist. He decided to look for alternative employment. It was at this time that he learned from his sister's husband in Cebu about a vacancy at his place of work, a large Filipino manufacturing company. He applied and got himself a job. Because he knows some English, and also because of his industriousness, he "rose up" in the company very quickly to become the personal chauffeur of Mr. Quirino, the owner of the company. He was well liked by his boss's family, and his relationship with the company owner took on the quality of a "patron-client" relationship. The nature of their relationship is best captured by his wife's statement:

> The house in Basak [where they stayed for three years after they moved from Manila to Cebu] was just as large as this *sala* [living room]. We divided it into two, for Lucio's family [HuBr] and ours. We shared a little space like that doorway for the kitchen. Lucio's children all had the measles and we all got it. When Mr. Quirino heard that I followed people's advice that measles is not a case to bring to a doctor and so caused the death of my baby, he scolded me and my husband. He came with a doctor to see us. The doctor continued to see us until we were all well. [He was paid by the Quirinos.] Then, two children were born [to us] in Basak. Pregnancies are nothing remarkable or new to our relatives. *They said anyway, we could afford many children* [emphasis added]. This time, not a *mananabang* but a head nurse delivered our babies per instruction of Mr. Quirino. One more baby [was] born in Hipodromo [where they eventually moved and established an independent household], [and] was delivered by a head nurse paid for by Mr. Quirino. At that time, Quirino had no hospitalization plan for his workers and there were some complaints [from Cesar's co-workers] that we were receiving special attention. But when my husband had to be operated, Quirino spent for everything at the Velez Hospital and continued to pay my husband's salary until he could work again. Later, the factory already provided for some hospitalization for the employees.

This warm, personal relationship made him the envy of their relatives on both sides of the family. To them, he is a man with great economic stability who has the proper "connections" to influential individuals, especially since he has been employed by the Quirinos since 1953. Cesar is the first person they approach when they are looking for a job or when they get into trouble with the police (for traffic violations, or loss of license due to careless driving in their capacity as chauffeurs). Their kinship interaction is characteristically one-sided. Apart from his cousin, Cesar avoids seeking the help of his better-off relatives, especially his father's stepsibling's stepchildren who had "insulted" them by refusing to lend them two pesos in an emergency. According to Cesar's wife:

> My husband does not go to any of these relatives for any kind of help. You see, my husband is . . . er . . . *ma-ulawon*" [a man with great sensitivity and

> feelings of shame]. And we have nothing to return for help we receive [*walay ikabalos*]. Also, you can never know what they'll say to others about you. Good if they'll just refuse you but if they give [assistance] and then say to others: "Just because I have plenty (*abi kay adunahan ako*], they keep coming to me." My husband tries to avoid this. Good if you could know whether the person you go to knows how to pity you; whether he can think thus: "Let's just give this one because he is *makalulu-oy* [to be pitied]. He has many children. We should give because we have bigger salaries." Good if it is like this, but if not. . . . That is why when we are in need, my husband just begs help from others [*maghangyo nalang sa uban*]. We have to pay these people, yes, but little by little, as we can afford.

Because of their large family size (thirteen pregnancies, twelve live births), the husband's work, and a certain degree of economic independence, the family seldom pays social visits to their relatives. This is how the wife describes their kinship interaction:

> I don't go visiting, and neither does my husband. He would rather stay home, tinker with his radio, teach the children and just read [the Bible, and old reading material which he picks up from his employer's trash]. Not that we feel superior to others. I, for example, have too much work with so many children. There is no time to visit people. . . . Fiestas, we have no celebration. On Christmas, we do go to Camp Lapu-Lapu [where Cesar's cousin lives]. That's all.

Both husband and wife have been able to cultivate friendship ties, which later developed into fictive kinship ties as these friends became the godparents of their twelve living children. The wife feels that their life has been very satisfactory and their hardships minimal (despite some reverses in health and finances) because her husband possesses an enviable trait: "the durability of the meek and friendly," as she puts it. In other words, he knows his position in life and is friendly to others.

On top of that, the husband feels that there is an inherent order in the nature of things: man can only do so much, and the rest is up to Divine Providence. For this reason, the husband never thought of contraception. Children, he feels, should be accepted as they come. They are a part of marriage, and besides he likes the idea of having many children. His wife did not offer much resistance, since she came from a big family and all her relatives desire a large family for themselves and for her. The following dialogue conveys the general perspective of the wife and her relatives:

> *Q:* During your first few years of marriage, how many children did your relatives think was a good number?
>
> *L:* Many. So that if some cannot help with farm work, there will still be others. Well, they [many children] are expensive, true, but even if life is not easy, *mabuhay man din* [we managed to live happily].

> *Q:* After you had three or four children, did you feel an additional burden with the coming of the next one? Were there new difficulties experienced in money or chores with the coming of a new baby?
>
> *L:* Perla, my younger sister was with me until two months after [my] delivery. My mother and father decided [that Perla should do] this so that I won't have a hard time. After that, there's not much to do. Wash, cook. Nothing. *Basta busog lang ang mga bata* [so long as the children's stomachs are full], they are no trouble. We managed to keep them full, yes. I did not have to buy milk. Only milk for coffee. When we [adults] ate, all [the children] ate. When Perla returned home I did almost everything myself. There was nothing to it. Unlike others here, they get maids even if they cannot pay. You know, it is different here in Cebu. In our place, we don't hire maids. We do things ourselves. Here even those who cannot pay have maids.

Thus, a supportive kinship system and a preference for a large family, along with the wife's positive attitude toward housework, made her feel there was no need to limit their number of children. Only after a succession of births did the idea of contraception enter her mind. That idea was introduced by her attending physician, who suggested a ligation:

> After delivering the seventh child, the doctor [told me about ligation and] advised me that for some time after the operation, I should abstain from having sexual relations with my husband until my wounds heal, otherwise I would get sick. Upon telling this to my husband, he told me to "go ahead, *but if I cannot endure it* [abstinence], *you are going to get really sick.*"

As a result, the wife did not heed the doctor's advice. It was not until her eighth pregnancy that she started worrying about having too many children:

> When I discovered I was pregnant again, with the eighth, I said to my husband—but calmly, without anger or blame, "We have many children already." He said: "Why should you be afraid? You have a husband. *Even others who have no husband got pregnant!*"

The husband's reply is revealing: as long as there is a husband, the woman should not worry about having too many children, since the husband—as is congruent with his male role—will provide for them economically. This is all the more true if the husband is "responsible" and economically productive by lower-class standards. By asking his wife to compare herself with women who became pregnant out of wedlock, the husband provided her with a reference against which her pregnancy appears most fortunate, and her anxiety about large family size unfounded. After all, as the family breadwinner, he has never been remiss.

This attitude finds parallel expression in another lower-class family, the Cabahugs. The husband works as an auto mechanic. Both the husband and wife come from families of fishermen; she from Leyte, he from Da-an Bantayan, 128 kilometers north of Cebu. In fourteen years of marriage, they have had six pregnancies, of which one child died from bronchitis. Compared to many of his friends, the husband is "economically capable." His wife feels economically secure with him and reiterated on several occasions that she chose her husband over another suitor precisely because he was more economically stable. In recent years, he has developed a drinking habit, "acquired" (according to his wife) from constantly mingling with his *barkada*. The wife's negative reactions to his drinking did not help to change him. As a matter of fact, it might have made his drinking worse. She candidly described the problem to us:

> I sometimes would go after him, especially on weekends, as he and his friends usually go to a bar in the Pier once a week, and have a happy time with the hostesses there, dancing and drinking. I cannot help myself, maybe it is my pride as a wife, so that I would go after him, and once there, I would try to tell him that it was very late already, but he would not hear me out. So I would come home alone, burning with anger. Once he gets home, I would quarrel with him right away. *He always tells me that I shame him in front of his friends by trying to drag him home*, as if he is *under-the-saya* [henpecked]. I would try to reason out with him but the fight would just grow big, so I would keep quiet. Then for some few days, I would not talk to him, no matter how much he would try to comfort me, but with the children around, I would give in later.

The wife dislikes her husband's relatives, particularly two of his uncles (MoSiHu) who always stop by their place unannounced when they come from Da-an Bantayan. They not only stay for weeks at their place, but also take the husband out drinking—at his expense. The husband does not mind paying their drinking bills; on the contrary, he is proud of it. The wife, however, has openly shown her disgust to them and to her husband. It only increased her husband's displeasure with her. Her own relatives were not very supportive either. They felt that since she chose him herself, she has only herself to blame for making such a poor choice. As a result, the wife decided to take some measure against additional pregnancies after her last delivery (the sixth):

> *L:* I happened one day to mention to a friend who had attended a Mother's Class [a class supervised by midwives in a government clinic], her name is Sosing and what she told me was the rhythm, but she mentioned also something about the Pill . . . that I have to consult a doctor about it. After I had the name of one kind of Pill, given by the doctor, I then started to use it. I did not have any side effects, and I even grew fat because of it. The name of it is Lyndiol. I kept using it for almost two years. I never told anybody else except Tiya Piling [MoSi] and Tiya Dita [HuMoSi] because they are the only ones

whom I trust. I did not want my husband to know, because he does not approve of it. [R cautioned me not to tell the husband in the first few interviews before.] Until last May, I think I told you about what happened, he saw me taking one of the tablets and asked what it was for. I was stammering when I answered him that I had a headache, but he did not believe me. Instead [he] took the packet from my hand and read the directions, so he knew then. He threw it right out of the window and was so angry. I tried to explain why I was using it but he did not listen. We had a big fight over it and he was angry for days. Again and again I would tell him that I used it for *panagana* [for protection, in case something happens] in getting pregnant. He said: I come from a big family [thirteen siblings, with seven still alive at the time of the interview], and *if my father who was a fisherman was able to support us all, there is no reason for us not to have as many*. Besides, it is a sin to go against the teaching of the church.

Q: So how did you learn about the IUD then?

L: A distant cousin of my husband, who is a doctor, gave me advice on it. That is because I went there to ask for some other methods which I could keep from him, and because she [the doctor] is also using it, so she advised me to try using it also. My husband keeps on asking me why I am not getting pregnant anymore. He suspects [*nag-duda*] that I am using something. Sometimes in the middle of our intercourse, he would suddenly stand up and the next thing I know he already has a flashlight in [his] hand. He would use it on me, to look into the vagina. But he is not able to see anything inside. I feel so embarrassed every time he does it and at the same time afraid that, that . . . he could see it.

What is fascinating in the husband's reaction is that he is not religious at all, if one measures religiosity in terms of church attendance. He never went to church on Sundays. The only time he would go, if ever, is on major holidays of obligation (such as Christmas or Holy Days). Even that is done with great reluctance on his part, and with persistent prodding from his wife. Therefore, it is not so much the observation of church ritual that led to his resistance toward contraceptives as "unnatural," but his acquisition of a world view that is alien to human intrusions because of the assumption of a Divine Providence, and the perceived existence of an inherent order in the cosmos.

Beyond the question of religiosity is the crucial issue of economic competence. The husband feels that, compared to his father, who is "only" a fisherman, he has "achieved" some degree of economic security. If his father, with such a "lowly" occupation as fishing, could afford thirteen pregnancies and support the family without seeming difficulty, he, a mechanic at one of the largest automobile repair shops in Cebu, the second largest urban center of the country, should be able to support at least as many. Hence, there is no need for contraception. In fact, to use artificial birth control devices would simply imply that he is financially unable to support his children—an admission that would make him feel even more "under-the-*saya*." It is bad enough for his wife to go after him at the bar on weekends and reprimand him in front of his *barkada*, but to be considered as "economically unable" as well would be a blow to his masculinity; it would strike at the very foundation of his manhood. Note that the husband particularly relished paying for the drinks of his relatives even though he is not that well-off, for that gesture distinguishes him as "economically able."

Thus, we are reminded of the significance in the Cebuano culture of being a breadwinner, and what it means to a man who defines himself as *responsible* to say that he can support as many children as God wants him to have. For this type of man, using any contraceptive device would be considered an admission of his inability to fulfill the male role. In his eyes, it is the men who do not want to face the consequences of their behavior and who fail to follow God's will who will face *gaba* (divine retribution) later in life. Until family planners in the Philippines can convince this type of man that not to practice contraception is irresponsible—rather than a mark of responsibility—it will be very difficult for any contraceptive method that requires the husband's cooperation to work effectively.

Conjugal Conflict

Another way of evaluating the conjugal relationship is to examine the occurrence and resolution of marital conflict. In general, a husband who comes home late or goes somewhere without the wife's permission frequently sparks minor squabbles:

> *M:* Sometimes when he comes home late, I ask questions and when I persist and show I am jealous, he gets mad. He does not like [to hear] me insinuating. But I do not doubt his fidelity. When he is mad, he goes out of the house. He starts his motor, but I always manage to follow so that he does not leave the house anymore. But they [quarrels] are trifles compared to my joys. He still remembers my birthday and I do his. He gives me gifts. I am really happy and contented. I am grateful to God for giving me such a fine man.

> *L:* We seldom quarrel and we never had any serious conflict. Only once we did not speak to each other for two days. . . . When I went marketing I saw his things lying in a *sari-sari* [mixed goods] store and when I inquired about it, the storekeeper told me he went to a movie. I was hurt that he did not tell me about this. I did not talk to him. [How was it resolved?] He asked me why I was *naglu-od* [sulking] and I told him about the movie. He asked if I was jealous. I told him, "You should have told me. . . . We must tell each other." So he let me go to the movie and he stayed home with the children. [What other things do you quarrel about?] The children. I get mad when the children are dirty and he sides with them. But if I tell him about the children's disobedient behavior, he uses his belt on them.

> *M:* We argue about things we don't like . . . buying big items—whether we can afford them, and when [to buy them]; whether the children should be al-

lowed to go some place or not. We usually meet each other halfway. . . . Conflicts are limited to minor omissions as when he comes home late without notifying me that he would be late or where he would be. When I am deeply hurt, I just don't talk to him for days and he makes amends. . . . He makes amends by trying to talk to me more than usual. But I don't talk to him until I am ready. *Manglu-od ko* [I sulk]. For example, we planned to go out to a movie, and later he changed his mind. Then I don't talk to him, so he says: "Oh, all right, let's go." [Or] he doesn't want me to wear a particular dress and I insist. But I let him have his wish. He gets mad if his wishes are not followed. So to avoid arguing, especially in front of the children, I don't go against him. I know when to talk to him, when not to talk to him, when to leave him alone. I don't go near him when he is tired. I know. So I just pretend I am also busy. Then later on, when he is no longer tired, he will just start talking [to me]. When he is like that, I don't bother him with household affairs, like picking up the children at a party or needs of the house. When his schedule is tight, he throws his clothes when he's changing [garments], I just don't say anything and [don't] go near him. . . . I simply pick up after him.

L: We quarrel when he comes home late in the evening, especially if he goes along with the downtown express late at night, so that the following day, he cannot get up early in the morning to report to work. When I get angry, I nag and nag. But he remains cool-headed and says nothing. I continue to nag but he doesn't respond. Then I would refuse to talk to him for days but he talks to me first. He is very patient and enduring.

Only one (middle-class) woman admitted that a desire for physical affection sometimes creates minor conflict that is quickly resolved:

We don't quarrel in the real sense of the word, but we do exchange words sometimes. It is natural for every couple to have a spat once in a while. I believe that it adds more spice to a marriage, because usually after a quarrel, each would be more affectionate. . . . It is not that I am bad, but there are times when I feel a strong desire to have sex with him, and who would not be offended when he would just dismiss me by putting it off later after he has rested? I do wait, but once he is awake, he would seem to have forgotten his promise. That is the time that I would blow up, I had been nervous of waiting and then he would act like nothing happened, so I would start banging things and not answering him [whereupon] he would ask me what was wrong. Then later, he would remember and would start teasing me in a way that I couldn't get angry with him anymore and then I would get what I wanted. I know that he gets tired sometimes from his work, [and] I am just foolish, [but] I guess it is a bad habit of mine that when I want something, I must have it right away. I know this is wrong, but I can't control myself and sometimes forget that I am being unfair to him.

Money, gambling, and drinking are three more common areas of marital conflict. These problems are understandably more acute among lower-class than among middle-class respondents. Note, however, that in the following cases, wife-beating is not used as a resolution. The wife's most common reaction is to nag or scold the husband, while the latter remains silent until the wife's anger has dissipated:

L: We used to be very *bastos* [vulgar]. We would bring our fights into the streets or when we do it in the house, the whole neighborhoods turned into onlookers. I remember one time we came home late one evening. . . . He was very drunk. We had to pick our way into the house between sleeping children [in the living room] and since he was swaying unsteadily, I tried to hold him up every time he looked like he was going to stumble. That made him angry because he insisted that he was not drunk. This resulted in a big fight. I ordered the children to get up and move away. I jumped at him. Because he was drunk, I easily subdued him. My mother was with us then. I told her to go get me a rope because I was going to tie him up. My mother replied: "*Asa gud ta ug pise*" [Where would we get a rope?] I told her to get the clothesline downstairs. When we fight like that, the children would either cry or *mosiga ang mata* [their eyes would pop out]. This time they ran to their uncle's [HuBr] who came in and then I let go of my hand. I said to his brother, "You do something about your brother. He is impossible."

When he gets drunk, he throws everything, breaks chairs, my flowerpots. I get very angry at him. This has subsided through the years, probably because I got to thinking maybe he is like this *tungod sa akong pagkasaba-an* [because of my scolding or nagging]. Now when I am angry, he goes out and when he returns I don't say anything anymore.

L: He drinks, especially on payday. He gets very drunk. Last time, he spent five pesos in one sitting on drinks alone. He drinks with the guys he works with. . . . When he comes up the stairs, I can tell from his red eyes and his swaying [gait] that he is drunk. I would tell my son . . . "Look at that! Your father is drunk again!" He [son] would usually say: "*Tatay, oy!* Always getting drunk!" And my husband would always say: "No, *Do*, I am not drunk. . . ." *Sa ato pa, wala na'y ibayad sa mga utang.* [In other words, we won't have any more money to pay our debts.] And his line of defense is always: "*Saba! Saba!* [Be quiet! Be quiet!] I am going to sleep. Tomorrow we will *husay* [settle the matter]. . . . " No, I never shout at him and he never beats me. The next day, after he returns from work, he would show me a list of the debts that he just went to pay for. But that means that we have no more money left for our food and other expenses, and the rest of our debts would have to wait till the next pay check. Or, sometimes, if we are lucky, he may still have about five pesos left out of a wage of forty-seven pesos. And we would have to wait until the next payday. . . .

Another source of conflict also revolves around money. He is fond of coming home with food or other items bought on credit. It makes me mad and I would tell him: "*Ka daghan ba nimo'g utang!* [You have so many debts!] How are we going to pay for our debts if it is always like this!" His usual response is "Be quiet! Anyway, these are for everybody." Sometimes, I get so frustrated, but not angry. I just pinch him. He would holler so loud that you could hear him next door. Yes, my pinching is very painful. . . . We end up laughing at each other. No, we don't really quarrel. Only very seldom, when he gets drunk.

L: We don't exactly quarrel, because whenever I nag and nag him about his faults, he would just keep quiet and would not say anything. This fault is usually about his borrowing some money from his co-employee in the camp for his *sabong* [cockfighting]. I would come to know of it only on payday when the salary that he gives me is lacking. He never comes out and asks me if he

> wants to go cockfighting; he would just say he has to do some typing at the [police] station.
>
> *M:* [Husband's gambling] has mostly been the cause of our quarrels. While it is true that he never takes a single centavo from the paycheck he turns over to me, he keeps his overtime pay and travel expenses [travel allowances provided by his company]. I keep reminding him of his obligations to the children. It would be much better if he turned over his extra earnings so we could have some savings. As . . . the children are all growing up and they will be needing all the support we can give them. But he just dismisses me with a shrug.
>
> Our serious quarrels come about when he loses and runs out of money. So he does not have anything to gamble with anymore. Then he becomes temperamental and gets mad at the slightest provocation. This is also true in my case. There are times when I do run out of money, especially when there are unforeseen major expenses which must be met. All hell breaks loose. I blame him for all of this. *I blame his gambling and his irresponsibility.* He drinks, too, you know and that makes things worse. These are our main areas of disagreement. . . . I keep hammering on him [not to gamble, not to drink]. In better times . . . that is, when I am sure he is in good spirits and I do not have money, I just wait for him to sleep and then I run through his pockets and take out ten or twenty pesos. He doesn't mind. In the morning, he will invariably find out. In a joking spirit, he would say to me he will send his oldest son to a school in criminology [in order] to track down the thief in our house.

This constant conflict over the husband's gambling was finally resolved after about six months, for in one of our last visits, the woman confided:

> I no longer complain about his gambling. But we have mutually agreed on a condition: he does what he wants with his incidental earnings. Should an expense [for the family] come up unexpectedly, he answers for it. Like now, for instance, there is the graduation dress and new pair of shoes [needed] for ______ [daughter], these will have to be bought by him. On occasions when he runs out of money, he must find his own ways and means of solving his problem. He borrows from somebody and pays for it himself. I cannot allow my budget to be disrupted. I know that his commissions and overtime pay which he keeps amount to quite a sum. I don't take that away from him. So that now I have made it a point to tell the children to name all their necessities whenever I find out that he has won in his gambling. And when he loses, I never lend him any money. This he has to learn to live with, too.

Other families, from the lower class, are not so fortunate:

> It is usually about the amount of money that he should give me, and it happens almost every Sunday. He usually goes to the cockpit on Sundays. If ever he wins, he does not tell me about the amount [of money] he wins, but then I would find out from a friend or a neighbor who happened to be there and had come home earlier [than he did]. I would feel furious that he does not tell me the truth. Anyway, I don't ask him for the whole amount. What I usually ask for is just enough for the week's needs or sometimes a little more because of the children's tuition and other school expenses. Because I am al-

> ready angry before he arrives, I would start a fight right after he gets home. We would get into a heated argument and I am likely to say things which I regret later on. *I would insult him for being irresponsible*, but he would only become quiet and then I would come to realize that I was being cruel to him, and I would stop. In those cases where I feel gravely wronged, and talking with him has reached an impasse, I would confide in Mama Teria [HuMoSi], who would often call him in and reprimand him for what he has done wrong. [Did it help to change his ways?] No. He has not changed his ways, because he still continues on doing the things he did.

Middle-class wives, like their lower-class sisters, control the purse strings. The husband is expected to turn in his total earnings, or at least to hand in his regular paycheck and to disclose the amount he receives on the side from time to time, whether it be from gambling or legitimate sources, such as overtime pay and company traveling allowances. The wives report a twinge of disappointment—to say the least—when their husbands fail to disclose their incidental earnings, especially when such income could amount to as much as two or three hundred pesos. As long as the conflict remains unresolved, tensions persist in the conjugal bond and weaken it.

Conjugal Decision-Making Processes and Activity Styles

The woman's role in managing the household economy is supported by our survey data. Using Herbst's method (1952) of classifying conjugal decision-making processes and activity styles into seven areas (food preparation, family health care, household money spending, child control, family economic planning, children's schooling, and leisure-time social activities), we obtained the data in Table 7.1 from our urban sample in Cebu.

The most striking finding is the almost absolute control of the wife in at least three areas of household task performance: food preparation, family health care, and spending money. This finding is so uniform that in spite of the great disparity in the income and lifestyles of the rich and the poor, social class did not make any difference in decision and activity styles. In fact, from our intensive interview data, we are simply impressed by the extent of the woman's control over the family budget:

> *L:* [Hu] gives me all his salary, and he asks money from me only when he needs it. He does not have any *barkada*. Every night before he goes to bed, he drinks a bottle of beer.

> *M:* My husband turns over all his pay check to me. All he asks for is an allowance of a peso a day from which he takes his expenses for fare and snacks. In this area . . . I am proud to say that because of childhood poverty, my husband has learned to take care of his money. From his daily allow-

TABLE 7.1

CONJUGAL ROLE CONSTELLATION, CEBU URBAN FAMILIES, N = 1,521

Item	*Ha Hd*	*Ha Bd*	*Ha Wd*	*Ba Hd*	*Ba Bd*	*Ba Wd*	*Wa Hd*	*Wa Bd*	*Wa Wd*	*Social Class*
Food	—	—	—	—	—	*	*	5.7%	88.6%	upper
	*	—	*	—	*	*	*	*	83.8	middle
	—	—	—	*	—	*	*	*	85.8	lower
Health	*	*	12.0%	*	9.0%	25.0%	*	—	46.0	upper
	—	*	12.8	—	*	22.2	—	*	53.2	middle
	—	—	—	*	*	—	12.7%	24.7	53.8	lower
Spending money	*	*	6.2	5.2%	17.5	14.4	*	10.3	37.1	upper
	*	*	5.9	*	10.0	7.7	7.2	19.4	37.0	middle
	5.6%	*	6.5	*	8.3	14.5	8.6	6.8	43.9	lower
Child	18.4	—	*	7.1	33.7	12.2	*	*	23.5	upper
	11.4	*	*	*	18.0	5.4	12.0	6.8	38.7	middle
	12.6	*	10.5	*	17.0	5.1	*	5.1	14.2	lower
Economic planning	20.6	*	8.2	15.5	20.6	15.5	6.2	*	7.2	upper
	9.3	*	*	7.9	16.7	23.1	6.4	6.7	20.9	middle
	8.0	5.1%	7.6	*	15.4	6.9	*	25.6	25.0	lower
School	*	—	6.5	*	31.5	35.9	—	—	17.4	upper
	7.5	*	13.6	6.6	17.4	35.3	—	*	14.2	middle
	7.2	7.6	*	*	18.1	*	11.0	32.2	18.7	lower
Leisure	11.5	*	9.4	*	32.3	26.0	*	*	11.5	upper
	8.6	17.5	11.6	5.1	30.7	17.4	*	*	14.1	middle
	8.3	6.3	*	6.1	29.5	*	11.3	17.7	16.9	lower

Key: Ha = activity by husband alone
Wa = activity by wife alone
Ba = joint activity
Hd = decision by husband alone
Wd = decision by wife alone
Bd = joint decision

*less than 5 percent
—less than 1 percent

> ance, he [is able to] save enough to give me a birthday or Christmas gift. . . . Saturday is my husband's payday. He always asks me to see him in his office and after that we go out and buy the things we need. We do this together.
>
> *L:* My husband gives me all his salary, and he always takes his lunch at home even if he should be on duty at the [police] station.
>
> *M:* Since I get all of his pay, it is only just that I be held responsible for the budget. For small things like buying clothes and dresses for the children, I do not have to ask Undo [term of endearment for husband]. Meeting with the teachers, spending for contributions are well within the sphere of my decision-making. But when it comes to saying which school my children should go to, what course they are to take, or lending comparatively large amounts of money, I have to consult my husband. He has given me much leeway in the running of the household. He does not object to the companions I go out with. He even presses me to buy things for myself and to make myself trim and pretty and young-looking again. My husband is the romantic and caring type.
>
> *L:* He gives me all his salary. I don't inquire about his side earnings. He uses that for his allowance. He never audits the money he gives me. He only asks me to explain when I come home late, sometimes coming from downtown.

Examining our intensive interview data more closely, we found that the degree of conjugal harmony is positively associated with the wife's nearly total control of the husband's earnings. In these same families, contraception has been discussed and the husband's assessment of the desirability or undesirability of the methods known or agreed upon plays a crucial role in the couple's ultimate decision on whether or not to contracept, and on the type of methods deemed acceptable. In other words, barring ignorance of contraceptive methods, the decision *not* to contracept is born out of careful deliberation, as is the decision to contracept, and the husband's authority in the sexual and contraceptive sphere of marital activities parallels the wife's control over the budgetary management of the household economy. In cases where the wife does not have full control over the purse strings, the couple *also* has not agreed on whether or not to contracept, or on a choice of contraceptives. Even when the wife persists in wanting to prevent conception, the husband either refuses to cooperate (claiming that the method chosen could make him sick, or that he is embarrassed to purchase the contraceptives) or sabotages the woman's efforts (for example, by throwing away the Pill she is taking without his permission). In those few cases where the wife has been openly using a reliable contraceptive method, she clearly has full control over the purse strings, and her decision to contracept as well as the choice of contraceptive method was made at the urging of the husband, even though the wife on several occasions privately revealed a strong desire to have additional children. It might be worthwhile at this juncture to mention that this finding converges with Hutchison's findings from the revealed-difference method. Comparing couples who are effective contraceptive users to those who are noneffective users, he reported that the effective husbands rated significantly higher than the noneffective husbands on the quality of encouragement they give to their wives. He also found that positive affect in the interpersonal relationship between spouses did not significantly discriminate between families that are highly motivated to use contraceptives and those that are not highly motivated, nor did it differentiate the effective contraceptive users from the noneffective ones. Certainly, our intensive interview data show marked conjugal affectivity in most cases even though the couples vary in the strength of their motivation to use contraceptives, and in the effectiveness of their efforts.

The convergence of these observations, being associational rather than causal, cannot be interpreted as conclusive, but it provides interesting hypotheses for systematic verification in future studies. From our interview data, we are led to believe that a unique balance of power exists in Cebuano marital relationships whereby the cultural prescription of granting women control over the budget is matched almost evenly by the normative expectation that the husband has final authority over sexual and contraceptive matters—a power that is consonant with cultural values about sexuality and masculinity. It follows, then, that family planning education aimed only at the woman would not succeed as well as education designed to appeal to men and women, since the availability of modern contraception has the potential of corroding men's traditional control over their sexuality and this may be perceived as a threat to their self-concept. It can be argued that for lower-class husbands, whose fulfillment of the breadwinner role is contradicted by their undeniable poverty, this potential threat to their self-concept is far more real.

Returning to Table 7.1, in two other areas—economic planning (for future security) and children's schooling—the lower-class housewives display considerably more power than the women in the other two social classes in the sense that the most dominant pattern is for the wife to act on decisions jointly reached with the spouse. To illustrate, 25.6 percent of the lower-class wives act on joint decisions concerning economic planning, whereas only 6.7 percent of the middle class and less than 5 percent of the upper class have as much autonomy to act alone on joint economic planning decisions. With regard to children's schooling, 32.2 percent of the lower-class wives act on joint decisions with their spouses while less than 5 percent of the middle-class and less than 1 percent of the upper-class wives exhibit this activity style. The lower-class wife's prominence in carrying out the instrumental role in the conjugal partnership is further attested to by the large percentage of cases in which the wife alone acts and decides on matters pertaining to economic planning for future security. As a matter of fact, the difference between the dominant pattern and the major variant pattern (the second largest number of cases) in the economic planning category is extremely slight: less than 1 percent. It suggests that the dire poverty experienced by lower-class families demands a painfully deliberate budgeting of whatever meager income the husband earns. Since their incomes are almost totally expended on food and rent, with very little left over (and sometimes a list of unpaid debts) the wife acquires the power not only to act and decide on day-to-day spending, but also to act on economic planning for family security in the future, and on whether or not their children should continue schooling. For the middle and upper classes, the possibility of real and substantial savings in excess of their subsistence expenditures facilitated the husband's invasion of the wife's autonomous region, but only by acting jointly with his wife in the greatest percentage of cases on economic planning and schooling. The husband alone seldom acts and decides on these issues.

With respect to child care, both husbands and wives act jointly in the majority of the upper-class families and in a great number of the lower-class households, but for different reasons. The economic condition of the lower-class families makes joint actions and decisions necessary, since their household structure is nuclear by default. Coresidence with relatives often occurs immediately after marriage and while the babies are small. Subsequent births exert great demands for the attention of the couple since, by then, they usually have set up an independent household. Although lineal or collateral relatives may move into their hut at later stages of their family life cycle, such a coresidence pattern is constantly in flux and does not last forever. The sheer number of children born into lower-class households demands the cooperation of both husband and wife on child-care problems.

For the upper class, however, material wealth and the institution of housemaids has segregated the boring, day-to-day physical aspects of caring for children, leaving both husband and wife free to attend to "higher-order" aspects of child care, such as discipline. The couple could still act and decide on issues of child care by supervising their children's *yayas* (nursemaids) and other houseservants and by carefully screening the applicants for such roles. Children are driven by the family chauffeur or an assigned chauffeur (if there is more than one family chauffeur) to their violin or piano lessons, sports and recreational activities, or their orthodontist's, optometrist's, or family physician's office without straining the parents' energy and taking up their time. They could discipline their children's misbehavior by withholding the weekly or monthly allowance that they have agreed to provide them, or by forbidding them to take a trip to another city or to travel abroad. Thus, both husband and wife need not be involved in the mundane aspects of bringing up their children but may still be said to act and decide jointly on child care.

The financial capability of middle-class wives enables them to utilize the institution of housemaids just as upper-class people do. However, there is a limit to their financial capacity, so that the husband must constantly guard his family against slipping down the socioeconomic ladder by working very hard as a breadwinner. His sense of economic insecurity allows for greater autonomy on the part of the wife, especially in an area of household task performance that could very well be handled by the woman, rather than the man.

Finally, insofar as leisure is concerned, the dominant pattern for all three classes is for both husband and wife to act and decide on what they do. Thus, 29.5 percent of the lower-class, 30.7 percent of the middle-class, and 32.3 percent of the upper-class respondents reported that they shared decisions and actions on this aspect of household task performance. In spite of the parallel percentage figures across the different social strata, the types of leisure activities are dissimilar. For the lower class, going to a cheap moviehouse is the most common recreational activity. Middle-class respondents have a broader range of recreational choices, such as going to the beaches, nightclubbing, bowling, dining out, and other activities.

The Threat of "Other Women"

Along with money, drinking, and gambling problems, "other women," whether real or imagined, pose a constant threat to marital harmony, one that is a cause as well as a result of marital conflict. Depending on the strength of the marital bond, the conflict may be quickly resolved or may drag on for a long period, as is evident in the contrast provided by the following two cases:

> *L:* You know, we had a quarrel last night. I went to look for him at his place of work [a local radio station] and imagine what I saw, there was this young girl, not really pretty and was sitting very close to ______ [Hu]. I would not have minded if this were the first time I saw them together. Of course, I got suspicious. The girl did not look exactly like a decent girl plus all the stories I have heard about her flirtations with men in the studio, I could not wait to tell [him] about it. I confronted him right after the girl left. I'm sure she knew that I did not like her. As usual, [he] did not want to pick a fight. He just dismissed my questions by saying, "You know what's good for you? You should stop coming here to the studio. What do you get out of it? You hear gossips and you immediately believe it. You become unreasonably jealous. Had you

stayed home like I told you, this would not have happened." I said lots of things which I could not remember now and he just remained silent. If it was not this girl, it was somebody else. But somehow it is somebody connected with his job in one way or another. Most of the time, this is the cause of our quarrels.

You know this is one thing about my husband, he never says anything when we quarrel, either he goes to another room and keeps quiet or he leaves the house. Later on, after it's all over, he tells me he does not want to be bothered by fights. He would like me to understand his position. Being in radio, he says he has to reckon with the public, male or female, and that these girls don't mean anything to him. . . . In our quarrel last night I told him how *he should be grateful I got pregnant before we got married or I would have married this guy back home whom my parents approved of.*

L: During my first pregnancy, my husband had a relationship with a married woman. I do not want to mention her name because she is married and it is shameful. I knew he was carrying on with this woman, so when I learned that he was in her house, I rushed to her room and caught them making *paraeg* [overt gestures of wanting love]. We had a big fight and he knelt before me asking for forgiveness. I did not mind him for over a week.

We had another quarrel when my husband got jealous. I was selling fruits to a group of men and he accused me of having a relationship with one of them. We had, again, a big fight and he hit me on my face. I packed my things, took my two children along and went home to Argao (a town 66.7 kilometers south of Cebu City). I arrived at about four o'clock in the afternoon, and by seven o'clock in the evening he was already there asking me to come home with him. *His mother would not take him in if he could not bring back our children* [emphasis added]. I had to give in.

When I was pregnant with our fourth child, my husband was regularly seeing one of the maids of the Velascos. I caught them lying in the grass and the maid quickly jumped off the cliff. I was ready and willing to fight over my husband with a knife. She was dismissed from her work because I told her master [of] her affair with my husband. I heard that she gave birth to my husband's child.

During my fifth pregnancy, my husband had a prostitute named Manuela Caydo. She is a dirty woman and I got sick because of her. My husband and I were treated at St. Theresa's Charity Center. I still have her photos. She had the guts to have those shots taken with my husband. [R showed three pictures after she said this.] I got these photos because I caught my husband showing them to his friends. I tore most of the other [photos] to pieces.

Recently, my husband was visited by another prostitute while he was at work in Beverly Hills [an exclusive upper-upper class residential area]. I don't know why women like him. Maybe because he is generous with them. He does not give me all his salary. There was a time when he gave me only fifteen pesos a week. (Husband's actual income is fifty pesos a week). That is not even enough for food. It's a good thing the children can just go to my mother-in-law during mealtime. . . . This woman who used to visit my husband at Beverly Hills is not satisfied with one man. She also had [Ma] Noy Silo [HuBr], my own brother, Tomas, and two other workers.

He got sick again and so were my brother and I. My brother, Tomas, got the worst. His private part was rotten, while my husband had pus and blood dripping from his penis. I was already six months at that time. I am just afraid my baby might be born deformed or abnormal. [R is now eight months pregnant.] We had to go to the [St. Theresa's] Charity Center again. These last two months I have spent most of the time with my husband at Beverly Hills, so he won't have a chance to cheat on me. We built a small shack near the water pump [where husband works], where I could rest and prepare his lunch. Actually, my husband does this [fooling around with women] only when he is drunk and when I am pregnant and have just delivered [a baby]. Then there is also his *barkada*. He spends most of his time and money on them. I don't know why my husband is such a maniac!

Note that in one of their quarrels, this woman had taken her children home with her. This prompted an immediate reconciliation when the mother-in-law sent the husband ostensibly to fetch the children. Such a request carries the implication that the children after all "bind" the couple together, for better or for worse. By taking her children along with her, the wife was assured that the husband would come and fetch her, if for no other reason than to take the children with him. This would give them an opportunity to clear their differences, thus forcing the husband into a conciliatory position.

Neither the wife nor the husband tried to keep their conjugal conflict from the children's view. As a matter of fact, the wife had on several occasions "informed" her children about the "cause" of their husband-wife quarrels:

That little girl . . . [aged three]—she threw stones at her father. She tells her father: "*Gi-atay ka* [cuss word], you have another woman again! Why did you not come home early?" [Probe.] He was quiet. *He listens to this girl because she is his favorite.*

This strategy of using one's child or children to "cool off" a conjugal conflict is not unusual in the Cebuano setting. A milder case of a husband-wife squabble demonstrates once again how children can solder the conjugal bond:

L: We also have our little quarrels, especially when I am about two or three months pregnant. I am usually ill disposed at this time. It annoys me when he interferes with my work, or tells me to do this and that; don't do this and that. When I am angry, he keeps quiet. There are no loud or harsh words. He usually leaves the house when we quarrel. If he does not come home at night, I go out to look for him, and then we come home together, reconciled. Very often, *I bring along my eldest boy*, so that *in case he refuses to come home, I will just leave the boy with him, so he will have to come home on account of the boy* [emphasis added]. [Husband interjecting] We quarrel about little things, but we don't shout at each other. Usually a quarrel starts when she does not give me permission to go out. There is an exchange of words, but I cannot go out just the same.

At other times, the wife may align the husband's favorite child as a way of ventilating her dissatisfaction with what she suspects her husband of doing:

> *L*: When his bus had a breakdown [*aberia*] in some town once, and he could not come home that night, he knew I would be angry. When he finally came home, he explained that he sent a telegram to the station [bus depot] but the mechanic took his time in coming so the bus got stalled longer than was anticipated. The second time it happened, I confronted him with: "*Aberia, aberia!* In the same place?! Can you explain why this has to happen in the same place?" That afternoon, before he came home [at two o'clock], Jose [son, aged three] asked: "Where's Tatay [father]?" I told Jose: "Your *tatay* won't be coming home because he has a wife there." Jose mentioned this later to Mama [HuMo]. She was here [staying with R]. [She] said: "What's that you said?" That night, Jose asked again: "Tatay did not come home yet?" Then he answered himself: "Because he has a wife there." [R laughs as she says this.] But he added something very naughty. [Probe.] [R embarrassed] Jose said: "Because Taty has big *titin!*" [Probe.] *Daku kono'g lagay si Silo* [Father has big genitalia].

These interviews suggest that Cebuano women, particularly among the lower class, do not feel any need to keep conjugal conflicts from the view of their children, especially when they involve conflict over other women. The wives tend to feel that there is an added advantage in "informing" the children, or one particular child who is the husband's favorite, about the father's "faults."

On the surface, the Cebuano women's insecurity does not comport with the power they possess in household task performance and the legal protection they receive. Unlike Chinese women, who as daughters must obey their fathers, as wives obey their husbands, and as widows obey their male children (the so-called *three obediences*), Filipino women are not subjected to institutionalized subservience. There is more equality in Cebuano conjugal relationships. The law also affords women considerable protection. They are allowed to inherit equally with their siblings from their parents, and they have full control over the property they bring to their marriages. Hence, the Cebuano woman's constant worry about "other women" cannot be adequately explained by the low status of females in the family. It is better explained by the widespread acceptance of the double sexual standard and the institutionalized *querida* system. This is discussed in the next chapter.

8 / Extramarital Relationships

Because it is relatively easy to obtain data on marital fertility, and because pregnancy is assumed to occur "accidentally" to unmarried women, population studies have tended to focus exclusively on the number of children ever born to married couples. Of the few studies that examine the impact of extramarital relationships on fertility behavior, Blake's work in Jamaica is probably the best known (Blake, 1960). Her findings indicated that, contrary to popular belief, sexual intimacy out of wedlock reduces rather than increases fertility because the seasonal employment available to men requires distant travel, leaving lower-class women without mates for relatively long periods of time between one union and the next, and also because coitus is less regular in nonmarital unions. This finding was reiterated by Stycos and Back (1964).

Despite some seeming parallels between the Jamaican society described by Blake and the Philippine society we studied, we believe that extramarital relationships have a significantly different impact in Cebu, where keeping a woman outside marriage is so widely practiced that it transcends social class and ethnolinguistic differences, even though it is against the church's teachings. Thus, although we do not have any survey data on the prevalence of marital infidelity, it is worth discussing how and why nonmarital coitus and pregnancies in Cebu may substantially contribute to societal fertility.

The Querida System

Querida is a Spanish word which means "beloved." As it is widely used nowadays in the Philippines, it carries the connotation of "kept woman" or "mistress." The *querida* system, however, does not refer only to the institutionalization of any semipermanent relationship with "the other woman." It can—as sometimes happens—include a relationship with "the other man," in which case we may speak of that man as the wife's *querido* (or lover). In its most elemental form, the relationship is triadic, involving a legally contracted or socially recognized married couple and one other individual, either male or female, whether single, married, separated, divorced (abroad), or widowed. It does not necessarily exclude the possibility that this other person may be a *querida* (or *querido*) to someone else.[1] In terms of emotional involvement and financial commitment, *querida* relationships fall into a spectrum which ranges from very high to very low. Objective feelings of involvement are irrelevant here. What matters is that either one or both of the partners in the *querida* relationship subjectively feel that some kind of emotional bond exists, enough to distinguish it from a fleeting encounter between strangers.

Likewise, the absolute amount of financial commitment in the relationship is not important as long as the parties involved recognize that *some* form of financial commitment is made. Thus, a Cebuano wife is likely to use the word *querida* for any "other woman" who has caught her husband's fancy and with whom he has exchanged gifts of some kind, whereas disinterested observers are likely to identify a *querida* relationship only when the illicit affair has stabilized over time. At the very high end of the continuum, a *querida* relationship may entail not only deep emotional involvement but also such financial support as a house, complete with furnishings, for the *querida* (or on rare occasions, the *querido*), an automobile, and privileges such as maids and monthly stipends—plus, in a few instances, property or business assets negotiated in the *querida*'s name or in joint ownership. Where children are born into such unions, paternity is usually recognized as long as it was never in question in the first place.[2] The more stabilized the *querida* relationship, the more likely the children are to be treated as socially rightful children. The stronger the financial foundation of the *querida* relationship, the more likely the *querida* household and family relationships are to approach those of the normal Cebuano family, minus the constant presence of one parent.

From the wife's viewpoint, the *querida* system poses a threat to the security of her legally contracted marriage or socially recognized union, for it can corrode husband-wife affectivity and deplete her family budget.

The Legal Infrastructure of the Querida System

Inasmuch as the Philippines is a Catholic country where marriage is considered a sacrament and where sexual mores are restrictive, the question arises as to how the *querida* system can be reconciled with the existing legal structure and social values. To address this issue, we believe that it is important to understand three sets of laws that impinge on male-female relationships. The first has to do with the absence of legal divorce in the Philippines; the second concerns the technical distinction between adultery for women and concubinage for men; and the third ensures the inheritance rights of illegitimate children.

The Absence of Legal Divorce

During the U.S. protectorate, absolute divorce was permissible on the ground of adultery (on the part of the wife) or concubinage (on the part of the husband). This represented a drastic change from the *Siete Partidas* of the Spanish regime, which regulated marital dissolution and allowed only for legal separations (called "relative divorce"). However, in 1950, when the New Civil Code passed by the Philippine Congress took effect, absolute divorce was eliminated and legal separation became permissible only on two grounds: (1) adultery on the part of the wife or concubinage on the part of the husband, and (2) an attempt by one spouse against the life of the other, such as attempted or frustrated parricide. Furthermore, Article 15 of the Civil Code clearly states that divorces granted on foreign soil to Filipino nationals are neither valid nor recognized in the Philippines. Legal separation is most difficult to obtain and very easily revoked, even though it is allowed under the law. Juco (1966:69) explains how difficult it is:

> An action for legal separation must be filed within one year from the knowledge of the offended party of the cause thereof and in every case within five years from the time of occurrence of the cause for legal separation. In no case may the trial of the action for legal separation be held before six months shall have elapsed from the filing of the petition for legal separation. . . . If reconciliation occurs before the grant of the final decree of legal separation, the proceedings will stop immediately. If it takes place *after* the separation has already been decreed, then the decree is rescinded and without any effect.

Moreover, legal separation can be claimed only by the innocent spouse. If both parties are offenders, it cannot be claimed by either of them. Neither can it be granted if the innocent spouse condones or consents to the adultery or concubinage.[3]

According to the vital statistics published from year to year, formal separations are extremely few and remarriage for separated individuals is even rarer. When remarriages do appear on public records they more often involve separated males who marry single women than separated females who remarry at all. The statistical profile, however, distorts the observed reality, for it reflects not only inconsistent reporting by local civil registrars but also the legal inaccessibility of separation to the majority of poor Filipinos. The figures, therefore, do not necessarily conform to the reality.

Adultery Versus Concubinage

The double sexual standard in the Philippines is nowhere more obvious than in the concept of criminal adultery and fornication, which is defined differently for married people, depending on their sex. As Carale (1970:345) emphasized:

> In the Philippines, adultery is primarily a crime committed by married women. Her paramour becomes liable for adultery *only if* he knows that the woman is married [emphasis added]. . . .
>
> [It] does not require cohabitation, lewdness, openness, nor notoriety. . . . A single intercourse, regardless of how privately or discreetly done, would suffice to convict. . . . The parties may be held liable for as many crimes of adultery as the number of sexual intercourses, because, in the colorful language of the Court, adultery is "an instantaneous crime which is consummated and exhausted or completed at the moment of carnal union."

Moreover, circumstantial evidence is sufficient proof of adultery in the Philippine courts. This is justified on the ground that establishing carnal union by direct evidence is difficult. The penalty for adultery is imprisonment for a term ranging from two years and one day to six years (cf. Francisco, 1952:796).

In contrast, a married man can have sexual intercourse with a single woman and not be guilty of any crime at all, provided that the single woman enters into carnal union voluntarily and privately. Only if that sexual relationship is scandalous or stabilizes into cohabitation may the husband be guilty of a crime, concubinage, which is punishable by a prison term of six months and one day to four years and two months. In this case, his paramour is also liable, although her penalty is only *destierro* (banishment). Put differently, fornication per se is not considered a crime.[4] Only fornication committed under scandalous circumstances or cohabitation by a married man is penalized as concubinage.

Carale rightly argued that the juxtaposition of this differential treatment of adultery and the absence of divorce in the Philippines offers very tempting opportunities for blackmail and complicates the married couple's attempt to procure a legal separation, since any condonation or consent given by the innocent spouse to the erring one would void the claim for legal separation.

Inheritance Rights of Illegitimate Children

Provisions to grant successional rights to illegitimate children came with the passage of the Civil Code in 1950. By law, legitimate children are entitled to bear their parents' surnames, receive support, and inherit from them. Of interest here is that an illegitimate child whose parents were not disqualified to marry each other when he was conceived and who marry after the child was born are considered legitimate by fiction of law. They are called natural children proper. This type of illegitimate child is entitled to the same rights as legitimate children. Furthermore, illegitimate children who were born or conceived of a void marriage, or conceived of a voidable marriage, are called natural children by legal fiction. By law, such illegitimate children are considered compulsory heirs to that part of the testator's property (called legitime) which he cannot dispose of by will. Likewise, illegitimate children born out of an adulterous relationship are also compulsory heirs to the testator's legitime. According to Sison (1973:399):

> The widow or widower and the illegitimate children share in the inheritance concurrently with the legitimate children or with the legitimate parents in every case, but their shares are taken from the free portion of the estate.
>
> The legitime of the legitimate children and descendants consists of one-half of the entire estate of the father and of the mother. The other half, referred to as the free portion, may be disposed of by the testator family, subject to the rights of the widow or widower and the illegitimate children.

This is a roundabout way of assuring the succession rights of illegitimate children. By making such provisions, the legal system in effect recognizes the widespread practice of keeping a *querida*.

The Functional Significance of the Querida System

The operation of these laws suggests that inasmuch as divorce is not possible in the Philippines, the social system must provide alternative ways for unhappily married couples to satisfy their affective and sexual needs. The legal distinction between adultery and concubinage in effect gives men the freedom to establish extramarital liaisons, for if a man merely visits his mistress from time to time without openly cohabiting with her, or if he only has sexual intercourse with her discreetly, then the man's legitimate wife may not bring charges against him, since there is no legal ground for her to stop her husband's philandering. The man's behavior in this case "does not amount to concubinage" under the revised Penal Code (Juco, 1966). The law, in effect, sanctions the *querida* system. Herein lies the basis of every married woman's fear that her husband will have *queridas* elsewhere, if she is not watchful of his needs.

Supporting the institutionalization of the *querida* system is the repeated undercurrent of the double sexual standard. Thus, if one reviews the verbatim records of the Cebuano couples we presented in the preceding chapter, one finds that both men and women judge a good wife on the basis of two achievements: the ability to accomplish her household chores and other tasks culturally ascribed to housewives, such as controlling the family budget, overseeing family health care, and planning for the future economic security of the family; and a knowledge that she "has attended to her husband's needs" or "abided by his wishes." As we stated earlier, the phrase "to attend to his needs" is broad and includes the sexual needs of the husband. Yet, if one reexamines the statements made by the Cebuano women in marriages with a high degree of husband-wife cooperation in household chores and heightened conjugal affectivity, not a single wife in the sample ever stated "and he has attended to my needs," on top of all the commendations they have for their husbands, despite the fact that the latter have assisted them in many aspects of household task performance, such as chopping wood, fetching water, changing and washing diapers, cooking, and turning over their salary. Of all the wives we interviewed, only one woman manifested considerable egalitarianism in seeking affection from her husband. Whether this was due to her middle-class background or *querida* status (since the woman is separated from her first husband) is difficult to decide. The closest the other women came to admitting their sexual desires was to intimate dissatisfaction with their relationship with their husband, such as:

> *L:* He seems not to be very aggressive anymore. Maybe it is because he *tambok na* [has become fat]. And I guess fat men are less aggressive. Also, when we would have sex, I don't enjoy it fully. I have never had . . . what they said you would feel like floating in the air. It's because we not only have to do it in a hurry, for the children are sleeping with us, but also most of the time he would ejaculate so fast . . . sometimes [it] would last less than five minutes.

This, of course, is not unique to the Cebuanos. Women in many cultures have been known to express similar frustrations. However, it does show how one-sided the fulfillment of "needs" may be in the sexual relationships of some Cebuano married couples. The belief is widespread that men have sexual urges which must be released periodically; women do not. A man whose sexual needs are not fulfilled *could, would,* and *should* seek outlets with other women. For a man to store these sexual urges in his body for too long is believed to be harmful. He will get nervous, become sick, and may even have a "nervous breakdown." It is unhealthy, and it can cause tuberculosis—so say some of our respondents. The following case epitomizes this belief in the male need for sexual gratification:

> *M:* I suffer from nausea at the start of the conception. This is how I know that I am pregnant. And I am tired most of the time and easily, too. Which is why any sexual relationship must take a backseat during my pregnancy. And since O [Hu] is the aggressive type, he goes to prostitute houses. . . .

[Probe.] I don't mind that, either. I understand his problems. . . . And I get to know about his adventures later from him when he comes home.

Although this type of husband-wife communication is held by some to be the ideal goal of the male-female relationship, one devoid of jealousy and possessiveness, it would be difficult to argue that in this example the wife allows her husband to go to houses of ill repute because of liberal concepts of sexual equality. Far from it, for the woman herself cannot possibly have extramarital relationships (not even a fleeting encounter) without incurring the husband's wrath and the community's condemnation, and without leaving herself open to charges of adultery —as many counts as the number of times of intercourse.

The belief in the potency of male sexuality is supported further by the world view that the woman is the temptress, the seductress, whom the man, by virtue of his maleness, is physically unable to resist. In fact, a man who fails to respond to a woman's advances is considered abnormal. His *pagkalalaki* (manhood) is suspect: he would be a *bayot* (effeminate or homosexual) if he refused her. This kind of attitude comes across very clearly in the following interview with the husband of one of our respondents:

H: [After specifically requesting that I not reveal to his wife what he is about to say to me, the husband proceeded to narrate his *querida* experiences as follows.] When my wife was pregnant with our second child I had a sexual relationship with Pacita. And then, during her third pregnancy, I had Carla, and during the fourth, it was the maid of the Velascos [one of the families residing in Beverly Hills]. Then there was a burlesque dancer who used to come up to Beverly Hills to see me. I met her during one of our [*barkada*] drinking sprees in a restaurant downtown. This was the time when my wife was pregnant with our fifth child. In between, I went with my *barkada—mag-abang ug babaye—[literally, renting women]. I do this only when I am with my friends and after we have had some drinks. I pay for everything, because I am the only one who has money* [emphasis added].

Yes, I kissed my wife, but that was when we were newly married. I do not like to do that now. I kiss her on the cheeks and make *paraeg* [overt affection-seeking gestures] and tell her that she is the only one I really love—to appease her when I come home late. I also bring her something to eat so she won't get mad.

We used to go to the movies together. Once I brought her to a restaurant, but she kept on nagging me that I was wasting my money giving tips to the waitresses. That was the last time I brought her out.

When she starts a fight, I keep quiet and refrain from answering back. My mother takes sides with her and I cannot reason out because I am in the wrong. *But what can I do? The women are there for the asking and for a few pesos and I am a man* [you know].

Q: How many illegitimate children do you now have?

H: I am not sure if I have. I do not inquire from them. I heard that one woman was pregnant but it was not verified.

Q: Do you use any birth control method with any of them?

H: No.

Q: Do you know anything about contraception?

H: Yes, the condom. I used it for my wife [only]. I also had the jelly which I got from a friend, but I did not use it.

Q: Why did you use the condom with your wife?

H: I did not want to have more children. It is hard financially and it interferes with my work. Like now—she [got] that small baby. When I should be going about in my work, I am minding [taking care of] the baby.

Q: Why do you go to other women?

H: I have had my fill with my wife so I look for something different. There is no more warmth in my wife, we are just like brother and sister.

Q: Did you ever talk of separating from your wife?

H: Formally, no. I only say it when I am angry.

Q: Would you want to separate?

H: I cannot do it. There are children to consider. *Antus lang* [I just have to endure it]. I also cannot give her my word about the other women. *I would be a bayot [homosexual] if I refuse the others.*

Q: Did your wife ever refuse you sexually?

H: She never refused me.

Q: Did you ever refuse her?

H: I refuse her when I am tired. This is also a cause of our quarreling. She starts accusing me of having other women.

Q: Do you not try to satisfy her sexually?

H: I try to satisfy her—prolong it, so that she will get tired and won't bother me anymore.

The husband's attitude that "I am a man . . . I would be a *bayot* if I refused the others" is also shared by his wife, as our interviewer found when she questioned her at another interview session during the husband's absence—after the wife herself had divulged her knowledge of her husband's latest extramarital activities:

Q: How did you confront your husband about his last affair?

W: Well, you see I learned about this affair from a friend. This friend notified me when this girl came to Cebu to see ______ [husband], told me that they spent the night together in Mandawe [7.2 kilometers north of the city center] at the house of the girl's cousin. The following day I made inquiries at the pier about boats leaving for Bohol [an island southeast of Cebu]. Just my luck, I met a passenger who happened to be a relative of this girl. I told her what happened between this girl and my husband and got the address of the girl's parents. Immediately I sent a telegram to the girl's parents and followed it up with a letter. I am sure they got the message.

Q: What about your husband?

W: I confronted him with this information, as soon as I got back from the pier, but he denied everything. I talked to him quietly, I shouted at him, but he just kept quiet.

Q: And your in-laws?

W: Ah, now—they are all against him. Even his father and youngest sister who are usually on his side blamed him. They did not like the idea that ______ [husband] will support this woman. I overheard his father say, "What can you do with this woman—when you can hardly support your own children?"

Q: Do you think your husband has an obligation to support his child by the other woman?

W: Of course not! *It's her fault.* She knew very well that ______ [husband] is married. That's her responsibility. These maids around here—they are all man-hungry. This woman especially—she is not even pretty. Well, she's nice to look from the back, but face to face—*chonggo*! ["gorilla!"] flat nose and scarred legs. That's why she always wears stockings. And ______ [husband] is just the type who cannot keep his eyes off stockinged legs. Maybe that's what attracted him because if you look at this girl's face—*Susmariosep!* I look much better, modesty aside.

Q: What does ______ [husband] think about this child?

W: He does not seem to show concern about this woman anymore. There is so much opposition from his own family about this affair. He is probably afraid.

Q: Afraid of what?

W: Of the girl's parents. I heard they had relatives watch the harbor in Bohol. Anytime he shows his face at the girl's hometown—her relatives will finish him off. I told him how I notified the girl's parents.

Q: Has his behavior toward you changed much?

W: I don't know. He has been cooling off even before this happened. He is indifferent toward me about this last affair.

Q: How would you feel if the girl will abort?

W: Ha! that's *her* problem. And I don't care a wee bit.

Q: How do you think will your husband react if she aborts?

W: I have no way of knowing. Until now he has not admitted it openly. Maybe he will feel sorry about it, but he cannot really do much.

Q: I would like to ask you again, do you think ______ [husband] has no obligation to support this child?

W: My husband has no obligation at all. *It is her fault. My husband would be a bayot if he refused her advances.* I would not also allow him to support her.

Q: Do you think ______ [husband] has stopped seeing this woman?

W: He has no chance. I warned him sufficiently that if he goes to Bohol, that will be his end, and if the girl will come to Cebu, I have friends at the pier who will notify me. That would be the end of her.

Q: Are you still angry with him?

W: No more. When I learned about it for the first time, I was really mad. I bit him, I boxed him, but he did not fight back. His mother scolded him but he denied it.

Thus, we have a situation in which the wife on the one hand condemns the husband for engaging in illicit sexual intercourse with other women but, on the other hand, does not hold him responsible for his actions *because she sees it as the other woman's fault.* Her husband would be a homosexual were he to refuse her advances.

Insofar as the man is concerned, illicit sexual intercourse is a sign of his virility. The fact that he could impregnate a woman (especially after he had contracted a venereal disease, as our previous interview revealed) is the most solid evidence to him and his peer group that his sexual prowess has not been diminished. Furthermore, although it is not an occasion calling for joyful celebration, neither his wife nor society would blame him for his behavior, for "he is only a man."

When such attitudes are superimposed on an economic structure in which men work as breadwinners while women bear children and keep their husbands' total earnings, and a legal structure restricting separations and divorce, the outcome is the unique institution of the *querida* system.

The Prevalence and Duration of Querida Relationships

Among the fifteen lower-class families we interviewed intensively, five reported that the husband had maintained at least one *querida* relationship until it was discovered by the wife. The sixth case we uncovered in the lower class is a *querida* household. The woman (our respondent) is a *querida* to a married man whose family was not in our sample.

Of the five families in which the wives reported that their husbands had established *querida* relationships at least once, four of the husbands cut the extramarital tie at the wife's instigation. In one case, the husband's father was instrumental in breaking off the *querida* relationship after the wife appealed to him. In another case, the husband carried on a *querida* relationship with a *tindera* (salesgirl) at a store he frequented with his *barkada* for their drinks. The relationship ended as soon as the wife started going after her husband and had a quarrel with the *querida* when she saw them talking together. All this was stopped because of her determination, and she added:

> *L:* If I don't give in to his [sexual] aggressiveness, he would have another *querida.* So, in order to be always able to give in to his desire, I had an IUD fitted *without his knowledge.* . . . I am taking the risk of using a contraceptive method [which husband strongly disapproves]. . . . I am afraid of having more children. The more children there are the less likely for me to attend to his needs for I have to attend to the children first and so I would be very tired already in seeing to his needs.

In the third case, the husband's *querida* worked in the same company as he did. The wife and the children were living in Minganilla (far from the city) and the husband's company was in the city. The wife confronted this *querida* several times, but the relationship lingered on until, at the last confrontation, the *querida* revealed to her that her husband had invited her to elope with him to Davao and establish another household there. Upon hearing this, the wife threatened to hire someone to kill both of them. The *querida* found herself a job in another company and severed her ties with the husband.

In the fourth case, the husband had a *querida* when the wife was pregnant with her third child. According to the wife, she "by chance" went through her husband's locker at his place of work and found peso bills and stacks of loose change. Since for some time she had been having difficulty keeping track of her husband's income, she surmised that he had *babaye* (a woman or women) outside. She is of the opinion that "these women are after the man's money especially if he is married." In her own words, "Men, especially married men, do this [fooling around with women] *in order to be able to brag about their exploits, aron lang gayud ingnon*" (so people can say they are men about town). The wife's *tambal* (cure), as she said, was to make him search for her frantically when he came home by hiding underneath the house. That, she said, ended his affair.

The fifth case contains the most information on lower-class attitudes toward women and sex. The man has had serial *queridas*, and the wife has so far not been able to stop him. Although we have presented some material from this case already, other noteworthy remarks in earlier interviews provide additional insights:

> *Q:* Does your father-in-law say something about your conflicts with ______ [husband]?
>
> *L:* Ay, the man is *salbahis* [savage; bastard]. Like father, like son. He also used to go around with women when he was young; that's why he does not censure this son's extramarital doings. Why, he even laughed proudly when he saw those pictures [of his son with a prostitute]. He even said loud enough for me to hear: "Why did she marry my son and then get mad with him when he goes with other women? It is very clear that she is plain hungry for his . . ."
>
> *Q:* Did you answer him back?
>
> *L:* I told my husband angrily: "Tell your parents that they are doing this to me because I am alone here—with no relatives to turn to or to defend me; but someday they will see, I will get even.
>
> *Q:* Does your husband turn to his parents for support when you quarrel?
>
> *L:* Yes, he goes to talk to them after we quarrel.
>
> *Q:* What did you quarrel about the last time?
>
> *L:* Just a month after I gave birth I learned he was having an affair with the

laundry woman of ______ [a Beverly Hills resident]. The wife of their chauffeur told me because her husband was also having an affair with the cook. I came up in a taxi to Beverly Hills with a pistol and I caught them kissing and he just said to me: "No hard feelings." I fired at him but it just happened that the pistol was not properly loaded so it did not work.

Q: Have you always been sexually satisfied by him?

L: Not always. . . . But my husband always is. . . .

Q: Did you ever complain when you were not satisfied?

L: No, *how shameful* [emphasis added]. The neighbors will hear us. We do not quarrel about that.

Q: When do you resume sexual intercourse after childbirth?

L: Two or three months. The doctor told him that because I am not healthy.

Q: And when do you stop sexual intercourse during pregnancy?

L: Usually at the eighth or ninth month. This last pregnancy we stopped at the sixth month because I got that sickness [VD] from him.

Q: Did you ever refuse him for other reasons?

L: No, so that he will understand that he does not have to go to other women.

Q: Why do you think your husband goes to other women?

L: Other women are more desirable to him while I am just like a sister to him. Also, *he cannot avoid the occasion, when the women go to him* [emphasis added].

Q: Does your husband give you his earnings now?

L: Only since January. From now on, I will see to it that I get all.

Q: How do you intend to go about this?

L: That's easy. I did not think of this before. I can just arrange it with Mrs. ______, the treasurer of the Beverly Hills Association, to give me his check. She knows me and she knows that ______ [Hu] is fooling around with other women. She advises him sometimes.

Our data suggest that among lower-class men who maintain *querida* relationships, the tie is often short-lived. Poverty limits the ability to parcel out earnings. It also forecloses any intention on the man's part to provide an independent household for his *querida* without the wife's knowledge. Thus, for lower-class men, *querida* relationships are seldom sustained over an extended period of time unless their own legally established family is being supported by someone else (such as the husband's or wife's relatives), or at least part of the family expenditure is supplemented by other kinsmen's earnings. At best, the man could establish extramarital ties serially whenever the "need" arises, as during the late stages of the wife's pregnancy.

This is not true, however, for the lower-class woman. She can always enter into a *querida* relationship without parceling out *her* earnings, if she has any. The culturally prescribed role for women as budgeteers assures them at least a nominal sum, however infrequent the monetary flow may be. This is not to say that the lower-class woman always enters into a *querida* relationship solely for financial gain, nor is it to deny that she suffers psychological loss or social stigma by entering into such relationships. Nevertheless, the potential and actual existence of an economic lifeline is a marked advantage that the lower-class *querida* has over the lower-class man whose role is to hand in his earnings to a woman.

The reader should bear in mind that in spite of their dire poverty, lower-class Cebuanos generally find a woman who served as a *querida* shameless (*walang hiya*), if not contemptible. There is thus a discrepancy in what the *querida* relationship means to the two sexes. For the man, having a *querida* does not necessarily lower his social standing in the community. The greater his wealth, the less affected he is by any negative attitudes toward such relations. It may even increase his status in some circles, especially among his *barkada*. For the woman, however, having a *querido* is "immoral" and being a *querida* is contemptible. Very rarely, if ever, are *querida* relationships celebrated and welcome. Legal marriages and a church ceremony are still the preferred form of formalizing male-female unions.

Most women who have accepted the *querida* relationship find that some of their significant relatives have severed ties with them precisely because of the social stigma attached to being a *querida*. Nevertheless, old wounds heal, and as the *querida* relationship becomes more or less permanent, kin opposition weakens—especially when the *querida*, by virtue of her financial stability, can offer monetary assistance to her needy relatives. This is illustrated in Luisa's case (abstracted from Liu, 1968:29ff.):

> Her relationship with Pablo began when she was 14 years old and terminated with his death almost 30 years later. He was almost 30 years her senior. They initially met when she went to him for professional services. . . . Her subsequent visits were attended by increasing familiarity . . . and finally to physical intimacies in a matter of months. At this point, the sexual aspect of their relationship was distasteful to her, but giving herself was an expression of gratitude and appreciation for the affluent world that he made available to her. This meant more to her than anything else and she meant to hold on to it at all costs. However, her grandfather quickly discovered the relationship through the new and unexplained possessions, and she was sent home. . . . Her mother was presented with the situation: marriage was out of the question, but her daughter would be treated as a "wife," and she would be adequately provided for. Shortly after this, her mother . . . received some money from Pablo and [was] apparently appeased. At this time, Pablo put Luisa up in a household of her own, complete with maid. *The following years saw one or another of her siblings coming to live with her, to be sent to schools [by her] until they obtained college degrees* [emphasis added]. . . . Her grandfather severed all ties with her but the bond with her immediate family was maintained.

> When they decided to have a child, it was for the explicit and mutually understood purpose of *making their relationship even more permanent.* Pablo built a house for her and opened a bank account in her name. The child meant security to them, giving each a stronger "hold" and "claim" upon the other, not only during their lifetime, but especially after the death of Pablo.

It is clear that, for the lower-class woman, the formation of a *querida* relationship could be a means of attaining aspirations she would otherwise have had a hard time achieving on her own merit. Although not all lower-class people approve of such a union, some have no choice but to accept it. The following pages provide a profile of one *querida:* her background, conjugal relationship, lifestyle, and kin interactions.

Profile of a Querida

Pacita's family had always lived in Villagonzalo (a lower-class district of Cebu City). Her father was an employee of a *maguey* (hemp) export-import firm. He died when she was only ten years old. To support them, her mother did laundry at her home for other families. Pacita helped her around the house, as well as with the laundry. Whatever income the mother obtained from such jobs, she spent on her children's school supplies. Pacita's brothers had to work at a young age, too, often by running errands for other families in the neighborhood, or accepting the menial job of loading or unloading goods at the wharf. Because of the great economic difficulties they faced, Pacita had to drop out of school after finishing the fifth grade. She got married at fourteen to a man named Fernando. That union produced three children: two girls and one boy.

Her husband, from whom she is now separated, came from a "better" family. They lived in Perrelos (35.1 kilometers south of Cebu). His father owned the land he tilled. Moreover, he was "rich" enough to hire other people to farm for him, while he supervised planting. His mother tended a big *sari-sari* [mixed goods] store they owned, which was annexed to their house. None of his sisters finished college because of the war. After the war, all except one sister married.

Pacita's husband's family had opposed their marriage from the beginning. They had hoped that Fernando would marry a teacher. Even after the marriage, Fernando's relatives continued to treat Pacita indifferently. Pacita had known for some time that her husband had a *querida*, but she never knew where the woman lived until he once failed to come home for two successive days. She decided to take a trip to Talisay (12.8 kilometers south of the city), where her husband was working as a builder. She couldn't find her husband, but his employer turned out to be a distant relative and decided to give her some information regarding her husband's whereabouts. Pacita's plan to confront her husband and his *querida* at the latter's house was not carried out because he was not there. She did the next best thing: she went to Perrelos, her husband's hometown, and revealed everything to her parents-in-law. They sent for their son to come home to settle the matter with Pacita, as they were not in favor of a separation because of the children. Pacita's mother, however, was agreeable to a separation. She was afraid that Pacita's brothers might take the matter into their own hands and "do something" violent to her husband should they ever hear how he mistreated their sister.

Fernando, however, did not show up before his parents. When the distant relative for whom he was working was notified of this, he tried to apply pressure on him by refusing to let him continue on his job unless he let Pacita personally collect all of his earnings. The case finally reached the "fiscal's office." Fernando was summoned and was made to promise that he would support the children at twenty pesos per child each month. He agreed to that. But things never worked out, as Pacita said:

> The next thing I knew, my husband together with that woman had left for Mindanao. I had no money, no husband, and no job. My parents-in-law felt sorry for me and asked me and my children to live with them. We had no other choice.
>
> I was planning to leave for Manila to look for a job. But I had to make sure first that my two daughters could adjust themselves to my parents-in-law. So I stayed with them at my parents-in-law's house in Perrelos for about three months. Then, I took my youngest child, a boy, to my mother's house in Villagonzalo and asked her to take care of my son. I then left for Manila.
>
> I stayed in Manila for one year working as a housemaid. I saved enough money to buy *pasalubong* [gifts] for my children, my mother and brothers, and for my in-laws. But then, my mother wrote me that my son was sick. I decided to return to Cebu to take care of my son.

In Cebu, Pacita found herself a job as a waitress at one of the restaurants along the waterfront and lived near her parents. Her monthly income was thirty pesos. Her youngest son stayed on with her mother, while her two daughters continued to live with her parents-in-law. Every Sunday, she visited her two children in Perrelos, and when she departed for the city, her parents-in-law would always give her some fruits and rootcrops to take along.

While working as a waitress, Pacita met a married man who was later to become her *querido*. From the start, her mother had disapproved of her becoming friendly with this man because of his marital status. He was very kind to her, however, and gave her money from time to time.

As their relationship became more friendly, and as her mother's objections became stronger, Pacita had to choose between her mother and Rolando (the lover). The outcome was: "I chose Rolando and told him to take me to find a house for me where we could live together with my son [from her previous marriage]."

Her mother found her newly rented house and scolded her severely for living as Rolando's *querida*. She was considered an outcast by her own family. She stopped working; she also stopped her regular visits to Perrelos (where her parents-in-law and two daughters still live). And when one of her daughters finally paid her a visit to let her know that she was getting married, Pacita felt so ashamed that she did not even attend the wedding. She felt that she could not face her parents-in-law and all the husband's relatives in Perrelos. She decided to cut herself off from her affines.

The few times that she had to visit her daughter, she did so secretly, without letting her parents-in-law know. Her daughter had assured her on several occasions that her parents-in-law held no grudge against her, but she still feels ashamed, and cannot bring herself to face them. Once when her mother-in-law saw her in the house, she talked to her and gave her money and gifts for her ("other") family. But it did not relieve her feelings of shame. There was a deliberate effort on both her and her mother-in-law's part to avoid mentioning her *querido* and her "new" family.

Pacita's natal kin have disinherited and disowned her now. When she last went to see her mother, who was near death, the latter refused to recognize her. She has not gone back to her mother's house since. In her own words:

> Even before my mother was ill, it was awful. She would see me in the marketplace or any place for that matter after I was already living with Rolando and she would shout unprintable words against me. So I tried my best never to cross her path anymore. My brothers have been more quiet in their objections. They would not talk to me, sure, but they don't do any physical harm to me either. Even until now they are civil with me but they still do not recognize my children by Rolando as their relatives. They would not even think of hugging my children. As far as these relatives of mine are concerned, my children by Rolando are not relatives of theirs.

The Conjugal Relationship

Owing to their peculiar relationship, Pacita and Rolando cannot have a legal marriage as long as Rolando's wife is still alive. Rolando spends most of his time with his legal family. He does not sleep at Pacita's house at night, but he visits her during the lunch hour and stays there for a short while thereafter. They have lived in this kind of arrangement for the last eleven years:

> Throughout all these years, we never miss eating together at noontime. Usually I let the children eat first. I always wait for him to come home because he likes it that way. He never hits me no matter how mad he becomes and he professes that he will share with me not only his sufferings but also his joys. If he has no money, we sacrifice together with what little we can afford. If he comes upon extra money, we also spend it together. On my part, I have adequately proved my love for him by sticking it out. He knows that there are a lot of things he cannot give me, for example: all his time and all his money. . . . One time my *querido* failed to come home for lunch. I took this as a danger signal, I immediately investigated him thoroughly and not until I was completely satisfied with the answer did I stop asking him for an explanation.
>
> There are times when the feeling of inadequacy practically overwhelms me. It is not natural that a woman is left to sleep in the house all by herself without a man beside her. And when problems come up which I cannot discuss with the neighbors, I have to wait for one whole day before I can ventilate these and confer with Rolando. In the meantime, I fret and turn and toss in bed and do not know what to do.

Conjugal interaction under such conditions is less diversified and more intense, with very little opportunity for greater involvement outside the conjugal unit. Pacita says it very well:

> We don't have any chance to go out together because first, we don't have extra money [for such expenses], and second, he is afraid that we would be seen by his wife [in public] and she would make a scandal. Whatever time we have together is spent at the house and this makes it doubly difficult for us to use abstinence for purposes of birth control. . . *the birth of our first child made us really closer to each other* [emphasis added].

The tentativeness of the relationship gives the *querida* a sense of keen competition with the wife. For instance, since learning from Rolando that his wife did not take care of him, she has tried hard to find out whether Rolando is tired or sickly or just not feeling well whenever he does not look well. And she massages him. Once she heard him complain that his children by his legal wife did not respect him, so she has also tried to teach their children to look up to their father and respect him.

Economic Arrangements

One of the distinguishing features of *querida* relationships is the existence of an economic tie binding the *querida* to her *querido*. The specific kind of economic arrangement, however, varies from couple to couple. In general, the man provides the woman with a place to live, whether rented or bought, in addition to a stipend of some sort. In Pacita's case, Rolando used to give her 40 pesos a week for living expenses when he was employed as an automobile painter by an American company that manufactures farm machinery and trucks. His salary then was 10.80 pesos a day. This stipend was considerably better than what she earned (30 pesos a month) while working as a waitress. At present he works independently, accepting contracts for auto-painting jobs from whoever needs the service. He still gives her money for living expenses, but the frequency and amount depend upon the size of his contracts and the number of jobs he is able to finish within a given period. According to Pacita, if he makes 200 pesos, she gets 50 and the rest of his earnings go to his legal wife. In her own words: "Rolando has been thoughtful; I do not have to ask for money. If only he had enough money he would be able to provide for us better. But as it is I don't have any complaints. I am sure that he is thinking of us all the time."

For her part, she says, she has managed to keep herself sexually attractive to her *querido*. She feels that one of the causes for her (legal) husband's leaving her was that she stopped caring for herself. She was negligent about her appearance, dirty, and unattractive, and she continually refused to give in to his sexual advances (for fear of having more children). When she did submit to her husband, she could not respond affectionately. She decided that she was not going to make the same mistake with Rolando:

> I wear lipstick all the time [to remain attractive in spite of all the household duties]. . . . *We have not used any birth control method because I don't want what happened to my husband and me to happen again.* We are leaving it up to God [the number of children]. I do not take tablets [the Pill] for fear of negative consequences. I don't have such a good heart and I heard that there can be side effects. Rhythm and withdrawal won't work under this kind of an arrangement. *I wouldn't want him not to be fully satisfied with every sex relation* and the rhythm method is just not applicable. *I am afraid that withdrawal, rhythm, and abstinence will drive my querido away to the arms of another woman,* as had happened to my husband. *Hilot* [folk curative massage] is too dangerous. Imagine, they play around with your internal organs.

Subsequent interviews revealed that Pacita was well aware of what she was getting into when she accepted her *querido*'s love. She knew the nature of his job, that he was married with children, and had no intention of leaving his wife and family:

> Besides, *I haven't asked him to leave his wife.* If I were in her shoes, how would I feel? After all, I am also a woman. *It is just that he has to divide whatever earnings he has into two* . . . one for us and the other for his other family. Since he has more children with his legal wife, and they are older, they get a bigger share of his earnings. I don't mind this arrangement. As a matter of fact, we never quarrel about money. He provides us and gives me

> what is my due. Sometimes this is not enough but I know that this is all that he can afford to give. When he sometimes has a bigger job [gets a bigger contract], and he earns more, he also gives me correspondingly more. He is not the kind that tries to forget his obligations. He is very sincere and I know he loves me, and I love him, too. I guess I love him very much for how could I bear all these difficulties and shame if I didn't? I could have found another man, why would I say "yes" to him?

Pacita is also aware that Rolando's wife knows of their relationship and has pleaded with him to discontinue it. But "my *querido* refused [to cut our relationship] *because we have been living* [in this *querida* relationship] *for eleven years now, and we have four children from this union.*"

Household Tasks and Major Decisions

The *querida* household, characterized by the absence of one parent, makes joint performance of household tasks very difficult, although co-operative decisions are possible and often made on important matters:

> Under this setup, decisions are left entirely to me. I stay in the house the whole day and Rolando comes only for lunch. I have the freedom to choose the friends I want and the places I go to and Rolando understands. We do not have any major purchases but if and when we have the chance to do so, the matter will have to be agreed upon by the two of us. . . . Questions such as what school our children would go to were talked over between Rolando and me. . . . My *querido* cannot spend as much time with the children as he should. My only regret is that he could not stay with us most of the time especially when the children get sick. . . . My position is such that I act as father and mother to the children. I attend the PTA meetings; I talk to the teacher; I sign my children's report cards; and they tell me their problems. I am the one who gives them their allowances.

The *querida* thus performs both the instrumental and expressive roles within the family.

Child-Rearing

In the process of overcoming uncertainty about the future, children represent an important source of mobility and security for the *querida*. They ensure a definite amount of cash inflow and continually bind the *querido* to her. The more children she has, the stronger is this extramarital bond.

Within the lower class, the nature of the *querida* relationship is such that the man has only a fleeting contact with the children that bind him to the *querida*. He shows his care by attending to the financial needs of her children. Only indirectly does he influence their upbringing, as is evident from the following remarks made by Pacita;

> Rolando shows us he loves us by little gestures of devotion. He wouldn't want the children left alone. He is against the children playing around with known bad elements. And whenever he sees them scratched, bruised, or otherwise hurt because of this or that he blames me for it and reminds me of my primary obligation to do right by them.

Since children and child care become the exclusive domain of the *querida*, child-rearing in this context takes on new significance. Egalitarian treatment is stressed because every child comes to be perceived as an "investment" in the future. Independence training is also emphasized more consciously, both to spread the cost of managing a family and to lighten the labor of household chores. The following remarks illustrate this point well:

> I made no distinction in sex when it comes to discipline . . . I don't play favorites. Everyone is treated equally. Like for example, in buying new dresses: since we are poor I make them understand that I cannot buy for all of them at one time. It has to be one at a time. Children should be taught to learn to do things. My children with my [legal] husband were spoiled. [They grew up with their relatives in Perrelos.] They were not made to do things, but now these children by my *querido* helped a lot. The oldest is only ten years old, and he sells ice candy [a fruit-flavored popsicle which consists mostly of water] in the morning . . . he turns over his earnings to me, usually one peso; the rest help in cleaning the house, fetching water, running errands . . . and I make it a point not to give money every time I ask them to do something. Otherwise, they might learn to help only for monetary reasons.

The *querida*'s expectations for the children's achievements are consequently raised, accompanied by heightened expectations of future aid that these children may give her. Pacita stated her expectations for her children as follows:

> I earnestly hope that in spite of my poverty I can educate my children so that I can give them equal chances [with others]. I believe that only education can open new horizons for opportunity and job placements. I do not want to see my sons use their strength and their hands to make a living. My heart just bleeds every time I see my oldest son [by Rolando] selling ice candy under the heat of the sun. My youngest child by my real husband [a boy] wasted his time and money. A cousin of mine spent for his school expenses but he refused to study. He has turned out to be a stevedore at the waterfront, a difficult job with very low pay. . . . I used him as an example to [let] my younger children [know what happens to them] if they don't study.
>
> *My children's success will also be mine in a very real sense. I expect them to help me out when they can. I know that I will be needing all the help I can get* [emphasis added]. Sometimes I find myself disappointed when my married daughter fails to offer to help me but I cannot also blame them since they grew up with their grandparents. . . . If I were made to decide for them [her children by Rolando] *I would not want to see them get married. I run the risks of their marrying selfish spouses who would not care for me* [emphasis added].

Neighbors Versus Relatives

In view of the social stigma attached to being a *querida*, the establishment of such relationships almost always invites keen disapproval from relatives. Sometimes, ostracism may give way to tacit acceptance. At other times, however, the *querida*'s socially significant kin may maintain their negative sanctions for a long time. As blood relatives recede into the background, neighbors become the best alternative source of emergency assistance and emotional support. Not having known the woman prior to her being a *querida*, the neighbors do not hold any expectations about her or experience any disappointment at the kind of union she establishes with a man. They are thus in a position to treat the *querida* for what she is, and are more willing to accept her love affair. The extent of assistance that Pacita's neighbors render may be gleaned from the following remarks:

> It's a good thing my neighbors understand my plight. They do not tease the children. As a matter of fact, they help. When one of my sons [by Rolando] died it was the neighbors who helped me through the ordeal. They attended to little minor details. They came for the wake. They went to the burial. You would think that Rolando would be here more of the time. But no. He had to maintain his once-a-day-at-lunch routine. If it were not for the neighbors, I would not have pulled through the difficulty. Thank God, I did. These are the things you will have to take with the good.

This does not mean, however, that the *querida* is always able to develop a network of intimate friends. The very nature of her relationship would caution her neighbors to keep their distance—even as they offer assistance. Moreover, the illegitimacy of *querida* relationships in general also means that the *querida* couple cannot publicly participate in social functions frequently, if at all. Nor can they engage in reciprocal exchanges with other conjugal dyads as a marital unit. Too much camaraderie with the neighbors would likely be perceived as a threat by the other married women, for a *querida* symbolizes the proverbial seductress, capable of luring a married man and "satisfying his needs" to the extent that he would be willing to provide for her economically. A *querida*'s best recourse is to mingle with other *queridas* or with unattached women who might sympathize with her plight. This is not always easy, however. And depending upon the husband's views on this matter, the *querida* may simply not be able to form any intimate same-sex friends. In Pacita's case, her *querido* refused to let her have any *barkada*, for the following reasons:

> I cannot possibly have any *barkada*. That would take me away from the house. I would also have to go on *paseos* [walks] or even useless activities together. Besides being expensive, the house and children will have to be

> abandoned for a time. And I know that Rolando is very much against this. On my own I also dislike the idea of having *barkada*. Now . . . there are times when I have visitors or when I stay in the yard for conversations with the neighbors, but that is all there is to that.

Christmas and birthdays are private rather than social events. For Pacita, Christmas is a minimal celebration. She and her *querido* do not even go to Christmas mass anymore. Instead, Pacita spends Christmas Day by taking the children to the zoo for a walk: "I do this for the sake of the children and for my own. The children have to be given something in exchange for the fact that their father cannot even share this day with us. He has his real family to care for."

Clothes for the children are bought in advance whenever she has some extra money and are kept for presents until Christmas Day. It is only then that these dresses are worn. She has to do this because she is never sure when she will have enough money to buy her children presents. To help her secure some savings for Christmas spending, she would stock empty soft-drink bottles for a long time and sell them just a few days before Christmas. The money would in turn be used for buying soft drinks. The children are made to understand that they must not touch these soft drinks before Christmas, so that when the holiday season comes, they will have something extraordinary to celebrate with.

Her birthday goes uncelebrated, although Rolando's and the children's birthdays are celebrated in a small way. On her children's birthdays she serves them rice cakes and gives portions of them to her relatives who live nearby, even though they have disowned her.

Future Uncertainty

The *querida* relationship is always volatile. The woman lives under the constant fear that her relationship with her *querido* will one day come to an end, and he will look for a younger woman. What would Pacita do if Rolando should decide to leave her and stay with his legal wife?

> I cannot hold him. Legally, it would be the wife who has the legal right to complain. After all, practically speaking, I am an intruder. I should be thankful that I have this much of him. *The only thing I will ask from him if he leaves me is that he keeps his promise to support his children.* Sure, I will be worried. But what can I do? . . . I am now taking up hair science. This is given free by the government and we have to show up two times a week. When Rolando leaves, I can either support myself [with this skill] *or I can use whatever extra money I will get from the children.* I hope and pray to God that this will not happen. I do love him.

One of Pacita's final statements was: "I am the other woman. I know how society looks upon our kind. But if people would only understand our plight. We are not really as bad as pictured. We just happened to fall in love with the wrong man, or the right man at the wrong time."

Implications for Cebuano Reproductive Behavior

In a country where divorce is not permissible and separation barely obtainable for large segments of the population, the *querida* system performs a double-edged function: it *undermines* but at the same time *strengthens* the institution of marriage and the family in the Philippines. By granting men the kind of sexual freedom implied in the legal distinction between concubinage and adultery, the law not only recognizes the double sexual standard and sanctions men's sexual adventures outside the marriage contract, it also shields them from being prosecuted for their sexual infractions. By inserting a qualifying statement which circumscribes the conditions under which the charge of concubinage may be made, and by imposing procedural obstacles to application for legal separation, the law ensures the permanence of legally contracted marriages and guarantees the stability of the family system. It forces men to remain "accountable" to their wives, but at the same time allows them some relief from unhappy or insufferable marital relationships. The *querida* system thus functions as a safety valve.

Although practically all the *queridas* long for the day when they alone will be the focus of their *querido*'s affection, they are cognizant of the fact that except in rare circumstances this hope is not likely to materialize. Caught in the precarious position of being without a valid marriage contract—and therefore vulnerable not only to social ostracism from all sources, but also to legal charges of adultery—the *querida* quickly realizes that having children with her *querido* is the best way of forging a commitment and alleviating her anxiety about being forsaken for another woman. If the *querido* leaves her for another *querida*, she can at least have a legitimate economic claim on him through the children he has fathered. The law, after all, protects her children, notwithstanding their illegitimacy.

Insofar as the legally married wife is concerned, unless she can put a stop to her husband's extramarital liaisons, she must live with the insecurity of having to share her husband's resources with the *querida*. This wife's insecurity stems from her role as budgeteer in the management of the household economy, and from the ever present possibility of a separation, procedural obstacles notwithstanding. Frequently, her main recourse is *not* to prevent further pregnancies in the hope that this will fulfill her wifely duty and that the burden of additional births will "siphon off" some of her husband's resources from that "other" woman, exhausting his capacity to support two families at once. In so doing, the wife also increases her "claim" on her husband, the breadwinner of the family. It is far easier to rally her kinsmen, and her husband's natal kin, to her side when she has many children to care for than when she has only one or two. Maintaining *queridas* can be condoned if the husband has the financial ability, but it is unforgivable if he cannot even support his own family.

In the absence of more systematic studies on extramarital liaisons in the Philippines, we would hazard a guess that, far from decreasing births—as multiple sexual liaisons between males and females in other societies reportedly do—the *querida* system in fact results in more births than if it were nonexistent and divorce permissible.

The importance of children in soldering marital and extramarital relationships cannot be overemphasized. For Cebuano wives, the performance of maternal and wifely duties—which include sexual cooperation, pregnancy, and child care—is the best way of expressing conjugal affection. For the man, the number of children he is able to support indicates his financial ability and economic competence. Contraceptives, though used principally by women, fall within the realm of Cebuano men's traditional prerogative over sexual matters in conjugal relationships. Although the ability to control the number of births can eventually augment the wife's ability to fulfill her budgetary role, it can also be interpreted by some men who define themselves as "responsible" husbands as an open admission of their inability to fulfill their male role as breadwinner. However, to men considered "irresponsible," who have *queridas* even though they can ill afford them, the number of children they father outside marriage is a testimony to their virility. Furthermore, these men have the advantage of being held "not responsible" for their actions since, as dictated by the double sexual standard, men by nature are believed to be incapable of resisting sexual overtures from women: only homosexuals can possibly resist such temptations.

For the *querida*, who is not afforded any direct legal protection for "falling in love with the wrong man," pregnancy, however shameful, can have positive consequences: it indicates a commitment, however ephemeral, and as long as paternity is not in question, it can assure her a legitimate claim on the resources of the man who fathered her child, through the legal provisions for illegitimate children. Hence, the different perspectives among husbands, wives, and *queridas* crisscross to produce reproductive outcomes that only a few Cebuanos are as yet able to control, but from which they can each attain some social rewards, self-fulfillment, and a sense of security. No doubt, the increasing availability and widespread use of contraceptives will have broad ramifications for marital and extramarital relationships.

9 / Parents and Children

In the traditional quantitative orientation which characterizes the field of demography, the topic of parents and children is seldom studied from the interactional perspective, unless it can be expressed in terms of rates or other tangible measures. Yet, in trying to understand Cebuano society, the processual dimension of the family attains such prominence that its relevance to fertility decisions or non-decisions cannot be ignored. In this chapter, we present a picture of the Cebuano family in both its structural and processual dimensions.

Household Composition Data from Cebu

Tabulations of household composition data indicate that the classic extended family is not widespread in Cebu. Table 9.1 gives a descriptive profile of the residential pattern of the families we interviewed.

This household information, obtained from sample survey, indicates that about two-thirds of all family structures are nuclear households. In terms of social class, the highest proportion of nuclear families is found in the rural lower-class category. At the time of the interviews, coresidence with relatives appeared to be uncommon.

A review of the anthropological literature reveals that such a small domestic unit is prominent in all societies characterized by bilateral descent, and is in fact one of the distinguishing features of bilateral social organization (Murdock, 1968:253; Fortes, 1953:33; Pehrson, 1957). It is, therefore, tempting to concur with the substance of existing literature without examining other important underlying factors that shape household composition in Cebu. However, to do so would be to overlook the significance of evaluating whether the nuclear family pattern was achieved in conformity with the cultural-normative *ideal* or by *default* as a result of a host of variables, most especially the stages of the family life cycle and the migration history of those who constitute the household. The reader will recall that in Chapter 4 we found that regardless of their social class or rural-urban differences, most of the Cebuanos had lived with some of their relatives at one time or another after their marriage. This is remarkable in light of the finding that a great majority

TABLE 9.1

COMPOSITION OF HOUSEHOLDS

Social Class	Type of Household					
	Nuclear[a]	*Nuclear Lateral*[b]	*Joint*[c]	*Nuclear Lineal*[d]	*Other*[e]	*Total*
Urban						
Upper ($N = 101$)	68.3%	4.0%	7.9%	18.8%	0.1%	100.0%
Middle ($N = 720$)	62.6	10.0	8.2	17.8	1.8	100.0
Lower ($N = 700$)	66.3	10.1	7.9	12.8	2.9	100.0
Rural						
Middle ($N = 179$)	70.4	6.7	6.2	15.6	1.1	100.0
Lower ($N = 403$)	78.6	4.3	4.8	10.4	1.9	100.0

[a]The nuclear family is defined in the commonly accepted way as consisting of parents and their unmarried children.

[b]The nuclear lateral type is a nuclear household plus unmarried kin who are laterally and *not* lineally related to the head of the household.

[c]Joint families consist of two or more nuclear families that are related either laterally or lineally.

[d]The nuclear lineal type consists of the nuclear core plus lineal relations of the head of the household whose parents are absent. Included in this category is the stem family.

[e]"Other" includes those in which our information on family composition is incomplete, or those for which information is available but difficult to decipher and classify into the preceding family types.

of the urban poor are first-generation migrants from surrounding rural barrios. Of the seven hundred cases in the urban lower-class category, for instance, only approximately one-fourth of the husbands and one-third of the wives were born in Cebu City.

Moreover, to accept the anthropological "explanation" that household structure is a consequence of kinship organization is to dismiss entirely certain ecological factors that are quite salient in Cebu. In the vast majority of the lower- and lower-middle-class dwellings, construction materials are not suitable for multiple units large enough to accommodate a classic extended family. Housing is very congested, especially in the "squatter" or slum areas throughout the city and on the urban fringe. Small structures are built beside or near larger buildings, since no zoning laws regulate their placement or construction. The lack of zoning laws, in turn, may have resulted from the impossibility of curtailing the increase in the number of houses inhabited by the widely scattered squatters in the city, some of whom have even penetrated into the upper class residential neighborhoods.

Thus, factors such as migration and the fragility and congestion of the available housing suggest that people live in nuclear households out of physical and economic necessity. Nonetheless, despite such factors, our finding that *most* couples had lived with relatives at some time or other after their marriage suggests that the "nuclear" composition of Cebuano households is not hard and fast. Given the problems with crowding numbers of people into a one-room *nipa* hut, and given that many well-to-do couples also lived with or near their relatives, the fact that there is as much coresidence as there is seems to indicate that the issue goes beyond one of mere financial means. We think that the fluidity of household composition indicated by our data points to underlying cultural patterns which encourage close relationships between parents and children—married and unmarried—that are far more important than the circumstances of their living arrangements. In the rest of the chapter we wish to take a more detailed look first at the fluidity of the Cebuano household and then at the factors which encourage continuing close relationships between parents and children.

The Fluidity of Cebuano Household Composition

Even after a married couple has established their own household, the composition of that household remains fluid. Coresidence with collateral or lineal relatives occurs intermittently for one reason or another. Thus, the exact composition of a Cebuano household is constantly changing, depending to a very significant extent on the specific stage of the life cycle. To illustrate, one of our (lower-class) respondents lived with the husband's mother, his two unmarried brothers, and an unmarried sister during the first seven years of married life. They decided to move from Pinamungahan (about 75 kilometers west of Cebu City) to Cebu City when the husband found a job as a *cargador* (longshoreman) at the wharf. Three years before we interviewed them, the husband returned to the mountains of Pinamungahan to live with his parents when he received an offer to tenant a corn field for a relative. Eventually, he moved back to Cebu City in search of a better livelihood. They now live in a one-room nipa hut with a very small cooking space in one corner. Their household appears to be nuclear, but the husband's sister often comes to the city to stay with them:

> *Q:* How often does she come to visit you?
>
> *L:* She is here regularly, because she buys and sells empty bottles like my husband. As soon as she saves a little money, she goes back to the mountain [Pinamungahan] and brings her savings to her parents. Then she comes down again and buys and sells.

In addition, another (married) sister of the husband lives next door. The wife describes their social interaction as follows:

> Luna [HuSi] comes to visit me regularly. Every year, before All Soul's Day [November 2], she brings me a bundle of strings to be made into candle wicks. She gets these from the Chinese candle factory where her husband is working, and she gives them to me so that I could earn a few pesos [the candles are in great demand during All Souls' Day]. She helps me now and then by giving me some food and medicine, and sometimes lends me some money.

A brother of the husband also lives in the neighborhood, within hearing distance of our respondent's nipa hut.

Lest this case be interpreted as extraordinary, consider the living arrangement of another family where the couple has never had their own house. Their monthly income is about sixty pesos, which is at least twice as much as the earnings of the family just mentioned. Yet, this family has been living with the wife's parents in a one-bedroom nipa hut. The wife's parents occupy the small bedroom. There is no other partition. In one corner of the "big space" is a native, improvised cooking area. Another corner has been designated as the eating area, although there is no dining set. Our respondent, her husband, and their six children sleep in the two remaining corners of this hut. Beside them, at the designated eating area a few inches away, sleep two other male cousins (R's FaBrSo) who are attending college.

In spite of the inconvenience of such crowded living conditions, parents almost never disapprove of such an arrangement. Many even express a strong preference for coresidence with their married children. They would accede to their establishing a neolocal household only in the face of overriding economic gains, such as when the married son or son-in-law has found a new job and needs to live near his place of work. For this reason, the decision to establish an independent domestic unit may sometimes be agonizing. The following remarks provided by one of our respondents convey the flavor of family tension surrounding such a move:

> We lived with my husband's parents for the first five years of our married life. When he found a job in Balamban [on the outskirts of Cebu City] and we decided to move here, my mother-in-law and my husband had a heated argument. She quarreled with him and said: "*Ngano, gipapahawa ba kamo?!*" [Why? Are you being chased out of the house?] I was silent all the time that they were arguing. When we left, they were very angry.

Thus, in the Cebuano context, it is not sufficient to rely solely on a single head count to infer household structure. What is necessary to complete the picture is information on the coresidence pattern over time. From a theoretical standpoint, to overemphasize the significance of household statistics is to mute the relevance of crystallized processes of kinship interaction that might transpire in spite of physically detached living arrangements. In the Cebuano culture, members of separate but related households often interact socially at a high level as a result of having to share a common yard, pathway, bath area, outhouse, or hand-powered water pump. Thus the predominance of nuclear family structures in the Cebu data does not imply the social isolation of the members of a "nuclear" family from their kin.

The Cebuano Family as an Open System

Using Weber's dichotomy between "open" and "closed" systems (1947:139–43), we may speak of the Cebuano family as an open system because "participation in the mutually oriented social action relevant to its subjective meaning is, according to its objective meaning and the binding rules of its order, not denied to anyone who wishes to participate and who is actually in a position to do so" (Weber, 1947:139). In other words, the status and obligations of parenthood are not vested solely in the married couple, but are shared with a wide circle of adult and elderly relatives. The openness of the Cebuano family is attested to by the authority of extended kin members in child discipline, as the following two respondents demonstrate:

> *M:* My husband scolds, punishes only once in a while. I do the disciplining mostly. The small faults, he gives to me. He simply "seconds the motion." . . . But one time my husband was really angry at his nephews [who are living with them], one of whom was then second-year high school, when they spent their school fees for gambling. My husband locked the two of them in the bedroom and whipped them hard.

> *L:* If ever she [referring to Dau, aged sixteen] is home, she comes in very late and her uncle [HuBr, who lives separately downstairs] usually scolds her for it. There are times when she would sleep with a neighbor whose daughter is also a classmate of hers, or sometimes she stays for a night in other people's houses. She knows that she is likely to get a spanking for it, but she won't listen to me. I think she is greatly influenced by her classmates. One Sunday, her uncle caught her in Cathedral Church with some male friends. She was dragged home by her uncle and given a good beating.

Thus, besides the survey findings presented earlier, our own observations and intensive interview data have bolstered our belief that family relations may be a more potent factor than household structure in the fertility behavior of the Cebuanos.

To understand the affectional ties that bind the nuclear family to some members of its kindred, it is important to realize how children are socialized and to appreciate the strength of sibling solidarity in Cebuano families. For it is the ideal values and actual applications of child-rearing methods among the Cebuanos which give their families a distinctive characterization that is not found among nuclear families in other cultural settings. The remainder of this chapter is devoted to a generalized description of these two important familial relationships.

Parent-Child Relationships: The Dependency Linkage

The intrusion of generational linkages into Cebuano husband-wife relationships gives the conjugal bond a sense of inclusivity rather than exclusivity. Parents and children of the married couple are never on the remote periphery of husband-wife interaction but rather constitute an essential part of it. This mutual interdependence between two potentially competing kinship dyads (husband-wife versus parent-child) exists because of the biological and social fact that every conjugal pair is linked bilaterally to a parent-child relationship, and because of a peculiar child socialization process which lays great emphasis on psychosocial dependence between parents and child while at the same time encouraging the economic independence of the young.

Our own observations and serendipitous findings from the intensive interview material indicate that in many ways, psychosocial dependence is nurtured from early infancy. Mothers who breastfeed their babies are often not very anxious to wean them early, either for economic or for alleged contraceptive reasons. This is especially pronounced in the lower-class neighborhoods, where women seldom possess the skills for gainful employment and the role of mother is not considered in any way counterproductive. Some mothers in our sample reportedly breastfed their babies for up to three years.

By and large, our interviewers' observation of parent-child interaction shows that Cebuano child-training consists of more prohibitions than demands for achievement or independence. At home, the infant is constantly asked to refrain from touching, throwing, or shaking objects, and is discouraged from such activities as climbing, jumping, or running inside the nipa hut for fear he might break things or sprain himself. Mothers also prohibit their children from exploring the outside environment too much lest they hurt themselves and incur medical expenses. Severe punishment often awaits the child who strays far from home:

> *L*: Yesterday, Arnel [age ten] and some of his friends walked all the way to San Carlos [Boys High School, only four blocks away] to get materials for sling shots. [They] went that far! Suppose he gets run over or something happens to him? Using a branch of the guava tree, *puerte g'yud nakong bunal* [I gave him a good lashing].

Consequently, children sometimes have no choice but to resort to deception in order to be able to play outside the house. The following thirty-minute observation of a family episode captures the kind of child-training that our interviewers frequently encountered among lower-class families:

2:45 P.M., July 7

Mother was reading comics. Marivi (aged five) was playing outside the house. Mother calls: "Marivi, come here. [Pause.] Don't stay under the rain." Marivi dallies. Mother: "I'm going to box you now [if you don't come into the house]. Where's Ruben?" Marivi: "He's shitting." Mother: "Call him [in]." Marivi goes out, comes back: "He's still shitting." Marivi then comes in and sits on a chair. Mother calls Evelyn (aged ten). Evelyn comes in, munching the seed of a green mango. Marivi runs to her, saying: "Give me, Evelyn." Evelyn gives it to her right away. It has very little flesh left. Mother (to Evelyn): "There's plenty of rainwater now, Evelyn. Get your [plastic school] bag and clean it." Evelyn to Marivi: "Get my bag upstairs, *Day*." Marivi runs up. Evelyn (to Marivi): "It's on the roof." Marivi comes down, bringing the bag. She puts it on the chair. Mother continues to read comics. Marivi and Evelyn play. A little girl comes in, looking for Romy (aged fourteen). Mother (to Marivi and Evelyn): "See whether Romy's upstairs." Evelyn: "He's not there. He's at Nang Tita's." Mother: "Call him." No response on the part of the children. Mother calls him herself.

Evelyn: "Ma, we'll go out now." Mother: "Clean your bag first. How can we go when it's raining?" Father comes in. Evelyn stiffens, saying in a whisper: "Papa's here." Marivi runs to Father and asks five centavos from him. Evelyn follows, then snuggles close to Mother. Mother to Evelyn: "Where's your bag?" No response. Then Marivi and Evelyn talk and play by themselves. After a few minutes, Evelyn starts to leave. Mother: "Wash it now, Evelyn, so it will dry. Use Tide." Evelyn: "It's clean." Mother: "You call that clean? Look at the dirt sticking to it. Clean it so it will look new, so the others will say you have a new bag." Mother hands Evelyn the money to buy Tide. Marivi: "I'll go with you, Evelyn." Mother: "Just to buy Tide. . . . I'll go with you? . . . How *kuyog-baboy* [piggy follower] you are!" Marivi stays inside the house, sulking. After a while, she goes outside. Evelyn comes back with her bag and a small amount of Tide. She washes the bag outside the house.

Mother: "Are Ruben [aged eight] and Dionisio [aged twelve] sleeping?" Evelyn: "I don't know. Where's Marivi? Let her call them." Mother whistles to call Marivi: "Look upstairs and see whether Dionisio and Ruben are there." Marivi goes up, and comes down again. Marivi: "They're not there." Mother: "So! Shitting was just an alibi they used to get out. The demons. . . . I wonder where they are. Even if it's very muddy, they go off wandering. Glance down the river."[1] Mother also tells Romy, who is now in the house, to look for them. Muttering to herself, Mother says: "So they really slipped out." Evelyn (who was washing her bag): "Ma, the water's gone inside [the house]." Mother: "Never mind." Romy: "They're not there [by the river]." Mother is not listening, goes on reading comics. After two minutes, she says: "Where are they? Romy says he didn't find them."

Mother tells Evelyn to look for Dionisio and Ruben. Mother whistles to call the boys. Marivi is in a store two houses away, where a young man is singing bawdy songs to a group of young men and women. Mother looks up, sees Marivi, calls her. Marivi does not move. Mother threatens to use her stick (to spank her). Marivi comes back.

> Dionisio and Ruben arrive, twenty minutes after Mother first started to ask the other children to look for them. Dionisio has a big sack of tin cans. Mother: "Why didn't you tell me where you were going? I've already told you that before you fly away you should ask my permission first." Dionisio goes outside again after depositing the tin cans in the family's small storeroom. Ruben tries to follow. Mother (to Ruben): "You stay here. Why do you follow him? It's raining." Ruben sits on bench. Mother (to Evelyn): "Put the Tide away, Evelyn, when you've finished with it." Evelyn: "I've finished." Mother: "The bottom [referring to the bag] . . . let me look at it." Evelyn brings the bag to Mother who hangs it on a hook suspended from the roof. Ruben goes out of the house. Evelyn tells Mother she wants to go to school to enroll for classes. Mother says: "Later only. It's raining. Besides, you'll only be told to scrub floors [in school today, if you do go]. Classes start formally on Monday only. This week, you'll only be cleaning rooms." Marivi lies on Evelyn's lap, flicking Evelyn's finger, looking up to Evelyn to see any effect. Marivi tweaks Evelyn's hair, and peeps into Evelyn's blouse. Marivi: "I can see your breasts, Evelyn. You also have moles. Do I have a mole?" Evelyn looks. A friend passes by. Evelyn: "She has a new dress. We don't have any. Our godparents did not give us. Don't move so." They talk about their neighbors. Evelyn mentions someone. She says they're rich; they have a radio and electric lights.
>
> I ask Marivi how old she is. Mother says four; Evelyn says five. Mother takes out the album, concludes Marivi really is five. She has the girls' pictures taken every year on their birthdays. The boys do not have any picture taken. Father comes in. I decided it is time to leave the house.

Space does not allow us to present similar episodes our field interviewers have faithfully recorded. But this observation should suffice to convey the nature of child-training in lower-class families, and the "chain of command" from parents to older children down to the youngest one. Although this episode took place on a rainy day, parental prohibitions in this family as well as in others are not significantly different on other days. If it is not the rain, it is "too late," "too hot," or "too close to mealtime." Moreover, our interviewers' observations show that such prohibitions start with infants as young as one year old.

The Significance of Parental Restrictions

If one accepts the premise of Winterbottom's argument (1958) regarding the importance of extracting more demands for independence training of children, then the logical outcome of Cebuano child socialization processes is not independence but dependence. For not only are more prohibitions than demands made on children, but also prohibitions appear to be imposed much earlier than demands. The former method of training starts as soon as the child begins to explore his surroundings, whereas demand training for the most part starts only after the child is allowed to cross the narrow path that separates slum houses from one another.

It is noteworthy that in the Cebuano language there is a special adjective not found in English which is used to describe children who must be constantly asked to refrain from doing things—*badlongon*. It has been loosely translated as "disobedient" but is really applied to any child who must constantly be cautioned *not* to do this or *not* to do that. The word is less often applied to children who have to be told to *do* something. It thus carries a prohibitive meaning and suggests the importance of tractability in Cebuano child socialization.

Demand Training

As soon as a child is able to understand his parents' instructions to serve as a minion, demand training takes place. For the most part, sending the child on an errand or commanding him to do household tasks is the most consistent form of demand training among lower-class families, and to a somewhat lesser extent, among middle-class families as well. (The latter are able to spare their children from burdensome household tasks because of the availability of housemaids.) For lower-class people, childhood is thus an extremely brief period in the life cycle:

> *Q:* Let's talk about your children. At what age do you think that they should be considered as adults?
>
> *L:* When they can do things by themselves, like cooking, fetching water, gathering fuel [by picking up branches or pieces of wood in the dumps].

Another respondent offered this answer:

> *L:* Before they go to school, I think children are still very young and cannot be sent on errands yet. But when they start school, yes, they can be sent on errands already. . . . With Rommel [aged three], I send him to buy things I need, like ingredients at the store [across the pathway from the respondent's house, no need to cross the street]. Others were not sent on these errands until they were nine or ten years old because all the stores were along the streets then.

Thus, it comes as no surprise that in all lower-class families, children perform one or a combination of household tasks. Because such performances are expected, children are *not* rewarded with verbal commendation for their accomplishments.

The "Good" Child in Cebuano Culture

An alternative way of looking at the Cebuano parent-child relationship is to examine the folk definition of a "good" child. Our intensive interviews with twenty-two families reveal that for both the middle and the lower classes, obedience is strongly demanded. Its ancillary, respect for parents and elders, is equally stressed:

Q: What is a good child?

L: Bu-otan, dili badlongon [obedient, someone who does not have to be corrected or asked to refrain from doing things]. Vir [aged three] is such a problem! He is very *badlongon*. . . . I tell him not to play in the dust and under the sun . . . almost every day he gets a horse whip and a pinch[2] from me. I really make him feel the pain. He cries. He cowers when he sees the whip . . . it [the whip] is really effective, but even then, when he is engrossed in playing with his friends in the dusty grounds, he doesn't hear a thing. No matter how loud I shout for him to come home. That's when I take out the whip again. . . .

Venerando [aged nine] is also very *badlongon*. He always goes out! We can't send him on errands or let him work in the house, nor [ask him to] fetch water, clean the floor. He pretends to do it for a few seconds, and then he would disappear. Junior [aged fifteen] was like that too when he was younger. I guess all boys are very *badlongon*.

M: [A good child is] one who is obedient, and who respects authority and the elders. *If they disobey, I punish them physically and shame them.* I scold them severely, sometimes I spank them with my slippers, in the presence of whoever is in the house, to shame them . . . ask them to kneel in the *sala* (living room). . . . Respect for the elders includes not only relatives but members of the household. It means that *even if they [the elders] are wrong, you must give in.*

L: A good child is one who listens to what you say, obeys you. First of all, they must respect the parents, *mahadlok* [fear them]. Children who are not cared for and looked after take to the streets. These criminals are so because they are not afraid of their parents. To me it is all right to talk back if it is to reason out. [But] Dante used to *musokol* [talk back defiantly]. I got him one day and *crushed his mouth until it bled* and from that time on, he never *musokol*.

It is clear that obedience is a prime value in Cebuano child socialization, a virtue that must be taught by any means and at a very tender age. This extreme emphasis on obedience gives the parent-child relationship a diffused authoritarian quality. In many instances, the distinction between respect for authority and fear of one's parents becomes blurred.

Not all parents use physical punishment to enforce obedience. Scolding or bribing are common sanctions as well. However, perhaps the most noteworthy form of nonphysical sanction used by Cebuano parents is to threaten or frighten the child into submissiveness. The advantage of this sanction is that it requires minimal linguistic competence on the part of the child. Hence, it may be employed at a considerably more tender age when the child is impressionable. After all, it does not take much verbiage to make the child realize that his mother would leave him "for good" if he misbehaves, or that unknown creatures will devour him or suck his blood if he goes out without parental permission. Ghost stories to the Cebuanos are what nursery rhymes are to American children. If one takes into consideration that sorcery and witchcraft are still very much a part of the cognitive world of the urban population in the Philippines, and that many of the folk tales transmitted orally depict fetuses, young infants, or children as the choicest victims, the potency of frightening or threatening the child into conformity becomes self-evident. Middle-class children likewise learn these tales through the servants who take care of them.

One effect of such psychological manipulation is to enhance parental or adult power by making the child increasingly dependent upon his parents to protect him from his environment. When this mode of non-physical sanction is used simultaneously with early prohibitions which stifle the child's efforts to explore and trust his surroundings, as well as constant teasing or foreboding epitomized in the phrase "*Hala! Hala!*" (a fear-provoking exclamation), the result is a strong attachment to one's parents and, by extension, to one's kinsmen. The dependency linkage between parents and child is thus sealed at a very early stage of the individual life cycle.

Parental Responsibility and Economic Reciprocity

For how long do children remain the responsibility of their parents? Most parents answer that there is no age limit. At the very minimum, parental responsibility continues as long as the child has not established an independent household. But even after the child has grown up and established a domestic unit of his own, he is not free from parental intrusion or assistance. A middle-class respondent aptly describes for us this attachment between parents and child: "I consider them my responsibility until they have a home of their own. I think even for as long as we are living and can see them [they are still our responsibility] because *we can't allow them to be miserable.*"

However, although the child is socially and psychologically dependent upon his parents, an effort is made to make him become as economically independent as possible. Older children no more than sixteen years of age often contribute to the family coffers or to their siblings' education by handing in a fraction, if not the total sum, of their earnings. When children live apart from their parents, the latter do not hesitate to pay regular visits on payday to collect some support money. In our interviews, we found that some parents take the boat from one province to another once a month precisely for that reason. The more children one has, the larger the total sum of support a parent can receive, other things being equal. A lower-class woman narrated her father's economic dependence on the children as follows:

> My father lives on what my brother Manuel [can afford to] give him. Every fifteenth of the month, when Manuel receives his share of the fishing earnings, my father gets a certain amount. The other [siblings], *Manang* Auring,

Opring, and Proceso, also contribute a little amount of money to support my old father. He supported us by fishing. Now it is our turn to support him. We would feel ashamed if we as children abandon him. Especially those of us who live near him have an obligation to support him.

We found that even housemaids working for upper-middle-class families in the city, with earnings as low as twenty-five pesos a month, give as much as fifteen pesos to their parents. In other families, girls as young as fourteen and sixteen hand in their entire wages to their parents. One couple conveyed lucidly the Cebuano emphasis on obedience and economic independence:

H: I want them [the children] to grow up *independent but obedient.* That is why when Diana [oldest daughter] wanted to work in a *chicaron* [fried pork rind] factory, I allowed her to do so, so that she will learn the value of money and the dignity of labor.

W: She is really very understanding and industrious. I pity her, because she is at an age when she should be enjoying her adolescence but instead is helping us. The money she earns is usually used to buy the things she and the other children need in school.

This kind of economic assistance is not restricted to the lower class but is common among middle-class families as well, although in the latter cases, child labor is rare and most parents let the older children finish their education before economic assistance is sought. A typical arrangement found in the middle class is as follows:

I expect Baby [oldest girl who is graduating in a few months' time, with a B.A. in education] to help out once she finds herself a job, which means that she is going to give me one-half of her monthly salary. This was our agreement while she was still studying. And she knows that I am doing this not for my sake but for that of the other children. *They must help in the education of their brothers and sisters.*

Boy [second oldest child], too. He has already finished his course [at the vocational school] in refrigeration, and he is going to take up an apprenticeship in one of the refrigeration shops. His father and myself have promised we would build him his own shop once he is ready for it. And the arrangement will be like that with Baby. We will get one-half of his profits.

I am quite happy with the way things turned out. Boy has promised that he will get married only when he turns twenty-five. I think that will be just fine. And Baby, well, she does not have a boyfriend as yet. There was a time when she had a boyfriend and she was still studying. It was one of the boys in the neighborhood. When I heard about it from the neighbors, I immediately called for her and scolded her. I reminded her of her obligations to finish her course before she can have any affairs of the heart. And her father, too, was very mad. We threatened we would force her to stop her schooling if she would continue seeing this boy. It's a good thing that she is a sensible young girl and she followed our advice. If she should find herself a boyfriend now that she is through with her studies, I will not mind. On one condition: that she chooses and picks the best—one who is professional, has a job,

> from a good family, well behaved and of good moral character. . . . There is the obligation to the younger children. *If they should get married now, they will still have to give me one-half of their monthly salary.*

This pattern of economic assistance is not uncommon in the Cebuano culture. It is for this reason that all the parents we interviewed expressed as their utmost desire to provide their children with an education. And as long as they feel that their financial condition allows educational expenditures for their children, they continually dream of a better education and a brighter future for the next generation. Such desires are so strong that only the respondents' own words can fully impart their undying dream:

> *L:* Although he [husband] is so concerned about not spending money for himself, *he does not hold back when it comes to the children.* Especially if these [expenditures] are for their studies. One time, the teacher required the child to buy an expensive material for the classroom. I had to consult with my husband first, thinking this was not terribly important anyhow, and we could postpone it. But he would not listen to me. He said: "If it's for the children's schooling, we must not make them wait. Who knows, we might jeopardize their studies because of our thoughtlessness."

> *L:* He [husband] firmly believes that education will open up the gates of opportunity for our children. *He is ambitious for them and he has big plans.* I think that I am more realistic than he is. . . . After all, I tell him, I have stopped wishing to become rich. I guess we will always be poor. . . . I know that *he is trying very hard. He even works overtime and on Sundays.* But why long for something that cannot be? The next best thing is to budget the income and expenses so there would be no problem about making ends meet. . . . [Two weeks after this interview, the husband had to be suspended without pay from his job because of exhaustion and fatigue from overworking.]

To all the lower-class parents whom we interviewed, happiness is seeing their children successful and well-to-do, but given the peculiar socioeconomic structure of the Philippines, it remains a farfetched dream. Nevertheless, that strong dependency relationship between parents and children remains indissoluble. And, to quote one respondent, "*even if the parents cannot send any of the children to school, still the [children's] obligation to help their parents, na-a gayud kana* [is always there]."

Sibling Solidarity

Next to the parent-child relationship, the sibling bond is the most binding kinship tie in the Cebuano culture. Over half of our respondents in each social class reported that their best friends in childhood were their own siblings. For many, the intimate, friendly relationship is not altered by spatial dispersion or by marriage. Concern for the well-being of the parents frequently keeps them in close touch with one another. Several women differentiated sibling solidarity from other collateral kinship sentiments in the following manner:

> *M:* Brothers and sisters are naturally deeper and *su-od* [closer] to one another due to the blood relationship and sentiments. Of course, we are related by blood to our cousins, but somehow there exists a gap. Brothers and sisters really feel for one another, perhaps by virtue of the fact that we have lived with one another in joy and in sorrow since we first saw light.

> *L:* Cousins are different from *igsu-on* [siblings]. There are family secrets which may be shared with our siblings, but not necessarily with cousins. . . . With our siblings, we feel for one another.

Regular correspondence is not necessary to sustain sibling affectivity. As one woman put it very well:

> *L:* I cannot say that I have been in touch with my brothers and sisters more often than with my cousins. But *I just know that I can depend on my brothers and sisters, and they on me.*

Many respondents, therefore, maintain that reciprocal exchange between siblings cannot be equated with other forms of social transactions, because "*they are about the only ones who can help one another fully without thought of any remuneration or any strings attached.*" Comments such as the following were frequently encountered during our interviews:

> *L:* It is obligatory for brothers and sisters to help each other in time of necessity like, for instance, when my younger brother wanted very much to study here in Cebu City, but my parents felt that they could not afford the expenses, because board and lodging are very expensive. I readily offered to have my younger brother stay in my house so they wouldn't have to pay for his board and lodging. *I feel that a favor done for a brother or sister is a favor done for my parents.* If it became necessary, I would offer to defray part of the school expenses of my *igsu-on* [siblings], something which I would not do for a cousin.

> *L:* Among my brothers and sisters, I have no favorite. I treat them equally. On payday each one receives his share [of money from my wages]. It was customary that they would expect allowances from me. Now that I am married, they don't ask me for the money anymore, but we are still very close to one another.

This strong sibling solidarity is not circumscribed by gender or class differences, although the nature of male sibling interaction may differ somewhat from that of female or cross-sex siblings. Thus, Cebuano women, by virtue of having to endure the hardship of managing a tight family budget, do have special experiences to share with their female siblings. Childbirth, children, and housework, not to mention a philandering husband, are uniquely female sufferings that only one's own sisters and mother can fully understand. Brothers interact in different ways. As breadwinners, they appreciate the difficulty of earning a living and readily extend to one another any monetary assistance they can offer. Occasionally, they may drown their sorrows together in a glass of *tuba* (coconut-fermented beverage) in the neighborhood *sari-sari* store. At other times, though less frequently, they may share the company of "other women," as some of the lower-class husbands we interviewed have done. Suffice it to say that a Cebuano, no matter how poor, is never alone in his struggle for survival. If he is young, he has many brothers and sisters who can help him by giving him a place to live, money for his pocket, and food for his stomach. If he is older, he can rest assured that his older children will take care of the other children in the family, as well as provide him with some form of subsistence.

Family and Fertility

The findings reported in this chapter demonstrate the difficulty of generating and substantiating theoretical propositions relating family systems to fertility behavior (cf. also Burch, 1967; Burch and Gendell, 1971; and Davis, 1955). Notwithstanding its popular appeal, high fertility is not exclusively associated with the existence of extended or corporate family systems. Our data from the Philippines show that, on the one hand, the country has had a long history of rapid population growth; but, on the other hand, the Filipino family system is not corporate or predominantly "extended." Contrary to widely held beliefs, the dominant household structure in Cebu is nuclear, a fact which is consonant with the bilateral kinship system of the Filipinos. (Detailed ramifications of this kinship structure will be discussed in the next chapter.)

Nevertheless, household statistics per se do not give a complete picture of the whole situation. They are a static measure—incapable of capturing the dynamics of family interaction and interpersonal processes over time. They fail to take into account the possible influence of the family life cycle on the patterning of household composition.

The hunch that fertility behavior may be differentially associated with various types of postmarital residence was put to rest in chapter 4 after we examined the length of time that elapsed between marriage and first birth, for couples who were living with different sets of relatives and by themselves. The entire range of variation was so slight that one is forced to conclude that other factors play a more important role in shaping the fertility behavior of the Cebuanos we studied. From a sociological perspective, however, this fact is consistent with the brunt of our survey findings which suggests that at the time of our study, the Cebuanos had universally high fertility, small variations by class and urban-rural backgrounds notwithstanding. It is, therefore, meaningless to manipulate "variables," as sociologists are prone to do. Rather, a more fruitful approach is to examine the flow of interpersonal and interfamilial assistance in order to have a better understanding of how the poor and the not-so-poor ever manage to cope with large numbers of children. In so doing, we have a better understanding of the "insider's" view of the world, rather than the "outsider's" attributions of cause and effect that social scientists sometimes cannot resist. And, indeed, what a difference the change of perspective makes! Now, instead of seeing the Filipinos as unconcerned about their children's future, we realize that they have shifted all their dreams of a better life to their children and would do everything they can to provide for their education. The larger the number of children, the better are the chances that one of them will someday succeed, and the more support money one can expect to receive from them, other things being equal. As a destitute respondent who has seven children once said to us: "*Pobre ang wala'y anak.* [Poor is the man who has no children at all.] Nobody to fetch you the things you need; nobody to run errands for you; nobody to cook for you when you get old."

It is not that the Cebuanos do not love their children. They do very much. But because of their extreme material deprivation and cultural distinctiveness, love between parents and children is not always verbally expressed. Rather, it must be extrapolated from the immense sacrifices that parents make for their children, and from the dreams they spin in the privacy of their fantasies. The parents' perceptions of the world are such that they feel the need to protect their children from the hazards of the environment, which changes daily as more and more modern technologies are transplanted from abroad. The discipline they give the child who crosses the "big" street without permission appears harsh only if we look at it from the "outsider's" point of view. But in their culture, and given their values, to punish the child is to protect him from being harmed by the environment. The heavier the punishment, the more they believe the child will remember to always ask for permission before venturing into the urban jungle. To punish, therefore, is to show how much one cares about the child's well-being and his future. It is love—in a different sense.

Furthermore, what distinguishes the Cebuano family from others is the importance attached to two potentially competing kinship dyads which, on the one hand, encourage economic independence but, on the other hand, foster the psychosocial dependence of children on parents and vice versa. Such a deep-rooted sense of dependence is nurtured by means of an intricate socialization process which gives parents and other adult family members tremendous authority to discipline the young and the "disobedient." Given that the Cebuano family is an open social system, the establishment of separate nuclear households does not necessarily sever kinship interaction, because the borderline between an individual's own nuclear family and a kinsman's family is not well defined. Relatives, especially one's own siblings, are never considered superfluous in Cebuano society. On the contrary, they provide the underprivileged a reliable source of mutual assistance and a support network which is not diminished by time or distance.

From the individual's vantage point, any change in fertility outcome produces a chain of reactions that can disrupt his probability for social advancement, sense of well-being, and the amount of aid that is potentially forthcoming. Whatever economic disadvantage exists with increasingly large numbers of children is easily offset by the economic gains of the older children who not only turn in their income to their parents, but are socialized to raise the rest of the children, to the extent possible. In an underdeveloped country with an extremely uneven distribution of wealth, having large numbers of children may thus be perceived as *functional*, rather than dysfunctional, by the poor masses.

10 / The Web of Kinship

As we shift our attention away from the antecedent variables which directly contribute to high fertility and concentrate instead on the ramifications of large family size for the individual Cebuano family, a number of sociocultural practices which have heretofore not been considered important in demographic research begin to take on greater significance. The preceding chapter emphasized the prominence of nuclear kinship dyads in the fertility-coping behavior of the Filipinos, and gave the impression that other extended-kin ties are of little importance. This perception, however, is *not* substantiated by our interview records. On the contrary, despite the insistence that cousins are emotionally less close than siblings, a complex web of kinship operates in wondrous ways as a fertility-coping mechanism. Precisely how it works has never been systematically studied before, much less documented. This chapter aims to present the beginning of a theoretical interpretation of Cebuano kinship and its significance in fertility-coping behavior.

Cebuano Kinship

In terms of descent, Cebuano kinship structure is bilateral rather than unilineal. Genealogical reckoning is traced through both the male and the female lines simultaneously from a focal individual often termed "Ego" by anthropologists. All those persons who are consanguineally related to Ego constitute his "kindred" (Rivers, 1924:16), or what Leach (1950:61–62) called "personal kindred."

Since kindred is not a spatially bounded, discrete unit but a *relational* concept, there is no concrete territorial manifestation of kindred groupings other than the household in which Ego and his nuclear kinsmen reside. Hence, it is not considered a descent group by anthropologists.[1] Theoretically, Cebuano kindred relations may be traced lineally and collaterally *ad infinitum*. In reality, however, the range of one's kindred is limited, although a sharp line is almost never drawn. The individual has considerable latitude in selecting from among his consanguineal kin those members whom he recognizes as his kindred. In contrast, this element of choice does not exist in the patrilineal kinship system, for instance.

The bilateral features of Cebuano kinship structure are manifested in various ways. Surnames, for example, are inherited bilaterally, with the father's surname appearing last and serving as the child's last name, preceded by the mother's surname which is used somewhat as a middle name is in the United States. Among prominent families, it is not unusual for both the father's and the mother's surnames to appear in hyphenated form as the child's last name.

Cebuano kinship structure does not specify a preference for either patrilocal or matrilocal residence. Depending on the socioeconomic background of the newly married couple, residence may be neolocal or bilocal. Coresidence with either the wife's or the husband's relatives is fairly common, as shown in chapter 4.

Cebuano kin terms likewise do not distinguish between paternal and maternal relatives. The borrowed Spanish words *tiyo* and *tiya* (often used interchangeably with the native Cebuano words, *iyo* and *iya*) are terms of address for uncles and aunts on both sides of the genealogical tree. Hence, *genealogical egalitarianism* is a distinguishing feature of Cebuano kinship (Brandewie, 1975). Moreover, terms of reference for uncles and aunts may be used for parents' cousins as well as parents' siblings. Such linguistic flexibility, we will argue, has an obvious advantage. It allows the individual to accentuate his remote consanguineal relations, if he so chooses, with any kindred member of the older generation, and to draw him closer socioemotionally. A more detailed discussion of the significance of Cebuano kin terms in use follows.

Cebuano Kin Terms

Although most sociologists pay very little attention to kinship terminologies, anthropologists consider them an essential source for understanding interpersonal and interfamilial relationships. For analytic purposes, we may distinguish three dimensions of kinship relationships: genealogical, social, and terminological (Bohannan, 1963). Traditionally, however, even some anthropologists have assumed that kinship terminologies are isomorphous with the exact genealogical reckoning of kin and the social network of interactions. It is only recently that this assumption has been criticized (Hunt, 1969:37).

Using a detailed listing of Cebuano kin terms of reference compiled by Brandewie (1975:93–95), we constructed Table 10.1 to show the Ce-

TABLE 10.1

CEBUANO KIN TERMS OF REFERENCE ACCORDING TO GENEALOGICAL CLASSIFICATION

Absolute Generation	*Direct or Lineal Relations*	*First-Degree Collaterals*	*Second-Degree Collaterals*	*Third-Degree Collaterals*
+ 2	*apuhán* (grandparents, great aunts, great uncles)		*apuhán*	
+ 1	*amahán* (m) / *inahán* (f) (father) (mother)		*uyu-án* (m / *iya-án* (f) (uncle) (aunt)	
− 1	*anák* (son/daughter)		*pag-umángkun** (nephew/niece)	
0	*igsúun* (siblings): *kamagulángan* (oldest sibling); *kamanghúran* (youngest sibling)	*ig-ágaw nga igtágsa* (cousin)	*ig-áwaw nga igtagúrha* (cousin)	*ig-ágaw nga igtagútlu* (cousin)
− 2	*apú* (grandchild)			
− 3	*apu sa súngkud* (great grandchild)		*kadúgu'* (blood relations); *paryinte* (relatives)	
− 4	*apu sa túhud* (great great grandchild)			
− 5	*apu sa káray* (great great great grandchild)			

Note: These kin terms are derived from the list supplied by Brandewie (1975).

*Occasionally, finer distinctions may be made between parent's sibling's grandchildren (*pag-umángkun sa pag-agáwan ig-tágsa*) and parent's sibling's great grandchildren (*pag-umángkun sa pag-agáwan ig-tagurha*).

buano system of encoding consanguineal relatives, if one were to use genealogy as the kinship referent. We note that in terms of classificatory principles, Cebuano kin terms differentiate: (1) absolute generations, (2) sex of referent in the first ascending generation, (3) linearity versus collaterality, (4) three degrees of collaterality, (5) relative age and seniority in the sibling generation, and (6) number of marriage or mating links.

Do we have reason to suspect that this system of nomenclature may be different *in practice*? None of our research colleagues in Cebu gave much thought to it. However, the interviewers and Elena Yu herself, all natives of Cebu, are aware of such discrepancies although they did not have any explanation for this anomalous observation at the time.

That nonrandom incongruities exist between the use of the terminological system and actual genealogical relations became apparent when we mapped the kinship charts of our respondents and asked them how they address the relatives they have come in contact with. Within the confines of nuclear family members, the vocative terms generally used are fairly consistent across the board. For those who are in the bottom socioeconomic stratum and who originated in rural areas, the Cebuano vocative terms *tatay* and *nanay* are most commonly used for addressing father and mother, respectively. Nevertheless, some changes are evident intergenerationally and as one moves from the bottom stratum to the middle class. For example, some lower-class respondents call their respective parents *tatay* and *nanay*, but their own children call them by the Spanish terms of address, *papa* and *mama*. Sometimes the change is not synchronous for both parents. In a number of families the father is addressed as *papa* but the mother is addressed as *nanay* for idiosyncratic reasons. Or the children call their mother (our respondent) *mama* but call their father *tatay*. One respondent explains the discrepant usage as follows:

> My husband does not like to be called *papa*. In Bohol where he is from, people believe that when someone is called *papa*, he is rich. And we are not rich. So the children call him *tatay*. But I do not like to be called *nanay*. I'm not used to it. So the children call me *mama*.

Apparently, kin terms are gradually being "modernized" in the Cebuano culture and the local vocative terms, *nanay* and *tatay*, are increasingly being devalued. To some urbanized people, the word *nanay* sounds too "provincial" or anachronistic, and conveys a picture of a poor, haggard woman, old and wrinkled well before her time. The change, however, is not always toward the Spanish form of address. The use of the U.S. vocative terms, *mommy* and *daddy*, is emerging among the middle class. But, regardless of whether one uses *tatay*, *papa*, or *daddy*, these terms of address when applied to one's own parents are fairly congruent with the normative system of genealogical reckoning. Once we shift our focus outside nuclear family members, however, some variability is evident. Not all aunts and uncles are consistently called *tiyo/tiya* or *iyo/iya*. Neither are grandparents uniformly addressed as *lolo/lola*. For lineally ascending relatives, the incongruity is striking.

For example, one of our respondents (and she is not the only one) calls her parents *mama* and *papa* and calls her parents' parents *nanay* and *tatay* instead of *lola* and *lolo*. Based on these terms of address, the respondent appears to have *four* parents instead of two, since the words *nanay* and *tatay* have the same meaning as *mama* and *papa*. When queried as to why she did not call her grandparents by the "proper" terms (from an outsider's point of view), the respondent explained that her mother had always taught them that the rich and more sophisticated families had other ways of addressing relatives. But since *they themselves are poor*, they had to stick to the simple ways of showing love and respect for elders. This answer, of course, did not satisfy our curiosity. We searched for other families who have also been inconsistent in their application of kin terminologies. The result was fascinating. One man calls his maternal grandmother (MoMo) Mama Inday. He explained that "perhaps this is because she owned some pieces of land." His maternal grandfather (MoFa), who also owned pieces of land, was called *tatay* instead of grandfather. Another respondent refers to all her uncles and aunts as *tiyo* and *tiya*, with two exceptions. One particular uncle (FaBr) was called *tatay* because, she said, "he assumed a position of influence in the whole kin group." Traveling kinsmen always stayed in his house when they stopped in Zamboanga, and he always attended to them. An aunt (FaSi) was called *nanay* or mother because this relative had "spent for" her and sent her to Cebu for her college degree. In still another family, the middle-class respondent who came from an upper-lower-class background reported a similar extension of paternal kin terms to uncles. Of her mother's five brothers, one was called *papa;* another was called *tatay*. Her explanation was:

> We call Papa Simon "*papa*" because when we were small, we were very close to them. They treated us like their own children. Tatay Basilio [also MoBr] was called "*tatay*" because he had no children. My sister was his godchild at confirmation. She called him "*tatay*," so we all did the same.

Likewise, a lower-class woman addresses one of her mother's three brothers as *papa* insted of *tiyo*. This favored uncle, Consuelo, is the person they turn to whenever there is a family crisis. For instance, when this woman's mother died, she and her siblings sought Papa Consuelo's help, because they did not have any money to pay for the funeral. It was Papa Suelo (as he is affectionately called) who borowed some money on his credit from a Chinese merchant in their hometown and arranged for the funeral. She added further:

> Papa Suelo gets things done and organizes things by virtue of respect and authority. He always acts as the big man during the *pamalaye* [marriage negotiation] of my brothers and sisters. He set the dowry for Manang Kosing and Deding [R's older sisters]. . . . When one of my brothers wanted to get married, he was the one who approached the girl's parents and bargained with the dowry. Ah! he is a good talker and a good man. He is respected by everyone in town. He was the one who told me not to have sixteen children like himself.

We should emphasize that not all esteemed uncles and aunts are brought genealogically closer by calling them "father" or "mother." In some cases, the kin terms used draw those relatives *even closer* (in age) —into the sibling's generation. For example, the husband of one of our respondents calls his mother's oldest sister *manay*, which is a term of address for older sisters. Similarly, he calls his paternal grandmother's sister (FaMoSi) *manang*, which has exactly the same meaning as *manay* or older sister (just as *Daddy* and *Dad* are the same in the English language). In another family, our interviewers found that the respondent called a paternal grandmother's brother's daughter (FaMoBrDau who is named Liling) *manay* because this relative's (Liling's) husband (FaMoBrDauHu) was a big farmer. He owned "a big land planted with lots of coconuts." Obviously, in this case, the specific nomenclature used indicates precisely through whom that kindred relationship was mediated. In the first example above, our respondent's husband's relationship with his paternal grandmother's sister (FaMoSi) is through his paternal grandmother. Since the latter (FaMo) called her sister (FaMoSi) *manay*, the respondent's husband was drawn into their generation by following his paternal grandmother's term of address. In the second example, the respondent's relationship with Liling (FaMoBrDau) was mediated through a "rich" relative, the paternal grandmother's brother (FaMoBr) whom she calls *iyo*, meaning uncle. Consequently, one cannot very well call the *iyo*'s daughter, Liling, *iya*. This, we believe, is the reason why Liling is called *manay* or older sister, even though she is actually the *youngest* child in her family.

Finally, we should also mention the fact that in some families, a relative may be addressed as older sister instead of mother for other reasons. Take the case of a woman whom we shall call Pacita Balagtas. Her mother's sister, Ingga, wanted to adopt Pacita when she was a child, but the offer was turned down because Pacita was the only girl in the family. As a compromise, Ingga always sent for Pacita during mealtimes, and she "spent for" her as well. What Pacita said about Ingga gives us a clue as to why the latter was called *mana(ng)* or older sister rather than *mama*:

> Mana Ingga was not rich, but she made sacrifices for my sake. I know it was a burden for her to buy me things but she wanted to. None of my relatives liked her at all. They have called her cranky and sarcastic. Ingga felt that somehow she wanted a small child and I filled that gap. All of her children were grown up then.

One wonders what the term of address might be if Ingga were rich and well liked by Pacita's parents.

There are, of course, other instances where the oldest girl in the family is called "mother" by the younger children in the family, instead of "older sister." Careful probing showed that often the oldest girl who is called *mama* by her brothers and sisters had undertaken the financial and psychological burden of raising the rest of the family after her marriage to a "rich" man.

Theoretical Interpretation

The alert reader will no doubt have noted that these illustrations converge on certain critical assumptions concerning Filipino family relationships. First and foremost in the conviction that the parent-child bond is the most permanent family relationship of all; that blood relationship is indissoluble. Parents have a moral obligation to raise their children and provide for them economically, to the limit of their capacity. Nevertheless, for many lower-class people, this fundamental value cannot always be fulfilled. In the face of extreme material deprivation and subsistent living conditions, they must find alternative modes of survival to provide a sense of security amidst all the uncertainties in life, and to spur them on with the hope that tomorrow will be better. A way of sheltering one's children against life's unforeseen exigencies is to reinforce existing blood ties by "doubling" the consanguineal relationship, for one of the most distinctive features of the bilateral kinship structure is its theoretically limitless genealogical reckoning. Since no human mind can possibly cope with an astronomical number of kindred, a selection process is undoubtedly necessary. Hence, the bilateral kinship structure is also inherently susceptible to genealogical amnesia. After all, there is no fixed rule for the inclusion or exclusion of kinsmen. By calling one's uncle as one's father, or an aunt as mother, Ego is in fact strengthening his consanguineal ties. The original uncle-nephew (or aunt-niece) tie is reinforced (or "doubled" for lack of a better word) by a second relationship, the (fictive) parent-child dependency linkage.

An uncle might perchance "forget" some of his nephews, but surely he cannot neglect a particular nephew who is *like* a son to him and who calls him "father."

It cannot be overemphasized that the parent-child bond in Cebuano society is culturally defined as permanent, immutable, indissoluble. An uncle (or an aunt) may choose not to extend assistance to most of his (or her) nephews, but he is *morally obliged* to aid his children to the last drop of his sweat. The need to engulf one's secondary relatives and mold a nuclear kinship bond is made more urgent by the very absence of any concrete territorial manifestation of kindred groupings other than the household. Extended or secondary (and more distant) kinsmen, therefore, cannot be held "captive" in the network of mutual assistance as they could be in unilineal kinship structures where rules of descent exist for the formation of clan associations or lineage as concrete manifestations of the kinship organization. Thus, in a society characterized by bilaterality, only the household and its essential (nuclear) members are "lasting." This explains why the maneuvering of Cebuano kinship nomenclature in use is almost always in the direction of the fundamental parent-child dependency linkage. "Rich" grandmothers are called "mother," prominent uncles are called "father," and an able older sister who marries into a "wealthy" family is called "mother"—all because the poor Cebuanos know that they are poor and recognize the potency of that parent-child relationship. Where such linguistic maneuverings are technically difficult or impossible to manipulate, a second-best compromise is struck by bringing esteemed secondary kinsmen into Ego's sibling generation. This is done, for instance, by calling one's FaMoSi *manang,* or one's FaMoBrDau *manay.* The terms used may be different, but the effect is the same. It draws an influential but distant relative into the second-most enduring kinship bond in the household, namely, the sibling relationship. It is, after all, these two sets of kinship dyads that distinguish nuclear relatives from the extended ones. As one respondent explains:

> *M:* There is a difference between *pamilya* [family] and *paryinte* [relatives]. *Pamilya* refers to *sulud bahay* [members of the household]. *Paryinte* is *layo* [far, distant] . . . [like] *ig-agaw* [cousins]. But a *paryinte* may be brought closer to the *pamilya* if there are frequent visits, regular contacts, and other exchanges.

Thus, the gap between nuclear and extended kinsmen can be narrowed by reciprocal exchange, and it is our position that the manipulation of kinship terminologies in use is but one way of inducing that interaction. Whether or not the use of nuclear kin terms on nonnuclear relatives in fact results in an extension of psychological sentiments commensurate with intimate family relationships is irrelevant here. What is crucial is the *perceived* expectation of a *possible* extension of familial sentiments. The observation that this practice is more prevalent among the lower class than in the middle class serves to validate our conclusion.

Implications

Rather than assume that all individuals address members of their kindred according to the demarcations drawn on the genealogical grid, our kinship material from Cebu indicates that some people may adjust the genealogical "given" to suit their preferred or expected interactions by manipulating the linguistic tags in their nomenclature system. Thus, *genealogically* distant relatives are *terminologically* transposed into "nuclear" kinsmen to symbolize the enduring relationship between parent and child, or the cohesive bond between siblings.

In a separate study based on kinship data from San Juan, Mexico, Hunt (1969:46) posited that one consequence of such a flexible mechanism for encoding kindred members is that it allows for the inclusive application of a genealogically exclusive kin term (such as *mama* as genetrix) to a variety of social network settings. In other words, a woman who fulfills the role demands for motherhood may be tagged "mother" even though she is not the biological parent. This is but additional evidence that the Cebuano family is indeed an *open* family system.

The next task is to examine whether there is any consonance between genealogy and social interaction among kinsmen. To accomplish this, we asked our respondents—housewives of child-bearing age—to supply us spontaneously with the names of those individuals whom they considered their relatives. The results are discussed below.

The Range of Kindred

Of the twenty-two families interviewed intensively, a lower-class respondent reported the largest number of kin, a total of 412 *paryinte* (relatives) spanning six generations and several cousinships. Added to this number is her husband, six living children, her daughter's spouse, and a grandchild-to-be. The smallest kindred size we obtained comes from a middle-class respondent who acknowledges only 50 relatives, going as far as her husband's grandparents' generation, and extending laterally to her husband's and her siblings, plus their respective children. This kind of comparison, of course, is misleading, since kindred size is a function, albeit not a unilinear function, of the family size of each relative and of the family life cycle. To control for variation in family size, we decided to examine the kin types enumerated by our respondents. This idea was inspired by an article written by Cumming and Schneider (1961:500).

In Table 10.2 we have classified kin types into different degrees of consanguinity: primary, secondary, tertiary, quaternary, and so forth. Primary kin are those which can be described by one word only: mother, father, brother, sister, son, daughter. Secondary kin are those

TABLE 10.2

RESPONDENTS' KNOWLEDGE OF KIN TYPES

Kin Types of Ego (Wi)	*Number of Respondents Who Enumerated This Type of Kin in Their Spontaneous Listing*		
	Total (N = 22)	*Lower-Class (N = 15)*	*Middle-Class (N = 7)*
Primary kin (Ego's parents and children)	22	15	7
Secondary ascendants (aunts, uncles, grandparents)	21	15	6
Secondary descendants (nephews and nieces)	22	15	7
Tertiary ascendants (great grandparents, great aunts and uncles)	4	4	0
Tertiary collaterals (first cousins)	18	14	4
Tertiary descendants (great grandchildren; cousins of grandchildren)	2	0	2
Quaternary ascendants (parent's first cousins)	2	2	0
Quaternary descendants (Ego's cousins' children)	15	11	4
Quinternary collaterals (Ego's third cousins)	4	4	0
Quinternary and sexternary ascendants and descendants and other more distant kin	1	1	0

which require the pairing of primary kin terms, for example, mother's father or father's sister. Tertiary kin are those which require three words, such as mother's brother's son. Within each degree of consanguinity we have, where possible, differentiated the generational affiliation of these relatives *vis-à-vis* Ego, the wife.

Table 10.2 shows that all of our respondents enumerated primary and secondary kin as part of their kindred. Among tertiary relatives, the collateral kin are more likely to be mentioned than the ascending or descending consanguines. This is most probably due to the life span of the Cebuanos, the age of our respondents, and the specific stage of their life cycle. Slightly over two-thirds of those interviewed consider their quaternary descendants as part of their kindred; a few were able to trace their quaternary ascendants and quinternary collaterals. One woman went as far as her mother's father's sister's daughter's son's daughter's son (MoFaSiDauSoDauSo) in her spontaneous listing.

Another remarkable feat is the inclusion of spouses of relatives and the husband's kindred (see Table 10.3). This inclusion, however, is somewhat more selective. Secondary descendants are always included as part of the husband's kindred and, hence, of Ego's kindred. A little less than half of the wives mentioned their husband's secondary ascendants (aunts, uncles, and grandparents) and tertiary collaterals (first cousins). Two women even traced their husband's kin beyond the fifth degree of consanguinity—as far as the husband's father's father's brother's son's wife's father's wife's brother's wife's brother (HuFaFaBrSoWiFaWiBrWiBr), who, as it turns out, also happens to be the husband's oldest sister's husband.

Although the total sample is much too small for any meaningful generalization regarding social-class differences in spontaneous kin listing, an interesting pattern emerges when one examines the aggregate figure broken down by social class. First of all, proportionally more lower-class women mention their tertiary collaterals, quaternary descendants, and quinternary collaterals than do middle-class respondents. Insofar as the husband's kindred is concerned, proportionally more lower-class women included their husbands' secondary ascendants (aunts, uncles, grandparents), secondary descendants, tertiary collaterals, and quaternary descendants than did middle-class housewives. If one assumes that interviewer variability occurred at random rather than systematically—and we have no reason to believe otherwise—then the data suggest that there may be a social-class difference in the recall of relatives. Might it not be possible that it is functionally more salient for the lower class to remember the entire expanse of their kindred because of their poverty, in the hope that they might be able to accentuate certain consanguineal or affinal ties to their advantage?

TABLE 10.3

RESPONDENTS' KNOWLEDGE OF HUSBAND'S KIN TYPES

Kin Types of Ego's Spouse	*Number of Respondents Who Enumerated This Type of Kin in Their Spontaneous Listing* Total (N = 21)	Lower-Class* (N = 14)	Middle-Class (N = 7)
Primary kin (parents and children)	21	14	7
Secondary ascendants (aunts, uncles, grandparents)	9	8	1
Secondary descendants (nephews and nieces)	21	14	7
Tertiary ascendants (great grandparents, great aunts and uncles)	1	1	0
Tertiary collaterals (first cousins)	9	8	1
Tertiary descendants (great grandchildren; cousins of grandchildren)	2	1	1
Quaternary ascendants (parent's first cousins)	1	1	0
Quaternary descendants (cousins' children)	6	6	0
Quinternary collaterals (third cousins)	1	1	0
Quinternary and sexternary ascendants and descendants and other more distant kin	2	2	0

*The total *N* for the lower class is only fourteen in this case because the data for one respondent's spouse were lost in transit.

Lower-class Cebuanos, after all, are painfully aware of their helplessness and cognizant of the absence of structures aside from kinship bonds which could offer them assistance without requiring immediate reciprocal exchange. By contrast, the middle-class family's struggle for upward mobility may intensify their dread of "slipping down" the social ladder through engaging in too many unilateral commitments which offer no immediate payoffs and may never be reciprocated in spite of profound appreciation. Hence, their pervasive genealogical amnesia. To test this hypothesis, we examined the interview records dealing with kinship interaction.

Lower-Class Kinship Interaction

Impressive though their spontaneous listing may be, the lower-class people are, in reality, able to sustain day-to-day interaction with only a small number of relatives. Extreme poverty, geographic dispersion of kinsmen, and the inaccessibility of communication channels render daily or regular contacts with relatives practically impossible. Even within the small circle of geographically accessible kinsmen, social interaction may be circumscribed by personal shame (*ulaw*), for the very poor resent being perceived as "so poor that they are unable to fend for themselves." Consequently, social visits with slightly better-off relatives are kept to a minimum for fear that "if I go out of my way to visit them, they might think I am asking for help." One woman looks at this matter philosophically: "All members of our family are resigned to the idea that they must fend for themselves. It would be futile to hope for assistance, whether material or psychological, from our relatives because each one has enough worries of his own."

Those who marry upwards often keep a certain social distance from their poorer relatives so as not to be importuned. As one respondent whose cousin married into a wealthy family said: "I recognize them as cousins. But *not them!* They *do* take notice of me when we meet, but just as if we were merely acquaintances."

Where interaction with kinsmen occurs, however, it tends to be very intimate and regular. We have a case, for instance, where the aunt babysits for our respondent in exchange for a few early morning drinks of *tuba* (a fermented coconut drink). A cousin (MoSiDau) from Jolo always brings some smuggled "stateside" goods such as soaps, blankets, and other items as gifts for the family whenever she is in Cebu to distribute these products in the black market. Two other relatives (FaSiSo) who own a merchandise store in Leyte also stay with our respondent whenever they are in Cebu to replenish their supply. Two more relatives (HuFaSiDau) are boarding with our respondent as they finish their college education. In turn, they perform some of the household chores in the family. A poor aunt (HuFaSi) who lives in Pasil (a slum district) constantly "borrows" money from our respondent. She is tolerated because "she is pitiful and, besides, she comes over to do the family's laundry." Thus, as long as the exchange is more or less balanced over time, lower-class kinship interaction can thrive without much disruption, although contacts cannot be sustained with all the relatives that are recognized.

Middle-Class Kinship Interaction

Middle-class kinship interaction contrasts vividly with lower-class interaction. Our interview data show that the number of *living* relatives they socially recognize is quite small—only between 47 and 145 individuals as compared to between 61 and 412 reported by the lower-class respondents. Genealogical amnesia, a nonchalant attitude toward kinship obligations, and less *ulaw* or shame about not reciprocating other people's gifts are characteristic of the middle-class people we interviewed. As one of them said, "We have many relatives, but *we are not really obligated to them.*" Another elaborated further:

> With regard to gift-giving among relatives, one is not obligated to give in return. Although out of respect, sometimes, one should give, as there are some relatives like, for example, a sister who is celebrating her birthday, and she knows that you can afford to give a little, she would be expecting something from you. . . . When it is services like somebody is ill . . . you are not really expected to help out *if you don't have time to spare*. . . . Financial help among family [members] is expected—that is, *if* one is also known to be financially well off.

These remarks sound especially callous when compared to those made by lower-class respondents. The latter generally feel that kinship obligation always exists and that assistance, once sought, must be rendered as long as one still has a few centavos to spare. The poor emphasized, "*Baslan man nato na, kon sila na sa'd ang magkalisud*" (we will also reciprocate when it is their turn to suffer difficulties).

Among middle-class people, activities that can lead to socioeconomic improvement receive top priority. Many couples find that they not only have to work in order to keep up with inflation and their growing taste for imported goods, but also have to hold more than one job in order to live the kind of life they want. Multiple occupations are thus quite common in the Philippines, as they are in other developing countries. For instance, a man may serve full time as an assistant manager of a big automobile dealership, sell insurance in his spare time, and operate a trucking and taxi service full time as well. We have one family where the husband, who has an M.B.A., teaches at a major university in the city, is the director of a local technical school, and operates an advertising firm—three full-time jobs. His wife teaches elementary school, operates a boarding house for twelve students and stewardesses, complete with food-catering service, and works as a bookkeeper in the family's advertising firm.

The almost complete mobilization of time and resources required for multiple occupations offers obvious economic advantages. The ambitious Filipino is able to spread the risk of financial commitments and maximize his income. Unfortunately, it also precludes the allocation of energy for kinship interaction, unless contacts with relatives facilitate social gains. To minimize social liability, the middle-class family is beginning to cultivate an impersonal attitude toward kindred relations. Remarks such as the following are commonly heard:

> *Q:* If a certain relative would come to you to ask for some kind of assistance like, for example, a job, since you have such a high position and many prosperous friends, would you help him?
>
> *H: No.* . . . As much as possible, I would not give any assistance, as there are some relatives who would take advantage of you and would be lax in their job, thereby endangering my prestige [reputation] and name. . . . I would rather give [the] vacancy to friends than to relatives.

However, even as they untangle themselves from their less fortunate kinsmen, the middle-class family often simultaneously cultivates extensive and intensive ties with others whom they perceive to be strategically important in their upward climb. As an example, we have one respondent who is in regular and close contact with seven relatives: (1) her mother, whose store she helps to tend during her free time and from whom she receives two pesos every day (sixty pesos a month) "in the name of the children"; (2) her "Mama" Inday, a maternal aunt who raised her and spent for her education; (3) her mother-in-law, whose house they stayed in after marriage, and to whom she continues to give monthly stipends; (4) "Papa" Magno, a "rich" maternal uncle who owns the lot on which the respondent's present house is built and for which they do not have to pay rent (in exchange, Papa Magno eats with the family once a week, on Sundays); (5) another uncle, who visits daily and plays with the children while the respondent tends her mother's store; (6) a female cousin who buys from her mother's store for all her needs and keeps our respondent company while she tends the store; and (7) a male cousin who is a lawyer and to whom the respondent turns every time her mother's store's license must be renewed. In addition, "all" her relatives gather at least on the following occasions every year: All Souls' Day (November 2), Fiesta (Our Lady of Guadalupe, December 12), and Christmas, besides occasional weddings, baptisms, and funerals.

The disparity in wealth between the lower-class and the middle-class families is also evident from the gifts they send their relatives. While the poor send bread, maize, dried fish (*buwad*), and perhaps a bottle of Tanduay or Siok-Thong (local liquor) to their beloved relatives via traveling townmates, the middle class exchange *kaseo* (cheese), *maha-real* (a delicious pastry), *piniatos* (peanut brittle), cloth, cash, and other items which are sometimes airfreighted from one city to another. Thus, the solid financial foundation of middle-class families is a distinct advantage over the shaky economic base of the lower-class households.

Ecological and technological factors, in addition to illiteracy, are formidable barriers to lower-class kinship interaction. In contrast, the middle class can sustain contact with geographically dispersed kin via long distance telephone and/or modern air transport systems. As a result, individuals have considerable latitude to decide who among their relatives will constitute the web of kinship. Note, however, that in terms of day-to-day kin interaction, there is very little *quantitative* difference between the two classes, as measured by the number of relatives in contact. But if one focuses on the general ability to recall the whereabouts of relatives, the lower-class respondents we interviewed demonstrated an impressive knowledge of the broad expanse of their kinship, even though they would not normally want to go out of their way to interact with inaccessible relatives. This, to us, suggests that the lower-class families attach far greater significance to "following up" their relatives than the middle class—probably with the hope of activating dormant kindred ties whenever absolutely necessary. After all, lower-class people cannot avail themselves of modern banking institutions to generate cash in emergencies. They must rely upon the kindness of relatives or engage in *prenda*.[2] Consequently, the ethos of mutual aid is far more pervasive among lower-class people than among middle-class individuals.

Kinship and Fertility

Our research findings thus far point to the importance of kinship among the Cebuanos even though their household structure is predominantly nuclear, and even though they do not maintain daily contacts with *all* their relatives. Given this insight, it seems only logical that we examine the relationship between kinship and fertility behavior. Does kinship pressure contribute positively or negatively to large family size?

Brandewie (1973) argued that the very structure of bilateral kinship itself may exert pressures on Filipino couples to bear children because the conjugal bond per se is weak. Hence, children are necessary —as we have argued as well—to solder marital relationships. To support his argument, Brandewie (1973:13) observed how mothers or mothers-in-law often rub the stomach of a newly married daughter or daughter-in-law to inquire casually whether she is "already conceiving." Our own observations indicate that such questions are asked as early as three months after the marriage has been formalized, and by individuals who may be just friends or distant relatives—a situation most American women would find terribly annoying. If the newly married woman answers negatively, peer teasing occurs which either accuses the husband of "already" dividing his attention with other women or hints at his ignorance in performing his role. In cases where some time has elapsed after marriage and the wife is still not pregnant, the man's "maleness" (*pagkalalaki*) may even come into question. Relatives do not hesitate to give unsolicited advice to the woman, ranging from asking her to visit a folk masseur (*hilot*) to "eating better." Certain foods, such as fish roe, are widely believed to be fertility stimulants.[3]

The hypothesis that kinship pressure induces large family size is further supported by other evidence. For instance, we have asked our respondents, "Who was happiest when your first child was born?"—to which many answered "my mother-in-law," "my father and my husband," or "my parents." However, one should not minimize the importance of children to the wife herself. In the early years of marriage, pregnancy confers "adult" status on both husband and wife, and gives them a legitimate social excuse for establishing "independence," residentially and economically. The following interview is informative in this regard:

> *Q:* How did you feel when your husband gave his earnings to his mother instead of you [even after your marriage]?
>
> *L:* It was my wish that he give it to Mama [HuMo with whom they were living then]. *Maikog man gud ta.* [I feel embarrassed not to do it.] I also pity Mama. What can she earn from her work [as a *manghihilot*]? And Papa [HuFa] has no work.
>
> *Q:* For how long did this go on? Why did it stop?
>
> *L:* For about one year—*until after we already had a baby.*

Having a baby thus gives the wife a valid claim over the mother-in-law on the husband's earnings. Unless the husband can still afford to share his earnings with two households—his parents' and his own—the birth of a child will hasten the delineation of nuclear household responsibilities. But even when the husband can afford to continue financial support to his parents, there will come a time when it must end, as in the following case:

> *M:* When my husband asked for permission from them [his parents] to settle down [at age twenty-three], he promised that he would not cut their allowance [the money he gives them out of his earnings]. He did just that when we were few, but now that I have three kids and another coming, we just can't be as generous.

True enough, the husband's parents finally agreed that they should turn to their younger children for support and spare the respondent's family from having to underwrite two separate households. We do not wish to suggest that Cebuano women deliberately conspire to frustrate the economic dependency of their parents-in-law. But the data attest to the importance of subtle and not-too-subtle kinship pressures on the conjugal unit that intentionally or unintentionally affect fertility outcome.

In view of the permeating influence of kinship in all aspects of Filipino life, the question should be raised as to whether kinship pressure does "suppress" large family size. We asked ourselves that question as we plowed through our in-depth interview records. We found to our surprise that they do exist as well. Perhaps the most colorful instance of such negative pressure on fertility is provided by the following woman. She herself wanted to have another baby besides the five children she had, because the children were in school and she wanted a "companion" in the house. She recounted how her older stepsister, who is living with her, feels about any additional children:

> Gracia [older half-sister] . . . is still single. We live together and fight furiously and frequently. But our proximity has also made us intimate in that we keep no secret from each other and she *interferes* with my life. She feels that she must have a say even [with regard to] the number of children that we should have. The reason for this is [based on] what past experience has shown. She becomes involved in the caring of [my] children so that she does not want us to have any more. Our house is small, we don't have any privacy. Whenever Undo [husband] returns from his trip to the provinces, she becomes watchful. [Respondent turns her head to make sure Gracia is not within hearing distance and then continues.] This sister of mine is the cranky and nagging type. . . . Each time my husband comes home from a trip, she becomes moody the next day. At the least provocation, she complains of a sleepless night. *She blames it on our love-making, that the house shook and there were all kinds of noises.* "All right," she says, "it is none of my business. But I'm making it my business because another child would bother me no end. After all, I help take care of the children." "And, besides, at your age," she says, "you should be ashamed of yourself [still making love]." I even refused sometimes the advances of my husband because of this. We understand her point since more children mean more work for her, but we also become irritated that she acts as though she were the only one concerned. In the first place, this is our primary obligation and our children are primarily our responsibilities. But . . . she not only lives with me, I owe her a debt of gratitude for serving me. Knowing that she does not have any means of livelihood, I treat her as one of my family. When I buy myself anything, she also gets her share.

Aside from such cases, the most common motivation for relatives to put pressure against having too many children is "health hazards." However, in most cases, that pressure was not evident until there were already five, six, seven, or eight children and the mother's health had obviously suffered from malnutrition. In fact, in one case, an uncle kept advising his niece (who is our respondent) "*not* to have *sixteen* children" as he had. At the time of our interview, the woman had had nine pregnancies, eight live births, and was only in her mid-thirties. Sixteen children seems "large" and undesirable, indeed.

To summarize, what is a "large" or "small" family is relative. At the time we did our study in Cebu, for instance, all the office staff were "quizzed" on their desired family size. Each unmarried woman insisted that she did *not* want too many. Six is enough, they maintained. Our Cebu data show that while kinship pressure to conceive is undeniable in the early stages of marriage, the admonition not to conceive also exists, but it is often expressed too late to be effective in reducing family size. Besides, the advice is not given for "population" reasons, but for health or medical reasons.

11 / Multiple Equivalent Bonds: Godparenthood and Fosterage

Every society develops a system of child care and adoption practices consistent with its cultural values and economic development. Thus, in the United States, the practice of allowing a total stranger to babysit for one's child at a fixed hourly rate is acceptable and widespread. So is the system of legal adoption, which transfers the exclusive right of parenting from the child's biological parents to others. From a sociological perspective, such practices are consistent with the closed family system in the United States which permits the transfer of parental rights only on a contractual basis. In the Philippines, however, child care and adoption practices can be informal as well as contractual, the latter being far less frequent than the former. We stumbled upon this finding in our effort to determine the precise number of children in the households sampled. Not infrequently, the number of children ever born and alive did not match the number of children actually residing with the mother, even though the children were not yet married. In no instance is the child's departure from his natural parents' home permanent, nor is the occurrence extremely regular, and yet it is of such duration and frequency that it cannot be considered as fleeting or random. Moreover, some households contain one or two junior members who perform certain functions more than the other children, and yet they cannot be classified unequivocally as housemaids or houseboys because they are not compensated for such chores in the same manner as most servants in the Philippines. These seemingly anomalous observations prompted us to examine how the Cebuano system of child care and fosterage actually serves to establish *multiple* equivalent bonds between adults and children.

Through intensive interviews, we found that aside from the entangling family assistance and kinship reciprocities that enmesh most lower-class households, two other culturally patterned and normatively prescribed social mechanisms are available to increase the likelihood that children will be looked after in case of emergency or death. Both mechanisms—godparenthood and kinship fosterage—establish coexisting multiple equivalent bonds between adults and children without displacing the biological parent-child relationship. The first is a legacy from Spanish Catholicism, the second probably evolved from necessity and indigenous cultural values. At any rate, both institutions are undoubtedly legitimated by the existence of an open family ideology and a strong socialization emphasis on obedience training. In some respects, they are also analogous to the concept of spiritual sponsorship.

Spiritual Sponsorship

The implantation of Spanish Catholicism in the Philippines over nearly four centuries resulted in the development of a folk syncretic belief system and practices which remain as salient to the masses of peasants and urban villagers today as they were a century ago. The concept of spiritual sponsorship obtainable through specific patron saints of the Catholic church is premised on a hierarchical order of powerful figures, with God at the apex as the ultimate source of mercy. As in Spain and other Hispanic cultures, this patronage practice begins from the moment of birth, when the infant is assigned the name of a saint to act as his patron or protector, and stretches to cover nearly every conceivable crisis situation when the individual petitions for the intervention of a powerful figure—human or divine—to deliver him from his earthly sufferings or to strike a solution to his predicaments. Among lower-class urban villagers, perhaps the most venerated patron is the bejeweled image of Santo Niño, enshrined in the Church of Santo Niño. Various miracles, interwoven with true historical events and characters, have been attributed to him, not only in folklore but also in college history books (cf. Molina, 1960).[1] Likewise, the Cross of Magellan[2] arouses intense devotion among the urban villagers who kneel around the barred enclosure that surrounds it, praying fervently amidst the noise of the cars, trucks, and jeepneys that whisk past them.

The majority of Cebuano peasants and urban villagers believe that urgent petitions may be granted by saints and spirits if the individual makes a sincere and persistent request—often through an act of contrition or by praying devoutly to a particular spiritual figure perceived to be most skilled and efficacious in handling his petitions. To ensure success in obtaining his request, the client-supplicant pledges a course of action—part of which he performs as he makes his request, the rest of which he promises to fulfill after his petitions are granted. These actions may include doing penance, saying the *novena,* walking on one's knees from the church entrance to the communion rail, carrying the heavy cross during Holy Week processions, donating generously to the church, and faithfully lighting a candle in front of a statue of a saint.

Since spiritual beings vary in their powers and functions, the individual may compartmentalize his relationship with them and "shop around" for the most "effective" figure. A person who feels that his petitions to a particular saint have been consistently granted may decide to become a devotee of that saint, believing that he has been spiritually "sponsored." He may even wear a votive of that saint to symbolize the protection he has received and hopes to receive. The supplicant's relationship with his spiritual sponsors is not monopolistic, for several individuals may establish similar relationships with the same figure. Neither is it monolithic, since the individual is free to enter into such relationships with more than one saint. By the same token, any individual who is a devotee of a particular saint becomes a more socially desirable and "powerful" person than his fellows who are not devotees of any saint, for the divine power is perceived as capable of "rubbing off" on him and he can thus intercede for the saint's mercy on behalf of others. The devotee thus becomes a much sought-after prospect for godparenthood.

Godparenthood and Coparenthood

As prescribed in the Catholic liturgy, baptism, confirmation, and marriage are the three major *rites de passage* which require sponsorship. Although variations in the preferred choice and functions of sponsors are discernible, each of these rituals formalizes at least three relationships. The first is the sponsor-child relationship called godparenthood; the second is the sponsor-parent relationship called coparenthood; and the third is the biological parent-child relationship. In the Philippines, however, a fourth relationship is discernible, that between the sponsored child and his sponsor's children. In this chapter, we will argue that aside from being liturgical necessities, godparenthood and coparenthood have socioeconomic functions as well.

Of the three religious sacraments, the choice of baptismal sponsors is perhaps the most critical in the sense that it is the first opportunity for any family to establish spiritual kinship ties with other households. An inauspicious choice means that one must wait for the confirmation ceremony or the birth of another child (and therefore another baptism) before the opportunity of establishing spiritual kinship ties arises again. Interestingly enough, the ceremonial requisites of baptism, confirmation, and marriage at once formalize and deformalize the relationship between coparents. On the one hand, by addressing each other as "*(kum)pare*" and "*(kum)mare*"—which means "cofather" and "co-mother" in a way—the coparents are normatively defined as equals in the task of parenting the child. There is an air of camaraderie and respect rather than social distance. Advice may be openly sought and assistance gladly rendered without the expectation of immediate reciprocal action. At the very least, Christmas and the sponsored child's birthday are occasions for renewing their fictive kinship bond through gift-giving. At the same time, the coparents are also bound to be less articulate about their negative feelings toward each other in their social and economic interactions. No matter how angry one feels, one must be forgiving toward one's coparents.

In Cebu, as in Spain, the incest taboo is extended to include the godparents' children. The sponsored child may never marry into his godparents' nuclear family or have sexual relations with any of them since he and his godparents' children, as spiritual brothers and sisters, are ritually children of the "same" parents.

Contrary to the hypothesis presented by Mintz and Wolf (1950), Foster (1961, 1963), and other scholars working in Latin America, who found that a certain mode of phrasing coparenthood relationships seems to predominate in each community, we found that among the Cebuanos, such ties can be either symmetrical or asymmetrical. Analytically speaking, symmetry exists whenever godparenthood links coparents who belong to the same socioeconomic class and exchange goods and services of approximately the same kind. Although it would be advantageous for lower-class Cebuanos to phrase the coparenthood relationship vertically in order to gain material benefits, only the most aspiring upper-lower-class family feels at ease in making such a calculating move, as the following respondent did:

> It is my husband who chooses the sponsors for my children. For instance, for our first child, he was being helped by his younger brother in the selection [of a sponsor]. The brother, being a lawyer, knows more people and better ones, too. While we would prefer personal friends, the first consideration must be [that the sponsor be] of good moral character *and if it would become necessary, we can ask help* [from him]. . . . Our youngest child had for a sponsor the chief engineer for All Broadcasting System, who is acknowledged to be quite influential.

While they would not voluntarily select a sponsor who is even poorer than they are, most lower-class Cebuanos prefer someone who is *kasagaran*, or average. In practice, this actually results in the selection of someone who is just slightly better off than the respondent. The danger of establishing coparenthood ties with "too rich" a sponsor is all too familiar to many of the lower-class families, as evidenced by the following remarks:

L: Ay! What can we do with those rich people? They will recognize you only during the baptism, at the baptismal party, but, afterwards, my goodness! They will not even recognize you even if you bump against them. . . . Look at that ______ [a rich man], he is the sponsor of ______ [Hu] at the wedding. Look at him now, he does not recognize [us], because he is rich and we are poor. I would rather have a poor man like us but who is good and can give good advice to my children later on.

M: Sus! I have had quite an experience [in having a sponsor who is wealthy]. As wedding sponsor for my husband, my parents-in-law selected an ex-mayor of Cebu City. He was mayor then when we were married. Now, when we meet each other anywhere, our supposed sponsor does not even recognize me. But I selected as [my] wedding sponsor one who is dear to me and whom I could run to in case of need. The experience I had with a prominent man for a wedding sponsor taught me a bitter lesson. A man may be poor, but if he is good-natured, that is good enough for us.

In most cases, both the lower- and middle-class respondents tend to stress the importance of character in their choice of godparents, in the hope that their children will model themselves after their godparents:

L: I always look at the *batasan* [manners], the *kinaiya* [character, personality], of the person because we know that *magliwat ang atong anak sa nagkugos nila* [our children will take after their godparents]. I would not take a gambler. I would take a good person, one who has no enemies, is understanding, and *mang-giluy-on sad* [also compassionate].

M: I want the godparent to be good in character. He may be poor, but as long as he recognizes my child as his own, that is good enough for me. I am not after the wealth of a man. . . . But I also see to it that the prospective godparent can afford to buy the baptismal dress, one who has the same standard of living as we have so there won't be feelings of unease between us.

Nevertheless, the importance of character in the choice of a sponsor seems to be related to the Cebuano belief that a man of good character would take on the responsibility of acting as surrogate parent to the sponsored child. Many of the respondents we interviewed unmistakably pinpoint this as the main function of a godparent, as illustrated in the following comments:

L: They [the godparents] should give them good advice, and I think that *they should take good care of them in the event the [natural] parents die.* [Do you really think that they will do that?] Yes. I know several who are doing that, but if the godparents cannot afford, of course, they will not do it.

L: The godparents have *dakung kahulugan* [great responsibility]. It is the godparents who have the obligation to act as parents in case of death or inability.

L: My children are generally intelligent ones, suppose we cannot afford to send them to school anymore, we can ask their [godparents'] help. [How do you know they will help you?] If they love the child and find something of value in the child that they can also gain, they will. If they find that the child is *bu-otan* [obedient] and would not in the future be ungrateful, they would help. . . . My own father grew up in the hands of a great uncle who was his godparent and he was made to finish his elementary education by them.

Expanding the Web of Kinship

The practice of having two sponsors per child for each Catholic ritual, though not studiously observed by all lower-class Cebuanos, enables each family to spread the fictive kinship network. The more children one has, the wider the spread of one's coparents. The following family we interviewed provided us with the best illustration. The numeral before each paragraph indicates the children's birth order.

1. For our first child, Junior, the godfather is attorney Santos ______, then mayor of ______. [Probe.] When Junior was born, *nag-ingon dayon si Mama* [HuMo], "*Si Santos ra'y atong kuhaon*" [Mama said right away we'll just pick Santos]. [Probe: Was Santos a friend of yours?] No, *dakung tawo gud* [big shots, you know]. Everybody called him Santos. It was my parents-in-law who knew them better because they were neighbors. Of course, when they *kugos* Junior, *nakahimamat-himamat na* [we got to know each other a bit]. [Probe.] *Mama* and *tatay* approached Santos themselves. [Probe.] We call him *Tiyo*, not *pare*. [HuMo interjected: *Sus! Pagkadaghan sa iyang Kinugos* (Jesus! He has so many godchildren) His wife became a mayor, too.] Godfather for Junior's confirmation is Bido, a *mananambal* [herb healer], friend and *kumpare* of Mama [HuMo]. . . . When Junior was nine months old he got seriously ill, and it was Noy Bido who saved him. So when Junior was to be confirmed [at age four], Mama said, "Let's get Bido. He is a good man. . . . I call him Noy Bido, not *pare*." [HuMo interjected: At the time Junior was confirmed, he was an employee at the highway construction. He is a *mananambal*, and he has land *pa gayud* (to top it all)! He has no children *raba* (emphatic).]

2. For Josefa, the godmother is Nisa [HuMoSiDau], then unmarried . . . school teacher. We were *suod* [close], yes, because we lived on the same street. We always met. They would come to visit Mama [HuMo], so we would meet. We used to live in Mama Inday's [HuMoMo] land then. I asked Mama [HuMo] who should be the godmother, she chose Nisa. [Probe.] We call her Nisa. No *manang*, no *tahud* [respect] term; not *mare* either because we are cousins. Mare Tinding, then unmarried, was second *madrina*. Nisa suggested that we ask Tinding to be a godmother also, as *katimbang* [balance]. We agreed with that idea.

For confirmation, the godmother is Mare Plising. She is a seamstress, her house was just next to ours. Pare Ising, her husband, was then an employee at the Lutupan mines. He was a friend of ______ [Hu]. Plising was my choice. I consulted Mama [HuMo] about my choice and she said: "*maayo sad*" [good also]. [HuMo interjected: Ising has a palm boat now (in a tone conveying "that's something!")!]

3. With Ester, [the baptismal sponsor] is Tinoy, then unmarried and a new

resident of ______. Worked as a public school teacher and lodged at Tacio's [HuMoSiSo] house; he was also a school teacher. Tinoy was already godfather for one of Tacio's children when my husband asked Tinoy to be the godfather for Ester. They were friends, yes, but not very close. He later married one of my husband's sisters. Tinoy looked for his own *kumare*. He got a Juling, then also unmarried and a teacher. We call Juling "Mare Juling." But we don't call Tinoy "Pare" [because he has since become an affine of the respondent's family].

Ester's confirmation sponsor is Felisa [HuMoSiDau], then unmarried, a college student. We were friends, of course, because our houses were lined up on the same street. They would visit Mama [HuMo] often, and we got to know each other. [Probe: Why did you choose her?] Confirmations were always like emergencies. When the archbishop happened to come to town, children—herds of them—would be lined up in church to have confirmation. We decided right away that we would take advantage of this opportunity and look for a *kugos* [sponsor] for our child. We decided Felisa would be a good person. We don't call her *mare*, just plain Felisa.

4. [With Veni, child no. 4] . . . it is Manang Vera, wife of a taxi driver. We were next-door neighbors when we moved into Calamba some years ago. She is much older than I am, and so I called her Manang ever since I first met her. It was she who asked to be *maninay* [godmother]. I said: "But you are a woman [how can you sponsor a boy?]" She said: "We'll just list my husband's name, that's all right." And so we did. We have became very close friends. . . . she had four children, didn't have any more.

For confirmation, [the godmother is] Mare Julia, my very close friend. She's now in Manila. But during the war, they lived across the street from our house; we'd gather firewood in the swamps together. . . . We selected her because ______ [Hu] and Julia's husband were the best of friends, yes, even before the confirmation. They would eat and sing together, *maghikay* [have little gatherings where food is served] and invite each other.

5. The fifth child . . . died shortly after birth. The sponsor was the midwife who attended the birth of the child. No, I do not call her Mare [because the child died soon after birth].

6. For Dani [child no. 6], Mare Laida is the baptismal sponsor. She lives two houses away, [is] a friend of ours. Laida and her husband are fish vendors. Laida *asked* to be Dani's sponsor.

[For confirmation], Mare Piling [laundry woman] and her husband, Carlos [gelatine refreshment vendor], our neighbors here. We were good friends: ______ [Hu], myself, and both of them. Actually, they first asked ______ [Hu] to be the godfather of their child, but I got pregnant before their child could be baptized. People say it is *ngil-ad* [ugly; not good; ominous] to *kugos* [sponsor] when one is pregnant. They say the children [the one in gestation and the one I sponsor] *mag-ilog ug kinabuhi* [will compete for life], and between the two, one is bound to lose and die. So, I could not become Piling's *kumare*. But when I delivered my child, we decided to ask Piling and her husband to be the sponsor. . . . That way, we become *kumare-kumpare*.

[Dani's confirmation sponsor is] Pare Soping, the youngest brother of Mare Julia's husband. He was then unmarried and lived with Mare Julia . . . worked as a driver of a bakery delivery truck. He was *ibog* [envious] because we were all *pare* with each other. He asked "Let me *kugos* Dani *na-*

lang [How about letting me be Dani's godparent?]" We were already very good friends so it was all right. Pare now lives near the highway with his family. He is so stout with his potbelly that he looks like he is nine months pregnant. Pare Soping's wife is the first cousin of Inse here. We [Inse and I] are very close. We give each other *utan* [vegetables].

7. Rose is Vir's [child no. 7] godparent. She is my best friend. We had agreed that whoever conceives first will let her child be *kugos* [sponsored] by the one who is not yet pregnant. *Magmare nalang ta aron magsuod gayud* [Let's become coparents so that we would be really close].

Vir has not been confirmed yet. We have been talking, Silo and I. . . . We thought we might ask you [the interviewer] to *kugos* him.

Thus, even concentrating on just one family, the circumstances under which the sponsors were selected for each ritual occasion are quite varied. They range from an impromptu decision, to careful consultation with elders, to a prior informal agreement for mutual sponsorship as a symbolic manifestation of deep friendship sentiments, even before the child is born. The choices are multifarious, not as uniform as some earlier anthropological literature suggests. Furthermore, both in this family and in the other cases we interviewed, one may also note that coparents are not consistently addressed as *kumpare* or *kumare*. Where age and status differences are great, the kinship term for uncle or aunt, *tiyo* or *tiya*, is often used instead, especially when no consanguineal or fictive kinship ties exist prior to the establishment of godparenthood relationships. At other times, where the coparent is already related to one's kinsman, the parent may simply adopt the genealogical term of address in lieu of *kumpare-kumare*.

Another interesting fact of godparenthood in the Philippines is that in a number of cases, the parents claim that the sponsors themselves asked to serve as sponsors. Moreover, the request for sponsorship is not always made to the child's biological parents. The fact that the request may be made to and granted by a mother-in-law, for example, attests to the openness of the Cebuano family:

L: We did not choose. He asked. I did not like Titing [the sponsor] because he is a drunkard, but we had given our word. He asked my mother-in-law first; they are good friends. And she agreed to it [on my behalf].

L: Most of them asked. They like to have many *kinugos* [godchildren]. [Probe.] *Simbako lang* [God forbid, but in case] they die, many godchildren will *du-aw* [visit the dead]. . . . [Plus] the happiness of having *mga inanak sa Dios* [spiritual children]; the right to teach and correct is also a *dungog* [an honor].

L: We did not choose them [as sponsors]. All of them asked to be the godparents of my children. [Probe: Which of these sponsors asked?] All of them. Enaluna and Edwin's godmothers asked even before the children were born. I was even ashamed when Manuela [Edwin's godmother] asked because she is older than I, but she started calling me *kumare* even before Edwin was born. [Probe: What was your relationship with Manuela?] She is my *suki*. I buy mostly from her, vinegar, corn grits, and others. [Probe: Why do you think did she ask to be sponsor of your child ?] I don't know. We are friends, that's why. [Probe: Has it ever happened that two persons asked to sponsor the same child?] Yes, with Enaluna. Danilo's [Hu] sister-in-law, the one who finally fostered her, wanted to be the baptismal sponsor, but my friend, Soling, asked first. So she said she would *kugos* [sponsor] her at confirmation but that she would wait until the child is old enough to eat with a spoon so she can bring her to a restaurant. And she really did.

What is perplexing here is that while these lower-class parents claimed that their coparents asked to serve as sponsors, they themselves maintained that they never asked to serve as sponsors for other people's children. Whether it is a consequence of the lower class's attempt to minimize costly obligations to other families (since they would have to engage in unilateral gift-giving to their godchild if they should serve as sponsors) or a manifestation of Cebuano *ulaw* (shame) at work, or both, is difficult to determine empirically. Certainly, it is conceivable that in the interest of maintaining "face" and self-respect, the lower-class families may want to give the impression that they had not "begged" to be a coparent of a slightly well-off kinsman or friend.

In sum, our intensive interview data provide some evidence that aside from its religious significance, godparenthood performs a vital role in establishing multiple equivalent bonds between children and adults. Where such fictive-spiritual relationships are claimed and validated, they may constitute additional sources of socioemotional support and economic assistance for the lower-class family. At the very least, they help to ease the psychic if not the economic burden of a large family by providing the parents with an expanded web of supportive kinship ties that they could draw upon in case of emergency or incapacitation. Another way of spreading the cost and responsibilities of childrearing is through fosterage.

Cebuano Fosterage

Fosterage in the Cebuano culture carries a different semantic load and social significance than adoption in North America. Carroll (1970: 5) noted that adoption in the United States, as a formal legal act, involves a host of assumptions and requirements, among which are: (1) The child is assumed to be unwanted. (2) The natural parents presumably agree to relinquish all their parental rights and duties to the adopters. (3) The identity of the child's biological parents is kept confidential by court order and cannot be revealed without the court's permission. (4) It is assumed and deemed desirable that the child "put up" for adoption "ordinarily will be placed in a home where the religion of the adoptive parent(s) is the same as that of his parents," unless otherwise specified (Child Welfare League of America, 1958:12). (5) Prospective adopters undergo a screening process. (6) Parents who voluntarily give up their children for adoption are not regarded highly, although mitigating circumstances may be sympathized with. (7) The act of adoption is perceived to be altruistic, particularly since the difficulties in adoptive relationships are generally recognized.

In the Cebuano culture—as in eastern Oceania (Carroll, 1970) and some parts of Western Africa—fosterage and adoption are generally simple kinship transactions unencumbered by formal legal procedures. In the families we interviewed, parents practically never "put up" their children for adoption and fosterage; children are seldom "unwanted" by their biological parents; the child is not "taken in" by strangers. In spite of fosterage or adoption, the natural parents generally do not relinquish their responsibilities and privileges completely. The adoptive parents are not necessarily childless or exactly wealthy. The fact of adoption or fosterage is not kept secret from the child or his kinsmen. The child is not always physically transferred from his natural parents' household; he may instead divide his time between his biological and adoptive parents' households. The natural parents are not stigmatized or accorded low regard for having allowed fosterage or adoption of one or several of their children. Furthermore, the children may be fostered by an individual, and the adopted children suffer no trauma or "genealogical bewilderment" (Sants, 1964) as they sometimes reportedly do in Anglo-American societies.

In contrast to the American practice, fosterage and adoption in Cebu are not always explicitly arranged or immediately identifiable. This is not to say that legal adoption does not exist in the Philippines. Rather, fosterage and informal adoption are more common. They represent a spectrum of social behavioral transactions whereby parent-child statuses and roles, rights and obligations, responsibilities and affection are casually, partially, and temporarily shared with one or a few of the child's senior or ascending kinsmen—by default, tacit consent, or importunate request. The circumstances under which such transactions are negotiated are complex and have so far not been described in the literature on Cebuano family and kinship.

Of the twenty-two families selected for intensive interviews, we found that fosterage is most prevalent among the lower class, although it is also found in middle- and upper-class households. Of the fifteen lower-class families in our intensive interview sample, fourteen reported at least one instance of fosterage in their households, involving either their children or the respondents themselves when they were young. Among the middle-class households sampled, five out of seven families reported at least one such practice. In none of these families was an adoption paper formally signed.

Three Ways of Circulating Children

A detailed analysis of our data suggests that, by and large, there are three ways of "fostering" or circulating children in Cebu. The first is what we call the "spend-for" pattern, where the child continues to reside with his biological parents but a part or all of his expenses are paid for *consistently* by a relative for one reason or another. A second way of circulating children—hence, establishing multiple equivalent bonds—is to "borrow" them regularly from another family or to "deposit" them periodically with a relative. Constant borrowing sometimes develops into a third pattern of fosterage called *gikuha* (taken) or *gi-angkon* (claimed). The subtle nuances of these practices are described below.

The "Spend-for" Pattern

Among the Cebuanos, "spending for" a child is not always an all-or-nothing proposition. It ranges from complete support for the child to partial assistance doled out irregularly but consistently. Complete support is generally prompted by the death or incapacitation of the child's natural parents, thereby forcing a grandparent or other relative to assume the responsibility of an adoptive parent. Partial assistance, however, is quite pervasive among the Cebuanos, even in the absence of emergencies or incapacitation. This is indicated by the fact that in practically all the families we interviewed, some or all of the children's expenses are being underwritten by relatives although the children are residing with their biological parents. Even a lower-class grandmother whose only occupational skill is repairing rice and flour sacks insists on providing for all her grandchildren's allowances in school. In another family, all of our respondent's four children eat their meals in their grandparents' nipa hut next door, but return home to sleep. In most cases, though, it is the children's schooling and clothing expenses, not their daily meals, that are being paid by their relatives. This helps to explain the high level of literacy among lower-class people in the Philippines, and their persistent dream of "making it" despite the burden of a large family.

"Borrowing" and "Depositing" Children

Borrowing or depositing children is an indirect way of establishing multiple equivalent bonds and fulfilling one's need for companionship and interdependencies. It may begin when a neighbor offers to babysit for a young infant in order to relieve the mother for gainful employment. The baby, however, is generally taken (hence, the word "borrowed") to the house of the "borrower" and not returned until the mother makes the specific request. Frequently, because of the neighbor's attachment to the baby, the mother may consent to let her assume the godmother role, as had happened with some of our respondents. Such borrowings, however, may stretch to as long as a week at a time, and can create ill feelings between the biological mother and the adoptive mother if either party feels the situation is forced upon her. One of our middle-class respondents, for instance, frequently has more children in her house than she has ever given birth to. When our interviewer finally inquired about it, the answer was as follows:

> They are the children of my brother. They were deposited here because the mother just had another baby. They are deposited here because they cannot be attended to at their own house. I say to them: "Go ahead, keep having more [babies] and then deposit them here. *Nagsalig lang kay manghud* [you think you can do this to me because you are the youngest child in the family]." They [the children] are brought here *aron sila mahayahay* [so that the parents can be relieved of the burden of child care]. I tell them that if this is the case, that they are only giving away their children to people, go to the World Neighbors [Organization] so that they could give them away and stop having babies. And they said to me: "It's *you* we are giving them to. You are not 'people.'" Sometimes, when I go to their house, they would tell me to take one of their kids home with me because they only have one maid. . . . I am not really serious when I said for them to go to the World Neighbors . . . they are used to me making such remarks. I'm always scolding [them].

Evidently, the depositing of children can be regarded as a burden by the family that has to take care of them, although it is a relief—physically, psychologically, and economically—to the family whose children are being deposited elsewhere. Because in the Cebuano culture, constant borrowing of a child may develop into a more permanent fosterage, some parents may feel a twinge of resentment, especially if the borrowed child is an only girl or an only boy. Among lineal relatives, however, any ill feelings are generally repressed.

Gikuha or Gi-angkon

Gikuha (taken) and *gi-angkon* (claimed) are the Cebuano words used to describe the status of children who are being physically removed from their biological parents' household or "claimed" by certain kinsmen as *their* child. The following is an example:

> *L:* When my sister, Saturnina, and mother came for a visit in 1967, Saturnina wanted to *kuha* [take] my second daughter to go along with them to

> Davao. Not to *sagop* [adopt], but just to stay there for a visit. If the visit is long enough, she could study there [at their expense].

Note that the respondent herself made a distinction between *kuha* (to take) and *sagop* (to adopt). She is also very clear on the distinction between "visiting" and *gikuha* (taken). That is, it is merely a difference of *duration*. Thus, no formal ceremony or special way of asking is needed for "taking" someone else's child. An informal invitation for a visit is enough. What if parents do not wish their child to be "taken"? Another lower-class respondent answered this question for us:

> Kumare Laida asks for Dani all the time. She keeps on saying to ______ [husband]: "Pare, now that my only child, Inday, is married, *diri nalang si Dani nako* [just let Dani stay over here at my house]. My husband usually answers by saying: "*Oo, Mare. Mahimo man sad kay na-a ra ta dinhi* [Yes, Mare, anyway we are all living right here—in this area]." But when we are alone and out of earshot, my husband would say to himself and to me: "*Asa man nako ihatag!*" [I would never give that child away!]

These remarks leave no doubt that to allow a child to be "taken" by some coparent or neighbor is in a sense tantamount to giving that child away. The fact that the husband was resistant but could not bring himself to refuse outright gives us an inkling of the social pressure he feels, since he and the neighbor are coparents—Dani being the godchild of Laida. The fact that the neighbor-godmother could openly make this request suggests how acceptable such practices are in the Cebuano culture. It should also be emphasized that Laida is not childless. But she wants a small child around the house. The following case illustrates why children are always in demand among the poor. The respondent in this case is an elderly woman whose son happens to be the husband of a lower-lower-class woman we were interviewing. The son, named Tino, was "circulated out" when he was a young boy.

> *Mo:* We let him [Tino] study until Grade IV. Then, Andres [her sister's son] asked that Tino stay with them. They promised to let him go to school. Andres was then an employee of his Tiyo Gonzales' lumber company. [A good job even then.] He is now a teacher.
>
> *Q:* What kind of work did Tino do for them?
>
> *Mo:* Tino's work was to cook and wash the *hapin* [cloth diapers] of their baby. [Tino's wife added] Tino would wake up at dawn, four o'clock in the morning, and he would fry fish [for the family's breakfast]. . . . [The mother continued] He would cook so many dishes. That's why he is always in the kitchen now. There were *three of them* living with Andres and his wife. Tino was twelve years old then. He stayed more than one year with them.
>
> [After a long silence] At another time, Fidel [Tino's oldest sister's husband] asked me to allow Tino to stay with them. There again, he learned to plant rice in the paddies, make kettles out of tin cans, to *guna*. He knows many kinds of work. He also washed the *lampin* [cloth diapers] which he

would iron immediately . . . he brought lunch to Maoling [Fidel's wife] who kept a store in the market . . . [and] he watched and took care of Maoling's children.

Q: Why did Fidel ask for Tino?

Mo: He had no grown child yet to help Maoling.

Q: Why [did Fidel ask for] Tino and not others—Tino's brothers and sisters, for example?

Mo: Because Tino was *abtik* [agile, quick]. The others were still very small. The older ones were girls and they married very early. Venacio [a brother of Tino] was always out of the house [hence, cannot be trusted to run errands].

It is our hypothesis that the process of "taking" someone else's child is not a random occurrence. There is a mutual selection process involved here. Certain characteristics of the person or the family who wish to "take" somebody's child determine to a great extent whether he or she will be successful. In addition, certain personality qualities of the child make it more probable for him rather than his siblings to be the "chosen" one. This becomes clear below:

L: Veni was almost *gikuha*. Whenever Mare Julia [Veni's confirmation godmother] sees Veni playing, gambling with rubber bands down there, she would say: "Mare, you let Veni stay here so he will become *but-an* [obedient]." I agree wholeheartedly with the idea. My husband also agrees because he says, "Anyway, Mare Julia lives right there. Veni can just come back and forth." Sometimes, Veni does do things for Mare Julia—runs errands for her, buys and carries things for her, helps in some repairs around her house. Julia in turn gives him fifty centavos or thirty centavos [for a job done]. He is having great fun at it, too! Mare Julia has asked me several times in his presence that he live there, and we encourage him that it is a nice idea. But Veni does not seem to take it seriously, so we don't force him either.

Q: Why Veni?

L: He's her godchild [at confirmation].

Q: Why do you agree to Veni's living with Mare Julia but not to Dani's stay with Mare Laida?

L: Mare Laida is *saba-an, yaw-yawan* [a grouch, a shrew]! She nags her husband, people, anybody! [Probe.] Oh, we are friends, yes, but she *yaw-yaw*'s a lot.

Q (addresses Husband's mother): How about you?

HuMo: That one [pointing to Veni]? I'll ask for that one to live with me? *Oy! Nagsigi la'g la-ag! Ay nalang ta.* [That's the one that is always roaming around. Thanks, but no thanks.]

The old woman's reply is significant for it narrows the parameters of characteristics that some relatives sought in deciding which child to "take." From the "adopted" family's viewpoint, the child who is *gikuha* has to have at least one characteristic: the ability to stay put around the house so that he will be there when you need him to run errands. Conversely, the decision to allow certain individuals but not others to "take" one's child is not a random process either. In this family, the explicit reason for turning down Kumare Laida's request is that she is such a "big mouth." A covert reason, which we uncovered after examining the socioeconomic background of the different families in that neighborhood, is that Kumare Laida and her husband are only fish vendors, poorer than our respondent's family, whereas Kumare Julia is at least *kasagaran* (comparable to the respondent's family). For this reason, the two families used to make frequent social visits and entertain each other before they each had so many children, whereas such reciprocal exchange never took place with Kumare Laida's family.

Finally, let us present another case which demonstrates how a child may be *gi-angkon* or claimed, more or less successfully. The respondent was a lower-class woman who had had six pregnancies in eleven years of marriage. Their oldest child was eleven years old, while the youngest was only four months old. Except for this newborn baby and a miscarriage, three of the remaining children were either *gikuha* (taken) or *gi-angkon* (claimed) by their relatives. Only the third child, Sara (aged seven), is living with them. The oldest child, Fernando, was *gi-angkon* by the husband's father. The second child, an eight-year-old boy, and the fourth one, a five-year-old girl, were *gikuha* by the husband's brother, who is childless. The lengthy interview record below shows how the respondent feels about giving her children away:

Q: Why did you let your children be taken away?

L: Because they [Hu's kinsmen] will *mahay* [regret and blame us] if we refuse. Also, *it is better for the children because Noy Berto [HuBr] promised to spend for their education up until high school.*

Q: Did you expect relief financially when you allowed them to be taken?

L: No. It is still the same. These children are clever. They ask from their "Mommy" and "Daddy" [adoptive parents] and they also ask from us. I still have to buy them school uniforms and supplies.

Q: What particular things do Alan and Luna [children taken by HuBr] ask from you?

L: The usual *baon* [pocket money] and sometimes paper and pencil and crayon.

Q: Are these not given by the one who has taken them?

L: Yes, but you know, these children are clever. They ask from their "Mommy" and they also ask from me.

Q: Why don't you censure them?

L: I cannot refuse them. . . . Yes, I do, now and then . . . but I seldom see them, so I give in sometimes.

Q: What about the discipline part?

L: I am glad Alan [aged eight] is gone. He is a naughty boy and does not obey me anymore. These children of mine—they are confident on account of their [paternal] grandmother [who lives next door] who always defends them.

Q: How do you feel if your children are punished by the other parents [referring to HuBr]?

L: It's all right with me. They behave better with their other parents because nobody will side with them. But if others will touch my children, my blood boils inside me. . . .

Q: What do you do if your children don't listen to you?

L: *Ay!* I tell them they will be punished by God—they will grow horns. Sometimes I whip them with anything I can lay my hands on, but then there is always my mother-in-law [interceding for them].

Q: How old were Alan and Luna when you let your brother-in-law take them?

L: Alan was three and Luna was one [they were "taken" separately]. But Luna came home last month. Her Mommy [HuBrWi] brought her back because she was sick. It was only last Sunday that her Mommy took her back.

Q: How do you feel about letting them *kuha* your children?

L: I felt the pain of separation at first as all mothers do, but I got used to it eventually. It is for the good of the children. *If we don't give them our children, they will adopt others who are not our relatives.* It is also painful for my brother-in-law if we refuse him. They have no children of their own. I pity them.

Q: How about your oldest son who is with your mother-in-law?

L: Fernando? . . . He has always been with them. He cannot even sleep without cuddling and tickling the armpits of his grandfather. He cannot do that with me because I spank his hands right away. It disturbs my sleep.

Q: How often do you see your children?

L: I see them every week. They come to the house and ask for this or that. . . .

Q: Why did your sister-in-law bring Luna back when she got sick?

L: They were afraid because many children in that area were seriously ill. They wanted to avoid further contamination.

Q: Does Fernando live with your parents-in-law or just spend most of his time with them?

L: He lives with them. He comes home only when his grandfather is not home.

Q: Why is Fernando close to his grandparents?

L: Because they love him more than the others, being their first grandson. Also, they were the ones who weaned him. We lived with them at the time [when Fernando was born].

Q: Do you encourage your children to go to your in-laws?

L: Yes, sometimes, *especially when they look for better food.*

This lower-class woman has lucidly described the reason she let her brother-in-law *kuha* two of her children. Her concern not to offend the brother-in-law is further reflected in another statement she made to our interviewer at a separate session:

> Alan used to cry and wanted to come home. *But we did not give in.* We did not want to disappoint Noy Berto. He would feel bad if he comes home and finds that the children are not there. *He will think we are being selfish with our children.*

Thus, children—like food, houses, clothing, medicine, and contraceptive pills—are resources to be shared with one's kinsmen. The ethic of sharing makes it very difficult to refuse a relative's request for one's child, especially when that relative is "in need." It is "selfish" to refuse since to do so is tantamount to negating the existing kinship tie. It also puts one in a precarious position where, in time of need, one may be all alone, never able to cull any assistance from others by virtue of a claim on kinship relations. By acceding to an importunate request for "taking" a child, the parents are able to personalize an existing kindred tie and maximize their possibilities for eliciting help in the future. As in Oceania, "'parenthood' is a complex of rights which may be shared, transferred, acceded to, delegated, surrendered, or otherwise circulated among social persons according to culturally specific rules" (Carroll, 1970:8).

Second, the material advantage to the children (and indirectly to the mother) cannot be overlooked. The promise of better living conditions and at least a high school education for the children is a relief from the economic and emotional burdens of child-rearing. The fact that the adoptive parents are addressed as "Mommy" and "Daddy" suggests that fosterage is seen as an addition to, and not a replacement of, the biological parent-child relationship. In another interview session, the mother revealed her reluctance to completely "give away" her children:

> *L:* The children are not really adopted [formally]. We are just giving them to him *for companionship* and in return Noy Berto will spend for their schooling. When they are big, they will decide with whom they wish to stay.

This remark is insightful, for it conveys the nebulous meaning of the Cebuano words *gikuha* and *gi-angkon,* both of which are in the passive voice. In practice, it is as close to the North American notion of adoption as it could be, except no formal papers are signed. Would the woman and her husband be willing to sign formal adoption papers? Out of curiosity, our interviewer posed this question one day and the husband answered emphatically: "*Signing papers would be like selling my children like animals*! Besides, they will not be ours anymore. But if we give them to Noy Berto [HuBr], they can still come to us and they will always know we are their real parents."

Beyond a doubt, the essence of the Cebuano practice of "giving away" children is to allow for the establishment of multiple equivalent bonds, but not to forfeit the duties and privileges of parenthood. Nevertheless, the question remains as to how the children themselves look at the situation. Luna is only five years old, far too young for us to assess her identity perception. Alan, however, is a little older. By coincidence our interviewer found out that because of Alan's ability to memorize, he has starred in a radio program, reciting verses. This brought him into the limelight when he was interviewed on that same program and asked about his parents. The boy gave the name of his foster parents, rather than that of his biological parents, as his "parents." If this piece of data is of any significance, it suggests how close the practice of *gikuha* is to a formal adoption.

These three patterns of circulating children—"spending for," "borrowing" or "depositing," and *gikuha* or *gi-angkon*—are not mutually exclusive. The first and the second pattern are likely to overlap. The third pattern implies the first one, and often develops after frequent "borrowing" has stabilized over time. Or "borrowing" may sometimes represent a compromise in those cases where the natural parents do not wish to "give away" their children but are also unable to make a flat refusal. Nevertheless, outright refusals *do* occur. One lower-class woman describes how her husband refused her mother's offer to *kuha* the oldest daughter, who is eleven years old, even though the mother had promised to pay for everything:

> At first I tried to convince him [husband]. There are several reasons I advanced for this. He wouldn't budge. And, if you know, he seldom opens his mouth to talk. But that time, he made every word count. He insisted on his objections. He did not want the children to live apart from one another and to be separated from us. He did not want this particular child spoiled by the grandparents. *He was also sure that he would be able to care for the children and teach them the right things.* This went on and on until finally, I saw how futile it would be to argue.

In this case, the mother lives in Toledo, fifty kilometers west of Cebu City. Poor and irregular public transportation makes frequent visits difficult. The city offers better school facilities. The husband also feels that he is financially capable and socially competent to serve as the child's parent. His sense of responsibility forbade him from acceding to the mother-in-law's request for companionship.

Fosterage and Reciprocity

The dynamics of fosterage is best understood by examining the long-range interaction between the households or individuals engaged in such mutual assistance. However, because of the length of time required to make longitudinal observations on fostered children, we must rely upon our respondents' own childhood experiences for illustration. One of them, for instance, was *gikuha* by her older sister, who married into a Chinese-Mestizo family:

> *M:* My father, Angel ______, made his livelihood as a *cochero* [rig driver]. He married twice. By his first wife, he had four children. By his second wife, he had five children and I am the youngest. Times became doubly difficult because none of my half-sisters were old enough when their mother died. So all of us lived together. My mother did not have any job and stayed home to take care of us—all nine of us! After a few years, my older half-sister, Mama Tina, got married to a Chinese Mestizo who was well off. She took me and my older brother . . . to live with them. She also helped my mother after my father died.

Upon the death of the Chinese-Mestizo merchant, the respondent and her brother dropped out of school and worked to support their "Mama" Tina who, by then, was suffering badly from tuberculosis. This kind of reciprocity between the "foster" parent and the "spent-for" child is quite common, we found out. The following case is another example:

> *M:* I used to stay with Mama Inday [a maternal aunt]. She does not have any children. She also spent for my high school education. She comes to our house almost daily now. She is newly widowed and when the need arises, like when she needs to see a doctor . . . I bring her to a doctor. She used to have a little *sari-sari* store and I tended it. It was only after my high school graduation that I returned to Mama [biological parent] because Mama Inday said that I should do so, to help her.

Although more women than men tend to seek a child to spend for, it is not unusual for men to assume the financial responsibility of raising a relative's child or children, particularly if that relative is a brother. Probably because of the egalitarian kinship system in the Philippines, we detected no marked preference for either sex in fosterage. Where necessary, intergenerational fosterage has occurred as well. The husband of one of our lower-class respondents is a case in point. Upon the death of his mother, he was raised by an unmarried aunt who asked to "foster" him. Now that he is married, this unmarried aunt continues to "spend for" his children as well. The significance of her assistance can be discerned from the following verbatim interview record:

> *Q:* With your income (sixty pesos a month), how do you manage to send your children to a private school?
>
> *L:* Mama Teria [HuMoSi] is helping us with the children's education, and also that of Elena [third child] who will be enrolled in kindergarten this coming school year.
>
> *Q:* Why is she helping you?

> *L:* Because my husband has no steady income and she was the one who offered to do so, too. She is a spinster and is not spending for anybody else, except for my husband. He had stayed with her ever since he was very young.
>
> *Q:* Why do you think that your husband among his other siblings was the choice of this aunt?
>
> *L:* He was the only boy in their family and ever since he was a baby, she was his *yaya* [nursemaid]. So that after the death of his mother, she felt that it was her obligation to look after them. The sister of Jesus [husband] was also living with her until she got married.
>
> *Q:* Do you think this aunt feels obligated to help your children because she sort of adopted Jesus before?
>
> *L:* It might be the reason, but I think she pities the children. For if it was not for her, my children would have only been studying at some public school rather than a private one.
>
> *Q:* Did she also spend for the other siblings of Jesus?
>
> *L:* No. Their father died in 1965 and the girls were with their father until he died, to take care of him. Jesus was specially requested by Mama Teria to stay with her as *she needed some companion.*

That fosterage may span more than one generation becomes self-evident when one considers another case we had, where three generations and several households are involved. Our interviewer had a challenging time untangling the web of kinship ties and following up on the children who have been "circulated" among different households. To begin with, the husband of one of our respondents—whom we shall call Cesar—has a cousin (MoSiDau) named Jacinta. The latter was raised by Cesar's mother upon the death of her mother. (Jacinta's two other siblings were raised by her father, who subsequently remarried.) Although Jacinta is only a year older than Cesar, she has taken care of him ever since they were children. Cesar called Jacinta *tiya* or aunt instead of cousin. "Tiya" Cinta later got married and had two daughters, Evangelina and Ging-ging. The former became a teacher and works in Palompon, Leyte. Ging-ging studied medicine and went to the United States to become a physician and the director of a hospital in Philadelphia. When Cesar got married, Evangelina and Ging-Ging gave him a house. Meanwhile, since neither of Jacinta's daughters could live with her, Jacinta requested one of Cesar's children, Talino (aged eighteen at the time of the interview), to live with her in Camp Lapu-lapu. This is how Cesar's wife describes the relationship:

> *L:* Evangelina stays in Tiya Cinta's house there in Palompon, Leyte, while Tiya Cinta stays in Evangelina's house here at Camp Lapu-lapu. But Tiya makes trips to her daughter's place in Leyte so often that Talino had to stay in Camp Lapu-lapu to have somebody in the house while Tiya is away. Jacinta pays for his tuition fee at the Abellana High School where he is now a fourth-year student. But all his other expenses come from us—clothing,

school miscellaneous expenses, transportation fare, and *baon* [small allowances for snacks in school]. . . . Joselito [aged thirteen at the time of the interview] lives with Evangelina in Palompon since two years ago. He was not able to enroll right away [having arrived in the middle of a school year]. Not having anything to do, Dodoy [Evangelina's husband] suggested that he just stay home to keep his wife company. He is now in school, first year high school. Evangelina pays for all his needs.

Q: How was this arrangement made?

L: Evangelina's husband simply told Joselito: "You stay here *nalang*. She has no companion here." Just like that.

Q: Did they say they were going to spend for Joselito, or how long he is to live with them?

L: Nothing. . . . They did not say how long Joselito was going to stay with Evangelina or what they will do or spend for him. I did not ask anything. [Probe.] Of course, since they took him, I *knew* they would let him study. All my children were and are studying.

Q: Did you feel that you were giving a child away?

L: No. I did not feel like that.

Q: What does Joselito do for the expenses that Evangelina paid?

L: Nothing. He just goes to school and helps in Evangelina's house just like he would if he were here living with me. But mostly he just plays.

Q: What does Joselito call Evangelina?

L: He calls Tiya Cinta "Tiya" but he calls Evangelina "Tiya" also. [Guffaws.]

Obviously, the respondent herself realizes the awkwardness of their terms of address. The complexity of the "fosterage" relationship in this case is shown further by the fact that it is not Cesar himself who is looking after his aging mother, but Tiya Cinta. As a matter of fact, at the time of our interview, Cesar's mother was living in Tiya Cinta's house in Camp Lapu-lapu where Talino—another son of Cesar—is also residing. The following verbatim record shows how the arrangement was struck:

Q: How did you and Tiya Cinta agree to let Talino stay with them?

L: On one of Jacinta's visits to our house here, she invited Talino by saying: "You stay in Camp Lapu-lapu *nalang* [entreating tag word]. There is nobody there." You see, Jacinta is always on the move. If she is not in Manila, she is in Leyte or at the movies. So Talino went.

Q: Was there any agreement of any sort?

L: No. Nothing. No spoken understandings. Nothing. . . . There's no difference his being there. It is exactly the same as if he were here. Only I don't see him [every day]. *He is not less my child.*

Q: How did it happen that Jacinta paid for Talino's tuition?

L: When classes opened in July, he came to ask me for his tuition fee. I gave him the money. But when the next installment was almost due, Tiya Cinta told me not to pay . . . said she will take care of it.

> *Q:* What kind of work does Talino do at Tiya Cinta's house?
>
> *L: Ay sus* [exclamatory expression indicating insignificance]. Fetch water, no more. To fetch water, all you do is draw out a hose [which is much less burdensome than the typical lower-class way of fetching water by walking several blocks to a public source and carrying heavy tin cans].

Apparently, it is an upward residential move for Talino to live with Tiya Cinta, her house being a far cry from his parents' house in the lower-class district of Hipodromo where noise, crowds, and dust abound. Tiya Cinta's house is well furnished with American electrical appliances since her son-in-law, Dodoy [Evangelina's husband], works with the Philippine Civic Action Group in Vietnam and apparently has easy access to the American PX stores. The new job trebled his previous salary in the Philippines and enabled them to live comfortably.

The manifest and latent functions of "circulating" children from one household to another become clear when one studies the pregnancy history of this family. Cesar has twelve children. The oldest is only twenty-two years old, the youngest is six. He himself is only forty-nine years old. By allowing his children to be circulated into another household, an existing kinship tie is reaffirmed and a debt of gratitude validated, since Jacinta herself is indebted to Cesar's mother for bringing her up. The children, as minions, are also performing certain functions around the house, however menial these chores may be. Most important of all is their role as *companions*. One does not have to stay in the Philippines very long before being impressed with the cultural belief in the need for companionship. It is unthinkable to many Cebuanos for a person to do things by himself, much less to live alone. Life is to be shared, so are one's joys and sorrows. Among our other respondents, we found that whenever the husband readies himself to take a trip out of the city, he almost always arranges for someone, usually a minion, to come and live with his wife and children, just for companionship. And as long as he has relatives to count on, he would never fail to call upon them when the need arises. Insofar as the parents are concerned, moving their children from one household to another helps cut the cost of child-rearing. Their meager income can be more easily stretched to meet their needs when some of the children's education, food, and incidental expenses are paid for by other relatives. Having a large family becomes less costly as a result. In fact, having more children may become an added advantage in this case, rather than a liability.

The intergenerational adult-child interdependencies in this family do not end here. Midway through our interview phase, new developments revealed some other latent functions of circulating children from household to household. Jacinta left for the United States to solve her physician-daughter's babysitting problem in Philadelphia. On our second-to-the-last visit with the respondent, we learned that their daughter named Tanya was undergoing a medical examination. Our interviewer probed further:

> *Q:* Why did you have a laboratory examination for Tanya [aged twenty]?
>
> *L* (hesitating): I'll tell you a piece of good news, that is . . . if, *ha!* [exclamatory expression indicating, "mind you, this is all it is, a conditional event"] . . . *if* God wills it to come true, Tanya is going to the States. Last week, his [Cesar's] mother brought a letter from Jacinta with her. [The letter says that] Jacinta has to come back after six months elapse [upon the expiration of her tourist visa] . . . the States will not let her stay longer. Ging-ging [Jacinta's physician-daughter in Philadelphia] said for us to find out about Tanya's citizenship situation. All our children until Salvador [child no. 6] are American citizens because Cesar was a member of the Philippine Scouts during World War II. . . . Ging-ging said she will place my daughter as a hospital attendant working for two dollars an hour [triumphant tone]!

On our last visit, we learned that Tanya's citizenship papers had been processed. She was getting ready to travel to the United States as a U.S. citizen, and will be working as a hospital attendant in Philadelphia while serving as Ging-ging's babysitter. Thus, for this particular family, having a large family has been amply rewarded. They can anticipate that someday their daughter Tanya will be earning a handsome income in the United States and may even send for the other children to serve as her companions or babysitters when she gets married. Insofar as our respondent and her husband are concerned, life has been good even though it was difficult to make ends meet, and cash is always short. Having large numbers of children has not exactly increased their liability, especially when three of their twelve children are being "spent for" by other relatives. As far as they and their neighbors are concerned, they have done well by following God's will and by staying away from the use of any contraceptive methods.

Fertility Implications

The actual incidence of fosterage in the Cebuano population may never be fully determined. Nevertheless, the three patterns of circulating children from one household to another ease the uneven flow of, supply of, and demand for children. Godparenthood and fosterage establish multiple equivalent bonds between generations in addition to gratifying the need for nurturance and the universal desire for minions. In the Cebuano culture, the practice is most prevalent among lower-class families, not without reason. By letting other relatives pay consistently for a particular child, or specific group of children, the parents are spreading the cost of child-rearing, thereby diffusing the financial responsibility and psychological burdens of a large family. Comparatively speaking, the cost of pregnancy is not as high to the Cebuanos as it is to women in a highly industrialized society where such adaptive mechanisms are absent, or are not fully exploited. Insofar as the senior relative who underwrites the children's expenses is concerned, his active participation in fostering the children provides a channel for nurturance and gives him an additional "dependency link" to count on, in case his own children—if he has any—are not able to take care of him either because they migrate to another city for better jobs, or because they die young, or for other reasons. By "acquiring" as many "dependents" as he can, the senior relative is able to spread his kinship network and can quickly mobilize resources in case of emergencies. In a society where care of the elderly is basically a family matter rather than a social problem, the elderly population simply cannot dismiss the importance of the chain of dependency links.

Furthermore, the possibility that the child who has been "circulated out" may attain socioeconomic status always exists. For the lower-class mother who possesses no occupational skill and who suffers under the constant threat of losing her husband, either through some occupational hazard or because of a *querida*, childbearing seems to be an expedient "enterprise." By not signing any formal papers of adoption, and yet letting another, more well-off family take care of her offspring, the lower-class woman can at least hope to draw upon her children's later success to lift her out of her dire poverty. Like godparenthood, fosterage is an outcome of choice, not chance. Beyond the triadic relationship among parents, adoptive parents, and children exists a fourth bond—the fosterchild-sibling relationship. Our data show how the practice of circulating children may span more than one generation, embrace foster sibling relationships, and ultimately pay off.

12 / Conclusion

A source of illumination throughout this study has been the pivotal role that family and kindred play in sustaining a high level of marital fertility in the central Philippines. Regardless of their socioeconomic standings and educational attainments, Filipinos are enmeshed in an ever-expandable web of kinship which impinges on and is, in turn, impinged upon by conjugal relationships and childbearing. Such an interpersonal environment is not easily described by the crude instruments that have been developed thus far in the social sciences, even though some economists have attempted to translate certain human factors into cost-benefit terms. Nevertheless, the significance of intra- and inter-familial dynamics in the reproductive behavior of the Cebuanos warrants careful study, with or without quantifiable measures. By integrating the large amount of demographic data obtained through our sample survey with the rich ethnographic materials collected from in-depth interviews, we have begun the task of documenting the complex set of factors which form part of the cultural context of Filipino reproduction.

The Cebu study demonstrates that although there is a fair amount of ignorance about family planning, it is erroneous to believe that Filipinos have no aspirations toward the ideal of a smaller family. However, in the daily lives of the Cebuanos, that ideal must take its place in a hierarchy of priorities, of which economic survival is highest. For a great many people, constant preoccupation with sheer survival has narrowed their view of the future and limited their sense of control over "fate." Absorbed in their struggle to make ends meet from one day to the next, a poor couple may find it difficult to foresee the day when present restraint would actually work to their benefit. At the same time, unlike economically independent couples living in developed countries, Filipino wives and husbands must consider, in bearing and raising children, the expectations and desires of those kin upon whose help they depend. Paradoxically, the result of such dependence is that having children is not as problematic for Filipino couples as it is for couples in wealthier lands. In fact, having a large number of children may not be a liability to a couple's pursuit of subsistence at all. Rather than creating a problem, children may often be the solution to some of the family's problems, depending on economic circumstances, the stage of the family's life-cycle, and the particular relationship between the woman and her man before and after conception. Given the highly institutionalized religious rituals and cultural sanctions that enable people outside the nuclear family to enter the network of *compadrazgo* as godparents and coparents, having a large number of children can actually increase a family's economic security, when those children serve a soldering function that extends beyond the conjugal union.

Moreover, in a sex-segregated society with clearly defined double sex standards, pregnancy can bring unmarried people together hastily to protect the young woman's reputation and to sustain the cultural ideal of virginity. In this context, premarital pregnancy may at times be exploited to "jell" an unstable relationship. From the male viewpoint, it certainly is a sure way for the suitor to discourage other competitors and secure his prize. From the woman's vantage point, it shows her willingness to sacrifice by giving away her most precious gift—her virginity—to the lover, in exchange for an honorable and binding commitment. In either case, the premarital act itself is a negation of the tight control of the family over the individual and a subtle indication of the social changes taking place in Philippine society.

In a similar vein, pregnancy outside of marriage has a distinctive significance in the Philippines. By being drawn into the married man's orbit of social and intimate relationships, the *querida* gives herself options that otherwise might be closed to her. The personal obligations of her lover increase proportionately with the number of children she bears with him, which, in turn, solidifies the network of support which is so critical in a society where secondary institutions for social security have not yet fully developed. Insofar as the man is concerned, sexual adventure outside of marriage is a symbol of social status and sexual prowess, some amount of community condemnation notwithstanding. Precisely because divorce is not permitted in a Catholic setting, the *querida* system functions to sustain the stability of the family even as it disrupts familial relationships in wedlock. Consequently, extramarital unions do not bring about a reduction in fertility, as happens in other societies. On the contrary, our limited evidence suggests that they may have the opposite effect, since children are the instruments through which both the wife and the mistress competitively assert their claims on the man—economically, socially, and romantically.

The Cebu study also casts doubt on the assumption that the Philippines, prior to the introduction of modern family planning methods, was a non-contraceptive society. The rich repertoire of folk methods of birth control and their continued practice by some segments of the Cebuano population have been carefully documented in this volume. That the delivery of these folk methods is transmitted through the most reliable circuitry—that of word of mouth—gives some indication of the strong sense of trust between the folk practitioners and their clients. Indeed, folk healers and midwives perform several meaningful functions which weave through the central fibers of peasant life and bring women together as allies in the control of their bodies and their lives.

In contrast, modern medicine and western contraceptive technology has little functional significance in the lives of the humble folk in the central Philippines. Physicians neither participate in neighborhood gossip nor engage in social exchanges with their patients as equals in human sufferance. Instead, they bring medicine and operations which, though "powerful," cost more and are less comprehensible. To use modern contraceptives effectively, the woman must first orient her thinking to the abstractions of modern science and technology. Unfortunately, biochemical notions of the hormonal suppression of ovulation are far too technical to be fully understood by ruralfolk and urban villagers. Moreover, modern contraceptives require the adoption of a concept of time and dosage based on precise measurements. Their dispensation is, further, regulated by impersonal norms and professional rules, rather than governed by compassion and personal wishes. Thus, for instance, to accept the IUD is not simply to believe in the "magic power" of the plastic loop once it is inserted into the uterus; it is to believe in the authority of a person who is accessible only during office hours on certain weekdays, who does not care to listen to intricate personal problems and, above all, who is not known to one's relatives and cannot, therefore, be drawn into the web of interlocking kinship reciprocities so essential in Cebuano culture.

In light of the cumulative experiences of our respondents, it is obvious that the cost-benefit ratio of children is loaded differently in underdeveloped countries compared to developed ones. Consequently, the motive to contracept does not derive simply from the high cost of childbearing *vis-à-vis* the low cost of contraception. Rather, the equation is much more complex. Because pregnancy carries a different meaning in different stages of the family life cycle, and because children are valued for what they are and for what they can be, couples facing the prospect of having children feel highly ambivalent about contraception. Aside from the interpersonal factors that shape family planning decisions, we note that the economies of contraception are often offset by the diseconomies of maternal illness from contraceptive consumption; the high returns of having a large number of children outweigh the uncertainty of having no children or only a few; and the need to purchase contraceptives is superseded by other more immediate needs, such as the demand for food. In short, by presenting poor Filipinos with the choice of actively using modern contraceptives to limit the number of births, family planners are in effect asking them to choose between an outcome with "known risks" (that of *not* using contraceptives) versus one which clearly spells "uncertainty" (that of using contraceptives), to borrow Schnaiberg and Goldenberg's terms (1974). It is not surprising, then, that the poor often feel they can better maintain their precarious existence by not tampering with "fate." After all, the risks and rewards of having many children are already known through the experiences of their parents and grandparents, and the mechanisms for coping with such circumstances are already entrenched in the culture. In this context, to opt for a drastic reduction in family size is to take enormous chances. For many Cebuanos, it generates tremendous uncertainty about their future, without the promise of known rewards.

Hence, the policy implications of our findings seem inescapable. The process of disseminating modern contraceptives goes beyond the mere transplantation of new methods. It involves numerous steps. At the very least, there is first the process of supplanting a bewilderingly rich and deeply entrenched body of folk beliefs about reproduction and contraception. Second, there is the process of involving folk healers and midwives in the campaign to improve rural health care and to spread scientific contraceptive methods. Third, there is the process of "modernization," with its myriad ramifications on social structures, cultural values, and interpersonal relationships. Each of these processes requires drastic changes in the social, economic, and cognitive systems, to mention only a few.

Population policies, therefore, cannot be formulated in a vacuum. It is our conviction that for the Philippines or any other Third World country to succeed in controlling its population growth, emphasis on disseminating contraceptive methods alone without accompanying changes in the masses' economic conditions, health care, sociocultural values, and psychological perceptions will be inadequate. Furthermore, if and when the masses collectively practice family planning, the traditional male-female relationships, family interactions, and kinship networks will also have undergone major changes. After all, modern contraceptive innovation does not merely introduce a set of techniques for limiting births that are more efficient than the folk methods; they ultimately have a "homogenizing" effect in Third World countries in that they break down traditional norms and values and implant "modern consciousness." We know of no society plagued with extreme poverty, traditionalism, and economic underdevelopment which has been able to reduce its birth rate *without* introducing other societal changes. Thus, for better or for worse, the transition from high to low fertility in the Philippines is bound to upset the status quo.

Notes

Note to the Preface

1. The first four volumes all bear the title *Population*, and were edited separately by George N. Shuster and Donald Barrett. The fifth volume, edited by William T. Liu, was entitled *Family and Fertility*, while the sixth volume, edited by Edward Manier, William T. Liu and David Solomon, was entitled *Abortion*. All were published by the University of Notre Dame Press.

Notes to Chapter 1

1. Our purpose in calling the reader's attention to this matter is not to deprecate the contributions made by Amos Hawley and Francis Madigan to Philippine fertility studies, but to discuss the turn of events that gradually resulted in a consensus among scholars in the field that a population problem indeed existed in the country. Both Hawley and Madigan have made substantial contributions to social scientific research in the Philippines, and they have since independently revised their perspective.

2. The same U.N. report did mention, however, that slightly lower estimates of the crude birth rate have been proposed by other researchers. It was noted that Cho and Retherford (1973:180) calculated 40.4 per thousand for 1960 and 38.6 for 1968. But the report also contrasted these estimates with that given by Lorimer (1966), which was higher and congruent with the figure supplied by Keyfitz and Flieger (1971:85), who placed the rate at 47 per thousand. Concepcion (1974:160) was also cited as having provided an estimate of 43.2 per thousand for 1970, thereby giving more credence to the estimated range of 45 and 50 per thousand than to the lower figures mentioned by Cho and Retherford.

3. Concepcion (1970a) subsequently adjusted her predictions downward to 110 million by the year 2001. The National Census and Statistics Office's projection is much lower—95 million by the year 2000.

4. These are the only comprehensive sources of nationwide fertility and mortality data in the Philippines. During census years, complete enumerations are required on population characteristics. Fertility, economic, and labor force data are also gathered, but on a systematic sampling basis. Between census years, surveys of households are conducted on a sample basis to obtain some knowledge of fertility and mortality trends.

5. Although efforts are now being made to remedy the situation, underregistration has been a major problem in the Philippines (cf. Morrison, 1956; Carroll, 1959; Flieger, 1974). In 1968, for example, only 908 out of 1,468 local civil registrars in the country submitted complete reports; 441 had incomplete reports; and 119 turned in no report at all. The magnitude of error that may occur was noted as early as 1939, when Jaramillo (1941) found the underregistration of

male births to be 29.2 percent and that of female births 32.2 percent. At the same time, the figures for underreporting were 14.6 percent for male deaths and 13.1 percent for female deaths. Dizon (1958, cited in Concepcion, 1970) disclosed that in Nueva Ecija Province there was an underreporting of births by 35 percent and of deaths by 11 percent. The Department of Health subsequently expanded their study in 1961–1962 to include all the provinces and cities of Luzon and one province each from eastern and western Visayas. They discovered that during the selected period (1959–1962), nearly three out of every ten deaths were missing from the death registers of the local civil registrars (Dizon, 1964). Madigan's study in Misamis Oriental for 1960 indicates that 59.5 percent of deaths and 55.4 percent of births were not registered. In another study, this time by the Bureau of Census and Statistics, Barretto (1965) revealed that the underregistration figure was 39.7 percent for births and 30 percent for deaths. Concepcion (1965) found that in Imus, Cavite, the local civil registrar underregistered 46 percent of all births and 15 percent of all deaths estimated to have occurred during 1960–1963. Using the randomized response technique, Madigan, Abernathy, Herrin, and Tan (1976) estimated that for the province of Misamis Oriental, 50 percent or more of deaths occurring in 1972 were not mentioned to the interviewers.

6. The figures are 16.5 percent in Imus, Cavite (1966); 19.1 percent in Calasiao, Pangasinan (1964); 23.4 percent in Tiwi, Albay (1964); and 53.4 percent in Miagao, Iloilo (1966).

7. The figures are 7.2 percent in Imus, 4.1 percent in Calasiao, 23.4 percent in Tiwi, and 23.8 percent in Miagao.

8. Eliminated were all chartered cities, municipal districts, and municipalities in which the dominant mother tongue was not one of the eight major languages: Cebuano, Tagalog, Iloko, Ilongo, Bikol, Waray, Kapampangan, and Pangasinan.

Notes to Chapter 2

1. The Chinese presence in the Philippines dates as far back as the tenth century (Sung dynasty), and by the thirteenth century, they began establishing themselves in the islands. After that, the number of Chinese in the Philippines fluctuated with the labor demand of the Spanish conquerors for building cathedrals and consumption demand for Chinese imports, not to mention political and economic conditions in China.

2. Phelan (1959:35–40) also mentioned disciplinary problems such as violations of clerical celibacy and infractions of the vow of poverty.

3. This is most evident in Lieban's perceptive description of Cebuano sorcery (1967), where Christian symbols and Latin concepts are combined with folk beliefs of malign magic to impute evil and also to obtain or receive miraculous power. The interested reader should also consult Arens (1956a, 1956b) for a description of syncretic rice and fishing ritual in Leyte and Samar.

4. Among these are the Payne-Aldrich Act of 1909, the Hare-Hawes Cutting Act and Tydings MacDuffie Law of 1933–1934, the Bell Trade Act of 1946, and, after Philippine independence, the Laurel-Langley Agreement of 1955.

5. Only in 1963 and 1966 did exports exceed imports, resulting in slight gains for the Philippines. But the "invisible items" of trade that accompanied this commerce offset the gains for the Philippine economy. Some of these invisible items of trade are tourist expenditures, Philippine government expenditures abroad, freight and insurance, and public and private donations (BCS, 1969).

6. This is based on the 1960 Philippine census data since the 1970 census data released so far do not contain any language breakdown.

7. The perpetuation of these different languages since pre-Hispanic times is due to a number of factors, of course, including geographic insularity; the Spanish colonial policy of *not* promoting a unifying language among the people, and their concept of elitist education obtainable only in the Spanish language; and the slow development of mass media in the hinterlands.

8. The word is sometimes generically employed for sorcery, but it also refers to a specific form of malign magic in which insects and other forms of tiny animals are "sent to" the intended victim; these creatures are believed to enter the victim's body through the orifices and bite his entrails. The stomach of the victim supposedly swells and becomes painful (Lieban, 1967:1–2, 50–53).

9. Lieban (1967:50) also cited another study (Aparece, 1960:28) which referred to *barang* in another Visayan province, Bohol.

10. This method entails massaging the woman's stomach with certain herbs.

11. The few who do not espouse these values and who hold "progressive" or "radical" ideas are by now safely closeted, or living abroad.

12. This arbitrary dividing line of 1,500 pesos was determined by multiplying the legally prescribed minimum wage (6 pesos) by the number of working days in a year based on a five-day work week, excluding holidays (BCSSH, 1968a).

13. In order not to overburden the reader with statistics, we have omitted the glaring urban-rural disparity. Suffice it to state that in 1965 the *median* income for all families in the Philippines was 1,648 pesos (2,636 for all urban families and 1,359 for all rural families). The *average* annual income for all families was 2,541 pesos (4,405 for all urban families and 1,755 for all rural ones).

14. They arrived at 400 pesos per capita by estimating that if a breadwinner earns 8 pesos per day for 303 days (52 Sundays and 10 holidays excluded), the family in 1971 would have had an income of 2,424 pesos a year. Dividing this by six, the share for each family member would be about 400 pesos a year.

15. This view of the Philippine economic conditions, widely shared by Filipino intellectuals, especially economists, is assailed by some writers as "professional criticisms." For instance, Averch et al. (1971) interpreted the same officially released unemployment figures rather optimistically by arguing that unemployment is concentrated in "quite specific groups of the population;" the inexperienced unemployed "have but an ambiguous commitment to the labor force, and the extended family shields them from the impact of joblessness;" most of the really seriously underemployed are rural females, and "most of those who want more work are already working 40 hours or more per week" (Averch et al., 1971:75). In the preface of their book, these writers emphasize the analogy between such widely held "misperceptions" of the Philippine economy to those pessimistic views held by scholars and intellectuals of Iran during the sixties even when events showed that country had built "strengths upon strengths." Unfortunately, the Shah's downfall in 1979 suggests that it is the optimistic, and not the pessimistic, views of Iranian society which were based on misperceptions.

Notes to Chapter 3

1. This will be discussed in greater detail in Chapter 6. Briefly, the method involves presenting two or more people with a problem and then asking them to reach a mutually acceptable solution. The subsequent interaction is observed and later evaluated on a variety of dimensions by a panel of judges.

2. The topics were: the *querida* or mistress system, the *bayot* ("effeminate,"

"homosexual") phenomenon, and the incidence of *couvade* (sympathetic pregnancy symptoms experienced by men) that we observed casually. However, owing to the reluctance of high-status *queridas* and *bayots* to be interviewed, the paucity of theoretical conceptualization on *couvade*, and the lack of budget, manpower, and time to pursue these three topics, our data-gathering efforts have mainly yielded anecdotal cases. We do believe, though, that these are significant social facts which deserve more thorough investigation. We also believe that they will unveil a wealth of data on folk conceptions of sex roles and health.

3. The rationale behind our decision to use these criteria for sampling rural barrios is obvious. For one thing, the social life of rural people is generally considered an adjustment to the economic environment. For another, in the Philippines access to transportation has been found to be associated with an above-average percentage of school-aged children actually in school, the presence of dwellings which have access to wells, and the availability of outhouses.

4. In many areas where the samples were designated, the houses were a considerable distance apart. The amount of time required to sample, say, every fourth house, would have been excessive.

5. This may have introduced a minor bias by excluding the most remote and isolated barrios. However, the demands of practicality permitted no alternative, and since this probably applied to very few barrios, the extent of error is minimal.

6. The barrios sampled were Atabay, Guiwang, and Daan Lungsod of the Alcoy municipality; Luka and Combado of Cantuud, which belong to the Balamban municipality; Cajel and La-aw of the Borbon municipality; Catarman and Cabadiangan of the Lilo-an municipality; Gun-ob and Pusok of the Lapu-lapu municipality; Poblacion and Cadwawan of the Tabogon municipality; Sangi, Lutupan, and Cantabaco of Toledo City; and Cogon, Colonia, Gimama-a, Manga, Maghanay, Bulwang, Poblacion, and Putat of the Tuburan municipality.

7. This procedure of selecting households was employed for the majority of the urban interviews, with one minor exception. Toward the completion of the survey phase, we were concerned that the middle-class families were so few. In order to obtain more middle-class respondents with our limited budget and manpower, interviews in the lower-class areas were terminated. The interviewers were instructed to concentrate instead on the middle-class neighborhoods, and to take every second residential structure. The number of completed interviews after this instruction change was less than two hundred. In retrospect, we believe that we might have been falsely alarmed by the small number of middle-class cases, because we did not realize until after the data were collected how insignificant the middle-class segment of the Philippine population was, compared to the lower class. Although the middle class has grown somewhat in recent years, their rapid "stateside" migration has kept their numbers small, as have the complex economic factors in the Philippines which have maintained the status quo for decades.

8. Jeepneys are war-surplus U.S. Army jeeps which have been converted into passenger vehicles, capable of seating as many as twelve under the most crowded arrangement. As the old vehicles wore out over the years, new jeep chassis were imported to replace the old ones.

9. Fortunately, the Chinese-speaking population of Cebu is only a very small fraction of the entire population, and almost all of them speak English or Cebuano; hence our decision to require bilingual English-Cebuano speakers. However, two of the project's staff members also speak Chinese fluently.

10. A principal difficulty in producing precise literal translations shouid be mentioned here. This problem arises from the structural differences between

Cebuano and English. For instance, a great number of action-oriented words are expressed in the passive voice in Cebuano, while English uses the active voice. In addition, any translation from one language to another, no matter how careful, is likely to suffer from some distortions in sentence construction. Cebuano is no exception, particularly since the dialect is much more limited in research-related concepts and terminologies than are many of the romance languages, for instance.

Notes to Chapter 4

1. Aside from Cebu Province, the Cebuanos also inhabit the islands of Bohol, Siquijor, Western Leyte, and Eastern Negros in the Visayas, and different parts of Mindanao to the south. However, because of political underrepresentation when the Philippine legislature was first convened to decide on a national language, Cebuano was not made the national language of the country.

2. A recent estimate places about forty percent of the population of Cebu Province in the city of Cebu. Available government statistics suggest that because of overpopulation in Cebu Province for several decades since the turn of the century, a steady outmigration has taken place for some time, about 45 percent of which end up in Mindanao to the south. Of the provinces that continue to experience an influx of Cebuano migrants, Davao, Cotabato, and Bukidnon rank among the highest. By 1980, the population of Davao City is expected to outpace that of Cebu City. The fact that Cebuano or Visayan is widely spoken in the south (probably because of earlier migration waves) makes Mindanao preferable for settlement. Unlike other Asian countries, where the migrants are usually men, in the Philippines women are as migratory as men. We believe this is due to the peculiar kinship system in the Philippines, where males and females are defined as structurally equal.

3. Because of nonresponse or refusals on certain items of our interview schedule, and because some questions were not asked of all respondents, the exact sample size will vary from table to table.

4. One of whom was Elena Yu.

5. See Chapter 8 for details on the distinction between adultery and concubinage under Philippine law, and the unequal sanctions imposed on men versus women who have had extramarital affairs.

Notes to Chapter 5

1. Data on foam, douche, sponge, and jelly are not included primarily because the percentage of respondents claiming to have knowledge of these devices and to have used them is quite small in every socioeconomic class.

2. One possibility is that there was some degree of ambiguity in the translation of the word "the Pill." Because of the absence of an equivalent word in Cebuano, a Spanish borrowed word, *tabletas*, was used which includes not only the Pill but also pills in general. This literally equivalent but phenomenally nonequivalent terminology might have produced a confounding effect because we later discovered a Cebuano folk contraceptive method in which *tabletas* are crushed and inserted into the woman's vagina before intercourse. Not too many women, however, knew what kind of *tabletas* should be used. We have learned that some people prescribed quinine while others believe *Cortal* (a locally produced aspirin) is just as effective.

3. Because of the cultural belief prevalent among the Cebuanos that it is harmful to take a bath or get wet during the menstrual period, bathday refers to the first day when the woman feels that her menstrual flow has ceased and she can wet herself with water without injuring her health. Hence, it is rather imprecise for rhythm purposes.

4. Translation: You know, every woman has two ovaries (*obario*). Every month it discharges an egg. This is called ovulation (*obulasyon*). The egg travels to the Fallopian tube (*palopiya*) and when it is seen by the sperm (*sperma*), this is called fertilization (*pertilisasyon*).

5. Sixty centavos at that time was equivalent to fifteen cents U.S. currency.

Notes to Chapter 6

1. Cf. Ruiz (1968) for a comprehensive description of Cebuano folk medicine and illness concepts.

2. Two of the physicians were from the Cebu Skin Clinic, and one was a popular general practitioner in the city.

3. The three *mananambals* surveyed were considered to be the most popular ones in the city.

4. In examining the province-by-province release of birth data from year to year, we found that in 1973 (the most recent data available so far), Manila (which is considered a province for statistical purposes only) and Rizal were the only two provinces in the whole country in which the largest proportion of births were attended by physicians. They assisted in 81.7 percent of the total reported births in Manila and 52.6 percent of those in Rizal—a fact which alone is sufficient to convey the extremely uneven development of the country.

5. This is a precautionary measure taken to protect the mother and newborn infant. According to one source (Damo, 1969:34), it is supposed to make subsequent deliveries easier. Unfortunately, native Cebuano researchers have taken it for granted that it is well understood, while nonindigenous investigators apparently failed to take note of it. Our only available information on *lihi* comes from an unpublished thesis housed at the University of San Carlos (Quisumbing, 1965:95–96). It describes *lihi* as "usually consisting of the pulverized shell of first laid egg of the pullet (*dumaga*) mixed with roasted ground cacao beans." What is done with this pulverized mixture—whether it is drunk or pasted on certain parts of the body—is not at all clear.

6. Coconut oil mixed with medicinal plants and stored in bottles. It is usually prepared on Good Friday. The kinds of plants used vary with the attributions of illness. Coughs, stomach aches, relapse, and sterility call for different substances of *hapas* (cf. Ruiz, 1968).

7. Poultice made from the leaves of plants. Again, the kinds of plants to use differ according to the type of illness they are supposed to treat (cf. Ruiz, 1968).

8. The first postpartum bath is given two weeks after delivery and consists of medicinal herbs in warm water. In primaparas, the mother gets the *lihi* together with the bath; in multiparas, only the child gets the *lihi* but the mother gets a bath with medicinal herbs just the same, minus the ritual (Damo, 1969:55).

9. In our discussion of these procedures, we have relied mainly on two unpublished sources: Demetria (1969) and Damo (1969), both of which were collected in consultation with the Cebu Family Health Project.

10. For this reason, Agnes Demetria, being female and unmarried at the time she was collecting these data, never had the opportunity to see one. Neither the *mananabangs* nor the women who sell them would show one to her.

11. Only three of the barrio *mananabangs* and four from the city sample admitted to using any of the folk contraceptive methods described here.

Note to Chapter 7

1. These constructs were operationally defined as follows: high motivation applies to spouses who have used at least one method of contraception, given the knowledge of how to use at least three methods; low motivation refers to spouses who have never used any method, given the knowledge of how to use at least two methods. Effectiveness had to be defined relatively rather than absolutely, since the majority of the respondents who were approaching menopause had relatively large families by U.S. standards. Hence, we considered a couple highly effective if they had had four or fewer children, conceived after marriage, while low-effective couples are those who had had seven or more children, conceived after marriage.

Notes to Chapter 8

1. In fact, some tragic stories serialized over the radio in Cebu have been known to include such chain (or double *querida*) relationships.

2. Paternal recognition, however, does not always mean that the father is able and willing to support his illegitimate children.

3. The separation, if and when granted, deprives the offending spouse of rights to any share in the profits earned by the conjugal partnership. It also disqualifies the spouse at fault from inheriting from the innocent spouse, whether it be an intestate succession or a testamentary one. Furthermore, under normal circumstances, remarriage is permitted only if an annulment was obtained from the church, or if one of the parties to the previous marriage contract dies, is mentally infirm, or is not heard from for seven consecutive years.

4. Carale (1970:351) noted that "voyeurism, lewdness, 'crime against nature,' sodomy and other abnormal sexual activities are not dealt with in the penal code of the Philippines. . . . Homosexuality is another sexual activity which is unknown to the penal code of the Philippines."

Notes to Chapter 9

1. This particular pocket of squatters is located alongside a river. Except during heavy rainfall, the river is dry. Children and many adults go to the dry riverbed to defecate.

2. Pinching is a disciplinary technique commonly used by women in the Cebuano culture. Any part of the child's body may be pinched, including the genitalia. Such disciplinary action is also reportedly used by female grade school teachers on male students. Although more boys than girls are pinched, the latter are not totally spared.

Notes to Chapter 10

1. Nevertheless, key members of an individual's personal kindred—or representatives thereof—may occasionally gather during certain stages of the indi-

vidual life cycle, such as baptism, marriage, or a funeral. Some kindred members may also agree to form a corporate group for business purposes or other forms of collective action. This activity, however, is a spontaneous and incidental occurrence rather than a structural requisite of bilateral kinship.

2. *Prenda* is an economic institution widely practiced since the Spanish Conquest. Through *prenda*, the impoverished peasant contracts a "temporary sale" of his land or other property for the *minimal* amount of money he needs to sustain his family during an emergency, such as tuition expenses or other fees demanded by an American-oriented bureaucracy. The rationale is that the less he *prendas* his land, the easier it will be for him to pay back the cash he borrowed in exchange. However, for the duration of the *prenda*, the poor farmer, while having lost the rightful ownership of his land, continues to pay taxes on it. And if he should be unable to pay back the money he borrowed, he automatically loses title. This means, in effect, that he has sold his land for a miserly sum of money. As a long-standing institution in the Philippines, *prenda* has provided the poor with just about the only means of acquiring liquid capital. Although the government has declared it illegal, many urban poor people still engage in it in order to generate cash for emergencies.

3. No doubt, the alternative of a childless marriage is unthinkable. The stigma of being *landay* (barren or sterile) is a social label most women want to avoid. Without sufficient medical evidence, most people tend to blame the woman for not bearing any children. It is she who must submit to "treatment."

Notes to Chapter 11

1. It is said that when Miguel Lopez de Legaspi landed in 1565 in Cebu Island (forty-five years after Magellan's death), he met with resistance from the local chieftain, Rajah Tupas. In the open fire that followed, one of Legaspi's detachments found an image of the Child Jesus in one of the houses they had raided. When it was brought to Legaspi, he reputedly revered it and on May 8, 1565, he was able officially to take possession of Cebu Island in the name of King Philip II of Spain. On January 1, 1571, Legaspi founded the city of Cebu, naming it Villa of the Holy Child (Molina, 1960). A chapel was built for the image of the Holy Child. It was later transferred to the Augustinian Church of Santo Niño in 1602. When a fire ravaged the church twenty years later, the Santo Niño was recovered among the wreckage. This was the second "miracle." Since then, legends have grown about how the Santo Niño has always resisted being transported out of Cebu.

2. This is the cross that Magellan placed in the center of the town square of Cebu on April 14, 1521, when Father Valderrama, Magellan's chaplain, baptized the chieftain of Cebu, Rajah Humabon, and five hundred others.

References

Adams, Edith
  1958 "New population estimates for the Philippines, 1948–1962." The Philippine Statistician 7 (3):134–166.

Aparece, Francisco
  1960 The Care of the Sick and the Burial of the Dead in the Rural Areas of Bohol and their Educational Implications. M. A. thesis, University of San Carlos, Cebu City, Philippines.

Arens, Richard
  1956a "Animism in the rice ritual of Leyte and Samar." Philippine Sociological Review IV (January):2–6.

  1956b "Animistic fishing ritual in Leyte and Samar." Philippine Sociological Review IV (October):24–28.

Aromin, Basilio
  1959 "Commentary on 'Some Filipino population characteristics and their relations to economic development.'" Philippine Sociological Review 7 (Jan.–Apr.):27–30.

  1961 "The trend of mortality in the Philippines: 1903–1960." The Statistical Reporter 5(3):1–7.

  1963 The Population Base of Economic Development Problems in the Philippines. M.A. thesis, University of North Carolina.

Averch, Harvey A., John E. Koehler, and Frank H. Denton
  1971 The Matrix of Policy in the Philippines. A Rand Corporation Research Study. Princeton, New Jersey: Princeton University Press.

Bales, Robert F.
  1950 Interaction Process Analysis: A Method of Study of Small Groups. Cambridge, Mass.: Addison-Wesley.

Bales, Robert F. and Fred L. Strodtbeck
  1951 "Phases in group problem solving." Journal of Abnormal and Social Psychology 46:485–495.

Ballweg, John A. and Donald W. MacCorquodale
  1974 "Family planning method change and dropouts in the Philippines." Social Biology 21, 1 (Spring):88–95.

Barreto, Felisa R.
1965 "Birth and death registration in the Philippines." The Philippine Statistician 14(4):224–64.

Blake, Judith
1961 Family Structure in Jamaica: The Social Context of Reproduction. New York: Free Press.

Bohannan, P. J.
1963 Social Anthropology. New York: Holt, Rinehart and Winston.

Brandewie, Ernest
1973 "Family size and kinship pressures in the Philippines." Philippine Quarterly of Culture and Society 1, 1:6–18.

1975 "The structure of kinship and family influence in Cebuano culture." Philippine Quarterly of Culture and Society 3 (June–Sept.):90–97.

Burch, T. K.
1967 "The size and structure of families." American Sociological Review 32 (June):347–363.

Burch, T. K. and Murray Gendell
1971 "Extended family structure and fertility." Pp. 87–104 in Steve Polgar (ed.), Culture and Population. A Collection of Current Studies. Monograph 9. Chapel Hill: University of North Carolina Press.

Bureau of Census and Statistics (BCS)
1969 "The central problems and issues of Philippine foreign trade." Journal of Philippine Statistics 20 (Jan.–March):vii–xix.

1973 Vital Statistics Report 1970. Manila.

Bureau of Census and Statistics Survey of Households (BCSSH)
1968a "Family income distribution and expenditure patterns in the Philippines: 1965." Journal of Philippine Statistics 19 (April–June):ix–xxix.

1968b "Implications of demographic factors on rural development." Journal of Philippine Statistics 19(Oct.–Dec.):xiii–xxi.

Carale, Bartolome S.
1970 "Criminal adultery and fornication in the Philippines: a reexamination." Philippine Law Journal 45, 3(July):344–52.

Carroll, John J.
1959 "Population increase and geographical distribution in the Philippines." The Philippine Statistician 8 (Sept.):154–173.

Carroll, Verne (ed.)
1970 Adoption in Eastern Oceania. Honolulu: University of Hawaii Press.

Child Welfare League of America

1958 Child Welfare League of America Standards for Adoption Service. New York: Child Welfare League of America Committee on Standards of Adoption Service.

Cho, Lee-Jay and Robert D. Retherford

1973 "Comparative analysis of recent fertility trends in East Asia." In International Union for the Scientific Study of Population, International Population Conference, vol. 2. Liege.

Christensen, Harold T.

1966 "Scandinavian and American sex norms: some comparisons with sociological implications." Journal of Social Issues 22 (April):60–75.

Christensen, Harold T. and George Carpenter

1962 "Timing patterns in the development of sexual intimacy: an attitudinal report on three modern western societies." Marriage and Family Living 24 (Feb.):30–34.

Concepcion, Mercedes

1963 Fertility Differences among Married Women in the Philippines. Ph. D. dissertation, University of Chicago.

1964 "Some socio-economic correlates of completed family size." Philippine Sociological Review 12:16–26.

1965 "Under-registration of births and deaths in a Philippine municipality." Philippine Sociological Review 13(4):277–31.

1966 "The population of the Philippines." Pp. 185–199 in Population Institute of the University of the Philippines, First Conference in Population, 1965. Quezon City: University of the Philippines Press.

1967 "The effect of current social and economic changes in the developing countries on differential fertility." Pp. 124–127 in United Nation's Department of Economic and Social Affairs, World Population Conferences 1965, II. N. Y.: United Nations.

1968 "Family building patterns of young Manila couples." Philippine Sociological Review 16 (3–4):

1969 "Changing fertility behavior of Filipino women." Third Conference on Population, December 11–12. Population Institute. Manila: University of the Philippines.

1970a "110 millions by the year 2001." Philippine Sociological Review 18 (July–Oct.):211–220.

1970b The Philippines, Country Profiles. New York: The Population Institute.

1974 "Philippines—East Asia review, 1973." Studies in Family Planning 5, 5(May):160–162.

Concepcion, Mercedes (ed.)
1969 Philippine Population in the Seventies. Proceedings of the Second Conference on Population, November 27–29. Manila: Community Publishers, Inc.

Concepcion, Mercedes B. and Gerry E. Hendershot
1969 "Prospects of a fertility decline in the seventies." Pp. 367–395 in Mercedes B. Concepcion (ed.), Philippine Population in the Seventies. Manila: Community Publishers, Inc.

Concepcion, Mercedes B. and Wilhelm Flieger
1968 "Studies of fertility and fertility planning in the Philippines." Demography 5(2):714–731.

Cortes, Irene R.
1973 "Population and law: the fundamental rights aspects in the Philippine setting." Philippine Law Journal 48, 3 (July):303–454.

Cumming, Elaine and David Schneider
1961 "Sibling solidarity: a property of American kinship." American Anthropologist LXIII (June):498–507.

Damo, Nieva Tan
1970 The Midwives: A Functional Analysis of Social Change. Uncompleted M. A. thesis, University of San Carlos, Cebu City, Philippines.

Davis, K.
1955 "Institutional patterns favoring high fertility in underdeveloped areas." Eugenics Quarterly 2(March):33–39.

De Los Angeles, Noli
1965 "Marriage and fertility patterns in the Philippines." Philippine Sociological Review 13(Oct.):232–248.

Demetria, Agnes M.
1969 Folk Methods of Birth Control. M. A. thesis, University of San Carlos, Cebu City, Philippines.

Dizon, Jacinto J.
1958 Unpublished report. Manila: Department of Health.

1964 Unpublished report. Manila: Disease Intelligence Center, Department of Health.

Duff, Robert W. and William T. Liu
1975 "The significance of the heterophilous structure in communication flows." Philippine Quarterly of Culture and Society 3 (June–Sept.):159–175.

Escultura, Edgar E.
1974 "The roots of backwardness: an analysis of the Philippine condition." Science and Society 38, 1(Spring):49–76.

Flavier, Juan M.
1970 "Comments on the Concepcion paper." Philippine Sociological Review 18(July–Oct.):224–225.

Flieger, Wilhelm
1974 "Some comments on current mortality information in the Philippines." Paper prepared for the Experts meeting on Philippine Population Research, Population Center Building, Makati, October 10–21.

Francisco, Vicente J.
1952 The Revised Penal Code (Act no. 3815). Annotated. Manila: East Publishing.

Fortes, Meyer
1953 "The structure of unilineal descent groups." American Anthropologist 55:17–41.

Foster, George M.
1961 "The dyadic contract: a model for the social structures of a Mexican peasant village." American Anthropologist 63: 1173–1192.

1963 "The dyadic contract in Tzintzuntzan, II: patron-client relationship." American Anthropologist 65 (Dec.):1280–1294.

Fox, Robert B.
1959 "The study of Filipino society and its significance to programs of economic and social development." Philippine Sociological Review VII (Jan.–Apr.):2–11.

Goldstein, S.
1967 "Pre-marital pregnancies in Denmark." Pp. 993–1000 in Sydney Conference of the International Union for the Study of Population, August.

Gustavus, S. O. and C. B. Nam
1970 "The formation and stability of ideal family size among young people." Demography 7(1):43–51.

Guthrie, George M.
1966 Child Rearing and Personality Development in the Philippines. University Park: University of Pennsylvania State Press.

Hart, Donn V.
1965 "From pregnancy through birth in a Bisayan Filipino village." Pp. 1–114 in Donn V. Hart, Phya numan Rejadhon, and Richard J. Coughlin, Southeast Asian Birth Customs. Human Relations Area Files Press. Behavioral Science Monographs. New Haven: Connecticut.

Hauser, Philip M.
1967 "Population and family planning programs: a review article." Demography 4,1:397–414.

Hawley, Amos H.

1954a "Differential population pressure in the Philippines." Philippine Sociological Review II(July):28–36.

1954b "The Philippine Census of 1948." Pp. 11–26 in Papers in Demography and Public Administration. University of the Philippines, revised edition.

1954c "Rural fertility in central Luzon." The Philippine Statistician 3(3):162–174.

Herbst, G.

1952 "The measurement of family relationships." Human Relations 5:3–35.

Hill, Reuben, J. M. Stycos, and K. Back

1959 The Family and Population Control. Chapel Hill: University of North Carolina Press.

Hollnsteiner, Mary R.

1970 "Reciprocity in the lowland Philippines." Pp. 65–88 in Frank Lynch and Alfonso de Guzman (eds.), Four Readings on Philippine Values. IPC Papers No. 2. Quezon City: Ateneo de Manila University Press.

Hsu, Francis L. K.

1969 The Study of Literate Civilization. N. Y.: Holt, Rinehart and Winston.

Hunt, Chester

1965 "Female occupational roles and urban sex ratios in the United States, Japan and the Philippines." Social Forces 43, 4 (March):407–417.

Hunt, Eva

1969 "The meaning of kinship in San Juan: genealogical and social models." Ethnology VIII:37–53.

Hutchison, Ira W. III

1970 Husband-Wife Interaction and Fertility Patterns in the Philippines. Ph. D. dissertation, University of Notre Dame, Indiana.

1974 "The functional significance of conjugal communication in a traditional society." Journal of Marriage and the Family 36, 3(August):580–587.

1975 "Conjugal relations and family planning." Philippine Quarterly of Culture and Society 3(June–Sept.):146–158.

Jacobson, Helga E.

1970 "Urbanization and family ties: a problem in the analysis of change." Journal of Asian and African Studies 5, 4(Oct.): 302–7.

Jaramillo, Trinidad J.

1941 "Statistical applications of the 1938 life table." Journal of Philippine Statistics 1(3–4):575–81.

Jimenez, Teresita T.
1955 "A study of health practices in the slums of barrio Bonifacio." Philippine Sociological Review III(July):28–31.

Jocano, F. Landa
1969 Growing up in a Philippine Barrio. N.Y.: Holt, Rinehart and Winston.

Juco, Jorge M.
1966 "Fault, consent and breakdown—the sociology of divorce legislation in the Philippines." Philippine Sociological Review XIV(April):67–75.

Jupp, Kathleen M.
1960 "Patterns of population change in the Philippines, 1939 to 1957." The Philippine Statistician 9(1):11–29.

Kaplan, Abraham
1964 The Conduct of Inquiry. N.Y.: Harper and Row.

Katz, Bonnie
1966 Manual for Training Interviewers. Mimeograph. Notre Dame: Social Science Training and Research Laboratory. University of Notre Dame.

Keeley, Charles B.
1973 "Philippine migration; internal movements and emigration to the U.S." International Migration Review 7,2(Summer):177–87.

Keyfitz, N. and W. Flieger
1971 Population: Facts and Methods of Demography. San Francisco: W. H. Freeman and Co.

Laing, John E.
1973 "Use effectiveness of family planning in the Philippines: 1970–1972." Philippine Sociological Review 21 (April):137–151.

Leach, E. R.
1950 Social Science Research in Sarawak. Colonial Research Studies No. 1. London, Colonial Office: His Majesty's Stationery Office.

Lewis-Faning, E.
1949 "Family limitation." Papers of the Royal Commission on Population 1:38–86.

Lieban, Richard W.
1967 Cebuano Sorcery. Malign Magic in the Philippines. Berkeley and Los Angeles: University of California Press.

Liu, William T.
1968 Quarterly Report of the Cebu Family Health Project, submitted to the National Economic Council of the Philippines and the Agency for International Development of the United States of America. Mimeo. University of Notre Dame, October 1.

1977 "The myths of the nuclear family and fertility in central Philippines." Pp. 35–62 in Luis Lenero (ed.), Beyond the Nuclear Family Model. N. Y.: Sage Publishing Co.

Liu, William T. and Ira W. Hutchison
1974 "Conjugal interaction and fertility behavior." Pp. 27–43 in Frank Bean and T. Y. Yuan (eds.), Family and Fertility. Holland: E. J. Brill.

Lorimer, Frank
1966 "Analysis and projections of the population of the Philippines." Pp. 200–314 in Population Institute, University of the Philippines, First Conference on Population 1965. Quezon City: University of the Philippines Press.

Lynch, Frank and Perla Q. Makil
1967 "The Brac 1967 Filipino Family Survey." Saint Louis Quarterly 6(3–4):293–330.

Madigan, Francis C.
1959 "Some Filipino population characteristics and their relation to economic development." Philippine Sociological Review VII (Jan.-Apr.):16–26.
1965 "Some recent vital rates and trends in the Philippines: estimates and evaluations." Demography 2:309–316.
1971 "Brief communications and research note: intensive population study in Mindanao." Philippine Sociological Review 19 (July–Oct.):255–256.

Madigan, Francis. C., James R. Abernathy, Alejandro N. Herrin and Clarita Tan
1976 "Purposive concealment of death in household surveys in Misamis Oriental Province." Population Studies 30(2):295–303.

Madigan, Francis C., Teresa B. Almonte, Eduardo B. Calica and Alejandro N. Herrin
1973 "Birth and death rates from a dual-record system in the Philippines." Philippine Sociological Review 21, 2(April):115–135.

Madigan, Francis and Rosalia O. Avancena
1964 "Philippine fertility and mortality with special reference to the northern Mindanao region: a critique of recent estimates. Part I: The Philippines in general." Philippine Sociological Review 12:35–42.

Malay, Paula C.
1957 "Some Tagalog folkways." University of Manila Journal of East Asiatic Studies 6:69–88.

Mathen, K. K.
1962 "Preliminary lessons learnt from the rural population control study of Singur." Pp. 33–49 in Clyde Kiser (ed.), Research in Family Planning. Princeton, N.J.: Princeton University Press.

McHale, Thomas R.
1952 "Economic development in the Philippines." Journal of East Asiatic Studies (University of Manila) 1, 3:1–10.

Mintz, Sidney W. and Eric R. Wolf
1950 "An analysis of ritual co-parenthood (compadrazgo)." Southwestern Journal of Anthropology 6 (Winter):341–368.

Molina, Antonio M.
1960 The Philippines Through the Centuries, vols. I and II. Manila: University of Santo Tomas Cooperative.

Monahan, Thomas P.
1960 "Pre-marital pregnancy in the United States." Eugenics Quarterly 7:133–147.

Morrison, Frank S.
1956 "Some comments on birth, death and infant mortality rates in the Philippines, and a suggested device for registration improvement." The Philippine Statistician 5(2):98–105.

1957 A Study of Vital Statistics in the Philippines for 1956 and Their Relation to the Annual Population Increase. Mimeo. Manila: International Cooperation Administration.

Mortel, Delores M. and Francisco V. Nazaret
1971 "A study of birth and death registration in Baloi, Lanao del Norte and Itogon, Benguet." Philippine Sociological Review 19 (July–Oct.):243–54.

Murdock, George P.
1949 Social Structure. N.Y.: Macmillan Co.

1968 "Cognatic forms of social organization." Pp. 235–53 in P. Bohannan and John Middleton (eds.), Kinship and Social Organization. N.Y.: The Natural History Press.

Murphy Edmund M. (ed.)
1968 Four Fertility Surveys. Quezon City: JMC Press.

National Census and Statistics Office (NCSO)
1973a "Foreign trade." Philippine Journal of Statistics 24 (April–June):64–66.

1973b "Foreign trade." Journal of Philippine Statistics 24 (July–Sept.):65–68.

1975a "Developments in the manufacturing industry of the Philippines: 1956–1973." Journal of Philippine Statistics 26 (July–Sept.):ix–xxi.

1975b "The family income of employed and unemployed persons." Journal of Philippine Statistics 26 (Jan.–March):ix–xix.

1975c "Foreign trade." Journal of Philippine Statistics 26 (April–June):89–91.

Nazaret, F. V. and H. V. Chaves
1964 "Fertility Survey of 1963 in the Philippines." Philippine Sociological Review 12(1-2):5-16.

Ortega, Manuel L.
1973 "Abortion and the right to privacy." Philippine Law Journal 48:653-695.

Pascual, Elvira Mendoza
1966 Population Redistribution in the Philippines. Mimeo. Manila: University of the Philippines.

Pehrson, Robert N.
1954 "Bilateral kin groupings as a structural type." Journal of East Asiatic Studies 3:199-202.

1957 The Bilateral Network of Social Relations in Konkama Lapp District. Indiana University Publications, Slavic and East European Series, vol. 5. Bloomington, Indiana.

Phelan, John
1959 The Hispanization of the Philippines. Madison: University of Wisconsin Press.

Pinard, Leo William II
1971 Heterosexual Relations in the Central Visayas. Ph. D. dissertation, University of Notre Dame, Indiana.

1975 "Courtship in an urban Visayan setting." Philippine Quarterly of Culture and Society 3(June-Sept.):98-113.

Piron, Georges
1972 "The educated unemployed." Philippine Sociological Review 20 (October):338-346.

Pratt, William F.
1967 "Family size and expectations in Manila." Saint Louis Quarterly 5, 1-2:153-184.

Quirino, Carlos and Mauro Garcia
1958 "The manners, customs and beliefs of the Philippine inhabitants of long ago; being chapters of a late 16th century Manila Manuscript." Transcribed, translated, and annotated. The Philippine Journal of Science 87, 4(December):325-454.

Quisumbing, Lourdes Reyes
1965 A Study of the Marriage Customs of the Rural Population of the Province of Cebu. M. A. thesis, University of San Carlos.

Rainwater, Lee
1960 And the Poor Get Children. Chicago: Quadrangle Books.

Rivers, William H.
1924 Social Organization, N.Y.: Alfred A. Knoph, Inc.

Rubel, Arthur J., William T. Liu, Mimi Trosdal and Virginia Pato
1971 "The traditional birth attendant in Metropolitan Cebu, the

Philippines." Pp. 176–188 in Steven Polgar (ed.), Culture and Population: A Collection of Current Studies. Carolina Population Center, University of North Carolina at Chapel Hill and Schenkman Publishing Co., Inc., Cambridge, Mass.

Rubel, Arthur J., Karen Weller-Fahy, and Mimi Trosdal
1975 "Conception, gestation, and delivery according to some *mananabang* of Cebu." Philippine Quarterly of Culture and Society 3 (June–Sept):131–145.

Ruiz, Angeles Llopes
1968 A Study of Cebuano Folk Medicine. M. A. thesis, University of San Carlos, Philippines.

Sants, H. J.
1964 "Genealogical bewilderment in children with substitute parents." British Journal of Medical Psychology 37(2):133–141.

Schnaiberg, Allan and Sheldon Goldenberg
1974 "Closing the circle: the impact of children on parental status." Draft.

Sison, Carmelo
1973 "Population laws of the Philippines." Philippine Law Journal 48, 3(July):356–428.

Strodtbeck, Fred L.
1951 "Husband-wife interaction over revealed differences." American Sociological Review 16:468–73.

1964 "A summary of current works on family interaction studies using revealed differences." Unpublished working paper 31, University of Chicago Social Psychology Laboratory.

Stycos, J. M.
1958 "Some directions for research on fertility control." Milbank Memorial Fund Quarterly 38 (April):126–148.

Stycos, J. M. and K. W. Back
1964 The Control of Human Fertility in Jamaica. Ithaca: Cornell University Press.

Taeuber, Irene
1960 "Bases of a population problem—the Philippines." Population Index 26(2):97–114.

Taylor, George E.
1964 The Philippines and the United States. Problems of Partnership. N.Y.: Frederick A. Praeger.

Terhune, Kenneth W.
1972 "The rewards and costs of family size: concepts and methods for a pilot study in the United States." Pp. 99–140 in James T. Fawcett (ed.), The Satisfaction and Costs of Children: Theories, Concepts and Methods. Honolulu, Hawaii: East-West Center.

United Nations

1959 The Population of Asia and the Far East, 1950–1980. N.Y.: United Nations.

1977 Levels and Trends of Fertility throughout the World, 1950–1970. Population Studies No. 59. N.Y.: United Nations Publications, Department of Economic and Social Affairs.

United Nations Statistical Office

1959 Handbook of Population Census Methods, Vol. III: Demographic and Social Characteristics of the Population, Studies in Methods Series F, no. 5, Rev. 1. N.Y.: United Nations.

University of the Philippines Statistical Center

1961 Demographic and Health Survey, 1960. Manila: University of the Philippines.

Valenzuela, Victor C.

1954 "Problems in the collection of birth and death statistics in the Philippines." The Philippine Statistician 3 (March):60–65.

Weber, Max

1947 The Theory of Social and Economic Organization. Ed. by Talcott Parsons. N.Y.: Oxford University Press.

Wickberg, Edgar

1965 The Chinese in Philippine Life. New Haven: Yale University Press.

Winterbottom, Marian R.

1958 "The relation of need for achievement to learning experiences in independence and mastery." Pp. 453–478 in John W. Atkinson (ed.), Motives in Fantasy, Action, and Society. Princeton, New Jersey: D. Van Nostrand.

Yoshihara, Kunio

1971 "A study of Philippine manufacturing corporations." The Developing Economies IX (Sept):268–89.